Christian Krettek (Ed.)

Dirk Aschemann (Ed.)

Positioning Techniques in Surgical Applications

Christian Krettek (Ed.)
Dirk Aschemann (Ed.)

Positioning Techniques in Surgical Applications

Thorax and Heart Surgery – Vascular Surgery –
Visceral and Transplantation Surgery – Urology –
Surgery to the Spinal Cord and Extremities –
Arthroscopy – Paediatric Surgery – Navigation/ISO-C 3D

Springer

Prof. Dr. Christian Krettek, MD, FRACS
Director of the Trauma Department,
Hannover Medical School (MHH)
Carl-Neuberg-Straße 1
30625 Hannover

Dirk Aschemann
Maquet GmbH & Co.KG,
Product Manager Mobile Operating Tables
Kehler Straße 31
76437 Rastatt

ISBN 3-540-25716-0
Springer Medizin Verlag Heidelberg

Bibliographic information by Deutschen Bibliothek
Deutsche Bibliothek has registered this publication in the German National Biography; detailed bibliographic details can be consulted on the internet under http://dnb.ddb.de.

This work is protected by copyright. The corresponding rights, particularly to translating, reprinting, presenting, extracting illustrations and tables, radio broadcasting, microfilming or duplicating by any other means and storing in data processing systems are reserved, even only for excerpts. Duplication of this work or parts of this work, even in isolated cases, is only permitted within the limits of the statutory regulations of the Copyright Law of the Federal Republic of Germany dated 9 September 1965 in the latest current version. Publication is always subject to a charge. Violations are subject to the penalties stated in the Copyright Law.

Springer Medizin Verlag
A company belonging to Springer Science+Business Media
springer.de

© Springer Medizin Verlag Heidelberg 2006
Printed in Germany

The reproduction of names, trade names etc. in this work even without special reference does not justify the presumption that such names were to be treated freely in accordance with the trade name and brand protection legislation and could therefore be used by anyone.

Product liability: the publishers cannot assume any liability for information referring to dosage instructions and types of application. Such details must be checked for correctness by the corresponding user in each and every case by comparing with other literature sources.

Planning: Dr. Fritz Kraemer, Heidelberg
Project management: Willi Bischoff, Heidelberg
Copy editing: Susan Peters, Hamburg

Cover design: deblik, Berlin
Layout: deblik, Berlin; W. Bischoff, Heidelberg
Typesetting and reproduction of the illustrations: Fotosatz-Service Köhler GmbH, Würzburg
Printing and binding: Universitätsdruckerei Stürtz, Würzburg

SPIN: 11420194   Printed on acid-free paper   2111/BF – 5 4 3 2 1 0

Foreword

The success of an operation depends not only on careful clarification of the indications, selection of the right time for operating and technically neat operating techniques, but also on correct preoperative preparation and positioning of the patient. But this aspect in particular is frequently neglected, particularly by young surgeons, because technical details of the operation assume far greater attention, underestimating the contribution made by optimum positioning to a time-saving operation which runs as perfectly as possible. How easy is it for an operation to develop complications out of all proportion because the surgeon forgot certain »minor matters« during preparations! Anyone who has witnessed this themselves will appreciate just how important exact preoperative planning and preparation is before an operation takes place.

It is therefore our great pleasure to present a work put together with the assistance of renowned expert co-authors about safe positioning techniques which are of great use to operating procedures and which cover the various different surgical disciplines.

Like no other surgical discipline, accident surgery clearly demonstrates the results of the dramatic rate of progress in medical development:
- new, gentler osteosynthesis techniques and new implants with a huge expansion in the range of possible operations
- introduction of navigation and new imaging procedures such as Iso-C3D imaging
- introduction of new operating tables with improved fluoroscopic properties
- new procedures for dealing with wound infections (vacuum sealing, new antiseptics).

The many new procedures in operative surgery – and also in the other medical disciplines – make it necessary to take stock of an effective approach to operation preparation. New techniques demand an increasingly intensive approach to dealing with new materials: completely new instruments and devices, developed for example for minimally invasive surgery, or concealed surgical procedures with direct visualisation techniques. Special instruments are only used for one specific purpose; a surgical needle today has its own anatomy. In addition, these aspects are joined by stricter safety conditions, increased demands made by patients, with the threat of legal consequences if something should go wrong in terms of »nihil nocere« …

We have therefore made an attempt to illustrate a procedure which has proven successful over many years at the Medical University Hannover. This does not mean that there are not other appropriate or even better suited procedures for specific situations, which would ideally supplement the procedure described here. We felt it was important to describe safe, practical positioning techniques to simplify each specific operation.

At this point we would like to extend our thanks to the years of intensive, trusting cooperation with Ms. Schröder, Ms. Conrad, Dr. Kraemer and Mr. Bischoff from Springer Verlag. Thanks also go to Susan Peters for her external copy editing.

Many thanks also to all the colleagues in the positioning and surgical teams in the various departments, to the MHH photo department, models Martina Prüser and Ute Gerber and to Maquet GmbH & Co.KG

Special thanks to Dr. Lutz Mahlke and Dr. Axel Gänsslen for their suggestions and corrections over the last few months, and naturally also to our families who have provided us with vital support day by day.

Rastatt/Hannover, October 2005
Dirk Aschemann
Prof. Dr. Christian Krettek

Many special thanks to my parents and, for all their personal sacrifices, to my wife Cornelia and our twins Lisa and Nils.

Hildesheim, October 2005
Dirk Aschemann

Contents

I General section

1	**Psychological management of children** ... 3	4.1.2.3	Radiation protection manager, radiation protection officer ... 24
	R. Sümpelmann	4.1.2.4	Obligations when operating an X-ray machine ... 24
1.1	Special aspects of childhood ... 4	4.1.2.5	Occupational exposure to radiation, personal dosimetry ... 25
1.2	Psychological and medication preparation ... 5	4.1.2.6	Helpers ... 27
1.3	Transport to the operating suite ... 5	4.1.2.7	Information and instruction procedures ... 27
1.4	Transfer of the patient and transport to the anaesthesia preparation room ... 5	4.1.2.8	Records ... 29
	References ... 6	4.1.2.9	Quality assurance according to the X-ray Ordinance ... 29
2	**Hygienic aspects** ... 7	4.1.3	Generating X-rays ... 30
	W. Kasperczyk	4.1.4	The image receiver system for surgical image intensifiers ... 32
2.1	Perioperative hygiene in accident surgery ... 8	4.1.5	The main components in surgical image intensifiers ... 32
2.2	Guidelines for formulating hygiene measures ... 8	4.1.6	Technical minimum requirements for examinations with surgical image intensifiers ... 32
2.3	Concrete measures ... 8	4.1.7	Application-related radiation protection in the operating suite ... 32
2.3.1	Clothing in the operating suite ... 9		
2.3.2	Cleaning and disinfecting hands ... 9	4.1.8	Correct positioning of the image receiver system ... 34
2.4	Preoperative patient preparation ... 10		
	References ... 11	4.1.9	Correct use of the automatic dose output control (ADR) ... 34
3	**Legal aspects** ... 13	4.2	Surgical image intensifier systems ... 35
	B. Debong	4.2.1	Expert inspection ... 36
3.1	Legal principles ... 14	4.2.2	X-ray radiation ... 36
3.2	Interdisciplinary cooperation in positioning the patient ... 14	4.2.3	Radiation protection ... 36
3.2.1	Preoperative phase ... 14	4.2.4	Structure and technique of a surgical image intensifier ... 37
3.2.2	Positioning for the operation ... 15	4.2.5	Application ... 38
3.2.3	Positioning on the operating table ... 15	4.2.6	Use of the surgical image intensifier ... 38
3.2.4	Changes in position ... 15	4.2.7	Tips and tricks for daily routine ... 38
3.2.5	Postoperative phase ... 15		References ... 39
3.3	Cooperation between doctors and nurses in positioning the patient ... 15	**5**	**High-frequency surgery** ... 41
3.4	Burden of proof ... 16		V. Hausmann
3.5	Documentation of patient positioning ... 16	5.1	General aspects ... 42
4	**Use of X-rays in the operating suite** ... 19	5.1.1	How it works/Definition ... 42
	General aspects and X-ray Ordinance, radiation generation and radiation protection ... 19	5.1.2	Incision ... 43
	H. Kreienfeld, H. Klimpel, V. Böttcher	5.1.3	Coagulation ... 44
4.1	Radiation protection in the operating suite ... 20	5.1.4	Influences on the surgical effect ... 45
4.1.1	Introduction ... 20	5.2	Neutral electrode ... 46
4.1.2	Legal principles for the use of X-rays in medicine ... 21	5.2.1	Task ... 46
4.1.2.1	X-ray Ordinance, Atomic Energy Law, Euratom Directives, ICRP recommendations ... 21	5.2.2	Safety systems ... 46
4.1.2.2	Use of X-rays on people ... 22	5.2.3	The neutral electrode, which, where, how? ... 46

5.2.4	Burns under the neutral electrode?	47	**8**	**Standard positioning**		91
5.3	Rules for safe use	48		*D. Aschemann, A. Gänsslen*		
5.3.1	General	48	8.1	Introduction		92
5.3.2	Use of high-frequency surgery in minimally invasive surgery	48	8.2	Preparation of the operating table		92
			8.2.1	Universal operating table Alphamaquet 1150.30 with water and gel mat for trauma surgery		92
5.3.3	Other information	49				
	Glossary	50	8.3	Supine position		93
	References	54	8.3.1	Head		93
			8.3.2	Shoulders and arms		93
6	**New technologies**	55	8.3.3	Back and pelvis		94
	D. Kendoff, L. Mahlke, T. Hüfner, C. Krettek, C. Priscoglio		8.3.4	Legs		95
			8.4	Lithotomy position		96
6.1	Navigation	56	8.4.1	Head, shoulders and arms		96
6.1.1	Equipment, arrangement and modalities	56	8.4.2	Back and pelvis		97
6.1.2	Iso-C3D general	57	8.4.3	Legs		97
6.1.3	Iso-C3D navigation	58	8.5	Beach-chair position		98
6.2	AWIGS/VIWAS – New systems for image-guided surgery	60	8.5.1	Head		98
			8.5.2	Shoulders and arms		99
6.2.1	Introduction	60	8.5.3	Back and pelvis		99
6.2.2	Overview of the system components	60	8.5.4	Legs		99
6.2.3	AWIGS	60	8.6	Prone position		99
6.2.3.1	Use and benefits of the system	60	8.6.1	Head		100
6.2.4	VIWAS	65	8.6.2	Arms		100
6.2.4.1	VIWAS in combination with an angiography system	65	8.6.3	Thorax and pelvis		102
			8.6.4	Legs		102
6.2.4.2	VIWAS in combination with a sliding gantry	66	8.7	The lateral position		102
6.2.5	Prospects	66	8.7.1	Head		103
	References	66	8.7.2	Shoulders and arms		103
			8.7.3	Thorax and pelvis		104
7	**Technical equipment**	67	8.7.4	Legs		104
	H. Colberg, D. Aschemann, B. Kulik, C. Rösinger		8.8	Final remarks		105
7.1	Operating table	68	**9**	**Function workflow in the operating suite**		107
7.1.1	Introduction	68		*D. Aschemann, A. Gänsslen, L. Mahlke*		
7.1.2	Historical development	68				
7.1.3	Classification criteria according to technical design	73	9.1	Standard steps in the elective programme		108
			9.1.1	Patient reception		108
7.1.3.1	Operating table systems	73	9.1.2	Selection of the operating table and placing the patient on it		108
7.1.3.2	Mobile operating tables	75				
7.1.4	Classification criteria according to purpose	78	9.1.3	Preparation of the patient in the anaesthesia induction room		108
7.1.5	Classification criteria according to the school of surgery	78				
			9.1.4	Definitive positioning		108
7.1.6	Production, production control and safety	78	9.1.5	Preparing the bed and measures at the end of the operation		109
7.2	Positioning accessories and aids	79				
7.2.1	Pads	79	9.2	Preparations in an emergency (under time pressure)		110
7.2.1.1	Pads with viscoelastic foam core	79				
7.2.1.2	Gel pads	81	9.3	Preparations for open fractures		110
7.2.2	Operating table accessories	82				
7.2.3	Extension table accessories	86	**10**	**Complications**		115
7.2.4	Special devices	88		*M. Bund, F. Logemann, H. Müller-Vahl*		
7.2.5	Vacuum mats	88				
7.2.6	Patient warming system	90	10.1	Positioning injuries as seen by the anaesthetist		116

10.1.1	Division of labour between surgeon and anaesthetist 116	10.3	Positioning injuries as seen by the neurologist	125
10.1.2	Occurrence of positioning injuries 116	10.3.1	Introduction	125
10.1.2.1	Frequency 116	10.3.2	Frequency	125
10.1.2.2	Kind of injuries 117	10.3.3	Pathophysiology	125
10.1.3	Supine position 119	10.3.4	Symptoms	126
10.1.3.1	Struma position 120	10.3.4.1	Diagnosis and differential diagnosis	126
10.1.3.2	Extension table 120	10.3.4.2	Therapy and progress	126
10.1.3.3	Lithotomy position 121	10.3.5	Special nerve injuries	127
10.1.3.4	Head-down position 121	10.3.5.1	Brachial plexus	127
10.1.4	Lateral position 121	10.3.5.2	Ulnar nerve	127
10.1.5	Prone position 122	10.3.5.3	Peroneal nerve	127
10.1.6	Sitting/half sitting position 123	10.3.6	Lesions of the lumbosacral plexus and its branches in the lithotomy position	128
10.1.7	Final remarks 123	10.3.6.1	Pudendal nerve	128
10.2	Patient positioning under resuscitation conditions 123	10.3.7	Compartment syndrome following surgical positioning	128
10.2.1	Necessary measures 124		References	128
10.2.2	Positioning injuries following resuscitation . . 125			

II Special section

D. Aschemann, C. Krettek, A. Becker, A. Gänsslen, T. Hüfner, D. Kendoff, T. Kofidis, J. Leonhardt, L. Mahlke, G. Scheumann, U. Schmidt, B. Ure
(Illustrations and picture processing: D. Aschemann, W. Mayrhofer, A. Lang, P. Lang, K. Adam; models: M. Prüser, U. Gerber)

11	**Thorax and heart surgery** 133	13.1.2	Supine position, neurosurgical head rest	160
11.1	Median thoracotomy (sternotomy) 134	13.2	Open laparotomy	162
11.1.1	Supine position 134	13.2.1	Supine position (median and transverse laparotomy, incision right or left parallel to the costal margin)	162
11.2	Bilateral thoracotomy 136			
11.2.1	Supine position 136			
11.3	Lateral thoracotomy 138	13.2.2	Lithotomy position	164
11.3.1	Lateral position 138	13.3	Laparoscopic operations	166
11.3.2	Modified lateral position 140	13.3.1	Supine position	166
11.4	Anterolateral thoracotomy 142	13.4	Heidelberg position (position for Kraske access)	168
11.4.1	Supine position 142			
11.5	Others 144	13.4.1	Modified prone position	168
11.5.1	Modified supine position 144	13.5	Lateral position	170
11.5.2	Supine position 146	13.5.1	Modified lateral position	170
12	**Vascular surgery** 149	**14**	**Urology**	173
12.1	Neck 150	14.1	Positioning techniques depending on various surgical indications	174
12.1.1	Supine position 150			
12.2	Upper extremities 152	14.1.1	Supine position	174
12.2.1	Supine position 152	14.1.2	Lithotomy position	176
12.3	Lower extremities 154	14.1.3	Flank position	178
12.3.1	Supine position 154	14.1.4	Modified supine position	180
		14.1.5	Prone position	182
13	**Visceral and transplantation surgery** 157			
13.1	Neck 158			
13.1.1	Supine position 158			

15	**Spine surgery**	185
15.1	Cervical spine	186
15.1.1	Supine position/CRP horseshoe headrest	186
15.1.2	Supine position/skull clamp	188
15.1.3	Supine position/spine holding unit MAQUET T554.0000	190
15.1.4	Prone position/CRP horseshoe headrest	192
15.1.5	Prone position/spine holding unit/skull clamp	194
15.2	Thoracic spine, lumbar spine	196
15.2.1	Prone position	196
15.2.2	Lateral position	198
15.2.3	Supine position	200
16	**Pelvis**	203
16.1	Pelvic girdle	204
16.1.1	Supine position	204
16.1.2	Lateral position	206
16.1.3	Prone position	208
16.2	Acetabulum	210
16.2.1	Supine position	210
16.2.2	Lateral position	212
16.2.3	Prone position	214
17	**Upper extremities**	217
17.1	Shoulder	218
17.1.1	Supine position	218
17.1.2	Beach-chair position	220
17.1.3	Prone position	222
17.2	Upper arm	224
17.2.1	Supine position	224
17.2.2	Prone position	226
17.3	Elbow	228
17.3.1	Supine position	228
17.3.2	Prone position	230
17.4	Lower arm and hand	232
17.4.1	Supine position	232
18	**Lower extremities**	235
18.1	Hips	236
18.1.1	Supine position	236
18.1.2	Lateral position	238
18.2	Thigh	240
18.2.1	Supine position	240
18.2.2	Modified supine position	242
18.2.3	Lateral position	244
18.3	Knee	246
18.3.1	Supine position	246
18.3.2	Prone position	248
18.4	Lower leg	250
18.4.1	Supine position	250
18.5	Foot	252
18.5.1	Supine position	252
18.5.2	Lateral position	254
18.5.3	Prone position	256
19	**Positioning on the extension table**	259
19.1	Extension table proximal femur	260
19.1.1	Supine position	260
19.2	Extension table thigh	262
19.2.1	Supine position	262
19.3	Extension table lower leg	264
19.3.1	Supine position	264
20	**Arthroscopic procedures**	267
20.1	Shoulder	268
20.1.1	Beach-chair position	268
20.1.2	Lateral position	270
20.2	Hips	272
20.2.1	Supine position on extension table	272
20.3	Knee	274
20.3.1	Supine position	274
20.4	Foot/ankle	276
20.4.1	Supine position	276
21	**Paediatric surgery**	279
21.1	Various positions	280
21.1.1	Supine position	280
21.1.2	Prone position	282
21.1.3	Lateral position	284
21.1.4	Lithotomy position	286
22	**Special aspects of Iso-C3D and navigation applications**	289
22.1	Iso-C3D applications with and without navigation	290
22.1.1	Spine	290
22.1.2	Pelvis/Acetabulum	294
22.1.3	Elbow/wrist	296
22.1.4	Hips/DHS/neck of the femur: screwed solutions	298
22.1.5	Head of the tibia and lower leg	300
22.1.6	Ankle/pilon/talus	302
22.1.7	Calcaneus fractures	304

Subject Index 307

Staff directory

Aschemann, Dirk
Maquet GmbH & Co.KG,
Product Manager Mobile
Operating Tables
Kehler Straße 31, 76437 Rastatt

Dr. Becker, Armin, MD
Urological Clinic,
Hannover Medical School
Carl-Neuberg-Straße 1, 30625 Hannover

Dr. Bund, Michael, MD
Medical Director, Clinic for
Anaesthesiology, Surgical Intensive
Care and Pain Therapy
Albert Schweitzer Hospital
Sturmbäume 8–10, 37154 Northeim

Böttcher, Volker, graduate engineer
Ziehm Imaging GmbH
Isarstraße 40, 90451 Nürnberg

Colberg, Heinz
Sternenstr. 16, 76473 Iffezheim

Dr- Debong, Bernhard,
Lawyer, Legal Practice for Medical Law,
Killisfeldstraße 62A, 76227 Karlsruhe
(Durlach)

Dr. Gänsslen, Axel, MD
Trauma Department,
Hannover Medical School
Carl-Neuberg-Straße 1, 30625 Hannover

Hausmann, Volker, graduate engineer
Electrical/communications enginee-
ring, Product Manager Electrosurgical
tyco Healthcare Deutschland GmbH
Auf der Höhe 15, 53859 Niederkassel

Dr. Hüfner, Tobias, MD
Trauma Department,
Hannover Medical School
Carl-Neuberg-Straße 1, 30625 Hannover

**Professor Dr. Kasperczyk,
Werner-J., MD**
Medical Director, Clinic for Trauma-
tology, Orthopaedic Surgery
Klinik St. Theresia Saarbrücken
Rheinstrasse 2, 66113 Saarbrücken

Dr. Kendoff, Daniel, MD
Trauma Department,
Hannover Medical School
Carl-Neuberg-Straße 1,
30625 Hannover

Klimpel, Herbert, graduate engineer
TÜV Nord X-Ray Technology
Am TÜV 1, 30519 Hannover

**Kreienfeld, Helmut,
graduate engineer**
TÜV Nord X-Ray Technology.
Head of Study Group
Am TÜV 1, 30519 Hannover

Professor Dr. Krettek, Christian, MD
FRACS, Director of the Trauma Department, Hannover Medical School
Carl-Neuberg-Straße 1,
30625 Hannover

Dr. Kofidis, Theo, MD
Clinic for Thorax, Heart and Vascular
Surgery, Hannover Medical School,
Carl-Neuberg-Straße 1,
30625 Hannover

Kulik, Bernhardt
Maquet GmbH & Co.KG,
Product Manager Operating
Table Sysems
Kehler Straße 31, 76437 Rastatt

Dr. Leonhardt, Johannes, MD
Paediatric Surgery Clinic,
Hannover Medical School
Carl-Neuberg-Straße 1,
30625 Hannover

Dr. Logemann, Frank, MD
Anaesthesiology Centre,
Hannover Medical School
Carl-Neuberg-Straße 1,
30625 Hannover

Dr. Mahlke, Lutz, MD
Trauma Department,
Hannover Medical School
Carl-Neuberg-Straße 1,
30625 Hannover

**Professor Dr. Müller-Vahl,
Hermann, MD**
Neurology Clinic with Clinical
Neurophysiology,
Hannover Medical School
Carl-Neuberg-Straße 1,
30625 Hannover

Priscoglio, Claudio
Maquet GmbH & Co.KG,
-Product Manager AWIGS/VIWAS
Kehler Straße 31, 76437 Rastatt

Rösinger, Charly
Maquet GmbH & Co.KG,
-Product Manager Accessories
Kehler Straße 31, 76437 Rastatt

**Professor Dr. Scheumann,
Georg, MD**
Clinic for Visceral and Transplantation
Surgery, Hannover Medical School
Carl-Neuberg-Straße 1, 30625 Hannover

Dr. Schmidt, Ulf, MD
Department for Traumatology,
Hospital of the Merciful Sisters,
Schlossberg 1, 4910 Ried/Innkreis,
Austria

Professor Dr.Sümpelmann, MD
Anaesthesiology Centre,
Medical University Hannover
Carl-Neuberg-Straße 1, 30625 Hannover

Professor Dr. Ure, Benno, MD
Director of the Paediatric Surgery
Clinic, Hannover Medical School
Carl-Neuberg-Straße 1, 30625 Hannover

Illustrations and picture processing
Dirk Aschemann, Armand Lang,
Philippe Lang, Katrin Adam

Walter Mayrhofer
Fotostudio Mayrhofer
Weingartener Straße 62,
75045 Walzbachtal/Jöhlingen

Models:
Martina Prüser and Ute Gerber

Note

The following text describes various positioning techniques used in our clinic. Naturally, procedures can vary from clinic to clinic. The aim must of course be to use positioning which gives the patient optimum protection and provides the surgeon with optimum exposure of the operating site.

In view of the fact that every institution has developed its own quality standards (QS) for positioning,
- we have not included any indications of quantities for positioning aids such as pads, safety belts, etc. in the »Preparation« sections
- the positioning techniques are illustrated for the most part by a model **without** any precautions against bed sores, given the wide range of different positioning aids used in each different institution.

Furthermore,
- the illustrations with models do not use any X-ray protection for C-arm use; these measures must be implemented according to the QS!
- the chapters do not feature all conceivable risks but deal specifically just with the risks involved with the specific position. General damage to skin and nerves must naturally still be expected from incorrect positioning.

We have made every effort to provide a comprehensive overview of possible positioning variations. But we do not make any claim to covering absolutely every kind of positioning, indication and risk. We feel it is important to stress once again that patient positioning is a joint task to be shared by the nursing staff and doctors both in the surgical and in the anaesthesia team, and must be implemented and monitored by the whole team.

Prof. Dr. Christian Krettek
Dr. Lutz Mahlke
Dirk Aschemann

I General Part

1 Psychological management of children

R. Sümpelmann

1.1 Special aspects of childhood – 4

1.2 Psychological and medication preparation – 5

1.3 Transport to the operating suite – 5

1.4 Transfer of the patient and transport to the anaesthesia preparation room – 5

References – 6

1.1 Special aspects of childhood

»A child is not a small adult«: this important rule applies not only to the special physiological aspects but also to the special psychological aspects of childhood. The reactions of young patients to surgery, anaesthetic and a stay in hospital depend on age, personality structure, the child's home environment, family background, previous experience of operations and the conditions in the hospital. The main objective of perioperative care of children should therefore consist in avoiding traumatic experiences in the perioperative phase for everyone involved. Particularly where children are involved, consideration should be given to the fact that this kind of trauma can have a negative effect on the attitude to the health system over a long period of time and make future treatment extremely difficult. Children are naturally flexible and can come to terms with even difficult situations. A successful approach to helping children to cope with the »operation crisis« can even promote their emotional development. But this is only possible if everyone involved knows the potential problems encountered with children and are willing to adjust to these individually. Unpleasant experiences are encountered with particular frequency in the immediate pre- and postoperative phase when the children are still awake or have woken up again. The weakest link in the chain of everyone involved has the greatest influence on the overall success.

Influence of age. Infants younger than 6 months rarely show resistance to a hospital environment. Even separation from the parents is tolerated for short periods if a »substitute mother« is available. There are greater problems with children between 6 months and 4–5 years. On the one hand, they are old enough to be aware of threatening situations and separation from their parents, but too young to understand rational explanations. Their reactions to an operation and stay in hospital can include separation anxiety, sleeping disorders, nightmares, eating disorders, estrangement or wetting the bed. Children of school age can cope better with being separated from their parents and are better able to come to terms with new surroundings. They are frequently afraid of their bodily integrity being violated, or have irrational ideas about what happens during an operation.

Influence of the parents. The parent/child relationship can vary greatly between being extremely overprotective and almost complete independence. Frequently the parents themselves have little or no experience in coping with operations and stays in hospital and are uncertain and anxious. Other parents have had negative experiences with hospitals themselves and are afraid that their children could undergo the same. Small children in particular cannot understand why their parents leave them in a critical situation. Even sensible parents often find it difficult to leave a sad, crying child in the hands of strangers. The anxieties of the parents can be transferred to the children with a negative effect on their behaviour.

The surroundings. Following drastic changes in recent decades, children's wards have made great adjustments even to the needs of younger children. On the other hand, the functional atmosphere of the operating suite still differs greatly from what children understand to be pleasant surroundings. All the technical equipment, the face masks and caps worn by the staff concealing their faces and the artificial light can trigger additional and irrational anxieties (ghosts, bad people in the operating theatre, fear of mutilation, ◘ Fig. 1.1).

Specific anxieties of children. Being separated from their parents and customary home surroundings is the main problem particularly for small children (1–3 years). Older children of preschool and primary school age have more concrete worries about the operation, anaesthetic and the actual disease itself. Many children do not want to take their own clothes off and put strange clothes on. In particular if they have had to go without food or drink for a long time, they will be hungry and thirsty. Almost all children are afraid of puncture pain, e.g. blood samples,

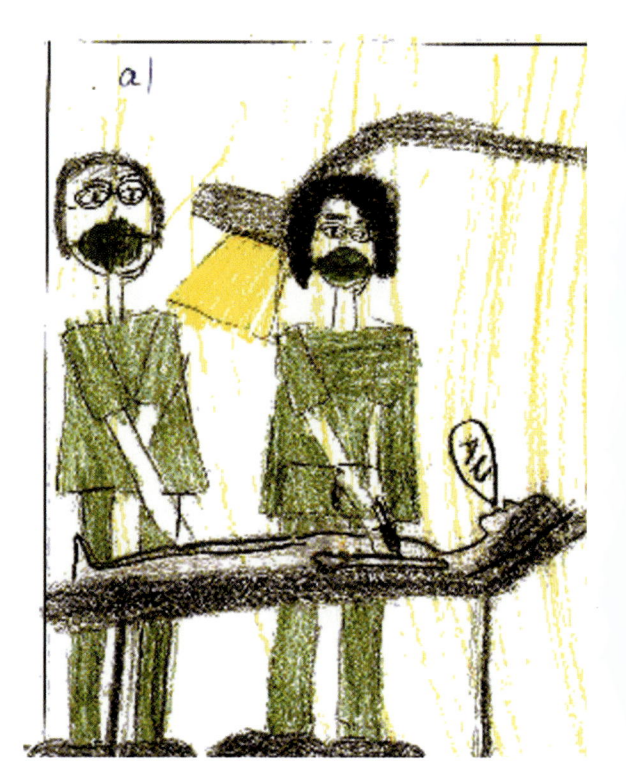

◘ **Fig. 1.1.** Children often find it difficult to be separated from their parents in the operation sluice. They are afraid of the strange surroundings and of the operating staff whose faces are concealed by face masks and caps

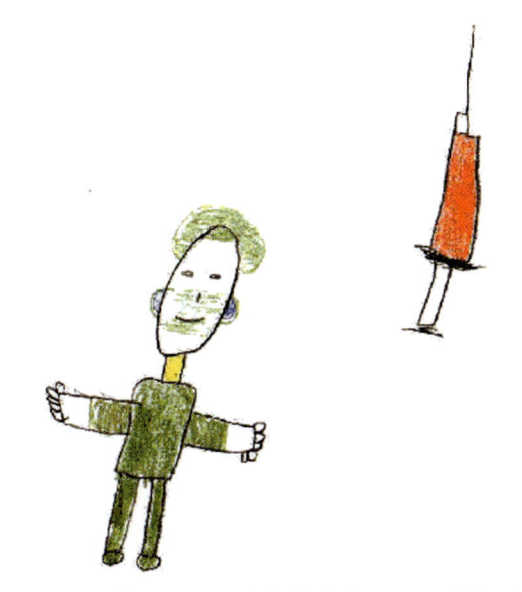

Fig. 1.2. Children are particularly afraid of puncture pain from injections or intravenous drips

injections or fitting intravenous drips (Fig. 1.2). After the operation, they will also be upset by all the strange material, e.g. wound drains, infusion drips or catheters.

1.2 Psychological and medication preparation

Usually the surgeon and anaesthetist will talk to the children and their parents to prepare them for the operation. This should happen as close as possible to the operation itself (on the day before) in a calm, relaxed atmosphere. What is discussed and how depends on the child's development status and previous experience. Some children's hospitals also provide video demonstrations or tours of the hospital for the families. The operation itself should then take place on the next day along the same lines as far as possible. False promises, misunderstandings arising from a lack of information and communication and short-term changes to the operating schedule mean that children and parents start to lose confidence and can make subsequent treatment extremely difficult. Long waiting times without food and drink increase anxieties and reduce compliance. This is why small children should be included right at the beginning of an operating schedule. It is usually a good idea to administer children with premedication about an hour before the operation while they are still on the ward, for example oral midazolam as medicine with adapted taste, or by rectal or nasal means. Painful injections are not suitable for children and should be avoided if at all possible.

1.3 Transport to the operating suite

Children should be brought to the operating suite in such a way that there will not be any unnecessarily long waits, and then preferably brought to the operating suite by a nurse in the company of the parents or someone they know and trust. Many children will be reassured if they can take a favourite soft toy or cuddly blanket with them. This should be treated carefully and must certainly not be lost. Older, cooperative children who have been well prepared for the operation in psychological and medication terms usually say goodbye to their parents without any problems and can be transferred to the operating table in the operation sluice. Preschool children find it much harder to be separated from their parents. Dramatic farewell scenes are traumatic for everyone involved and should be avoided at all costs. As a possible solution, in a calm preparatory room midazolam and ketamine or methohexital can be administered rectally to the child by an anaesthetist so that the child falls asleep while the parents are still there. In rare exceptions, intramuscular injections of ketamine are possible for extremely uncooperative children. If the child has already been provided with intravenous access, sedation is naturally administered this way. Many parents will want to know whether they can stay with their child while the anaesthetic is being induced. If compatible with the available space and staffing arrangements, there are no objections to this in the case of a routine anaesthetic. But another staff member should inform the parents about the rules of behaviour in the operating suite and look after them while in the operating suite. Most families are satisfied if they can be present in the operation sluice while their child is placed under deep sedation.

1.4 Transfer of the patient and transport to the anaesthesia preparation room

In the case of infants and small children, the anaesthetic is frequently induced in the operating theatre. The simplest method is for the children to be carried into the operating theatre. Nearly all children react positively to close bodily contact and being spoken to nicely. It also helps if the face mask is left off when the children are awake so that they can see into the faces. Children must never be left unattended on the operating table because of the risk of sudden, fast movements, resulting in them falling onto the floor. Children cool down more quickly than adults because their body surface is large in relation to the body volume, so they should always be covered well. Larger schoolchildren and teenagers can be transferred directly to the operating table like adults and then taken into the anaesthesia preparation room.

References

1. Büttner W, Breitkopf L, Engert J, Bilz M (1989) Das Psychotrauma ambulanter und stationärer operativer Eingriffe bei Kleinkindern. Anaesthesist 38: 597–603
2. Breitkopf L (1990) Emotionale Reaktionen von Kindern auf den Krankenhausaufenthalt. Z Kinderchir 45: 3–8
3. Pinkerton P (1981) Preventing Psychotrauma in childhood anaesthesia. In: Rees GJ, Gray TC (eds) Paediatric Anaesthesia. Butterworth, London
4. Steward DJ (1994) Preoperative evaluation and preparation for surgery. In: Gregory GA (ed) Pediatric Anesthesia. Churchill Livingstone, New York
5. Sümpelmann R, Wellendorf E, Krohn S, Strauß J (1994) Perioperatives Angsterleben von Kindern. Anästh Intensivbeh 35: 311

2 Hygienic aspects

W. Kasperczyk

2.1 Perioperative hygiene in traumatology – 8

2.2 Guidelines for formulating hygiene measures – 8

2.3 Concrete measures – 8
2.3.1 Clothing in the operating suite – 8
2.3.2 Cleaning and disinfecting hands – 9

2.4 Preoperative patient preparation – 10

References – 11

2.1 Perioperative hygiene in traumatology

Wound infection is the most frequent nosocomial infection in surgery. Medical literature describes a large number of factors triggering and promoting infections. The starting point for infections can be patients, staff, equipment and instruments, materials, surfaces and the air. *»The ten most important points for preventing infections are the ten fingers of every single person involved in the operation«*. This somewhat pithy statement does make it clear that personal hygiene measures must be given prime attention. The following descriptions refer to hygiene measures for preventing infections associated directly with the patient, the staff and the operation.

One of the first things a young surgeon experiences in the surgical department consists of all the instructions and warnings about »sterility«. It is clear to anyone that surgical medicine creates possibilities for the penetration of germs or for the release and spreading of germs, so that there is an increased risk of infection. Consequently there is a logical demand for special measures over and beyond the general hygiene requirements in a hospital, with high a priori acceptance of such surgical hygiene measures. Most people working in operating suites today are relatively well informed about the most important aspects of perioperative behaviour. But from time to time, drastic discrepancies emerge between required and actual behaviour. The causes of inadequate hygiene behaviour are frequently psychological in nature, resulting on the one hand from the contradictions between hygiene standards and recommendations and on the other hand from barriers to motivation [20].

2.2 Guidelines for formulating hygiene measures

Germany does not have a Federal Hygiene Law for comprehensive stipulation of how hygiene is to be monitored in the hospitals. It is up to the individual states to issue legal regulations referring to hygiene [22]. The (former) Federal Health Agency (now: Robert Koch Institute, Berlin) has appointed a committee for hospital hygiene and the prevention of infection. The committee regularly publishes guidelines for hospital hygiene and the prevention of infection (available through Fischer Verlag, Stuttgart). The hygiene guidelines have the status of expert recommendations. But this does not mean that the guidelines are without any essential significance in the case of legal disputes [22]. The guidelines are published in the Federal Health Gazette.

Other expert recommendations are issued by the German-Speaking Working Group for Hospital Hygiene (founded 1986). The group publishes its work in the magazine »Hygiene und Medizin« [Hygiene and Medicine]. The so-called BGA guidelines and the working group recommendations are also regularly featured in the »Mitteilungen und Nachrichten der Deutschen Gesellschaft für Unfallchirurgie« [Notifications and News from the German Society for traumatology].

Very interesting current monographs have been published by: Adam & Daschner, 1993 [1], Bennett & Bachmann, 1993 [3], Daschner, 1992 [6], Hansis, 1994 [10], Hierholzer & Hierholzer, 1990 [14], Sander & Sander, 1992 [18] and Bühler, 1992 [4].

2.3 Concrete measures

Wound infection is a treatment-specific risk of surgical operations. This risk must be minimised by methods corresponding to good medical practice and standards (hygiene status). In the event of any disputes, a medical expert decides whether avoidable hygiene violations were involved.

2.3.1 Clothing in the operating suite

Operating suite clothing. Everyone releases a large number of microorganisms all the time, particularly when walking. Normal hospital clothing (usually white healthcare workwear) is regularly affected by (facultative) pathogenic germs. This is joined by microorganisms released through the nose and throat when talking, coughing and sneezing. The hair of hospital staff has been proven to have a large number of germs, including in particular *Staphylococcus aureus* [9]. It is advisable to reduce the entrainment and release of germs in the operating suite as far as possible. The guidelines for hospital hygiene and the prevention of infections therefore require the staff to change their clothing completely in the staff sluice of an operating suite. The hospital clothing should be removed down to the underwear and replaced by germ-free surgical clothing (trousers, shirt, surgical shoes). The suite clothing must be disinfected and cleaned, and transported and stored with protection from contamination. Surgical clothing must not be worn outside the operating suite. This prohibition cannot be bypassed by wearing something else (e.g. white coat) on top. This strict rule makes it possible to monitor what goes into and out of the operating suite, underlining its special character.

Headgear and face mask. In the operating suite, everyone must wear hair covering which completely covers facial hair and hair on the head in order to prevent the exposure of the contaminated hair. The face mask fulfils two tasks: it prevents the transport of pathogenic germs into the sterile operating suite and into the wound, and protects the wearer from contamination with body fluids, e.g. sprays of blood. Protective goggles are also recommended as personal protection. Their meaningfulness or otherwise has been repeatedly discussed since the introduction of face masks. Already back in 1936, Riese [16] achieved the lowest wound infection rates during so-called silent operations without a mask. It is a known fact that the release of germs during speaking can be significantly reduced by wearing a mask [13]. Face masks should fit tightly over the mouth and nose. They should be worn in the operating theatre and, for disciplinary reasons, in the immediately adjacent ancillary rooms as well. Multi-layer masks with fleece and polyester inlays are superior to single-layer masks and gauze masks, because the latter are too permeable [13]. As the mask becomes increasingly damp, the filter resistance is increased. The so-called edge leak rate increases, i.e. the passage of germs between the edge of the mask and the face. Damp masks must therefore be replaced (between two surgical procedures). If the face mask has been loosened (e.g. in the day room), it must be replaced. This should be followed by hygiene disinfection of the hands to eliminate contamination of the hands from the used mask.

In the traumatology Department at the Medical University Hannover (UCH-MHH), hair covering is worn throughout the complete operating suite. The face mask is only obligatory in the operating theatre and is always disposed of on leaving the operating theatre after an operation. A face mask is not required in the operation preparation room, in the corridors or ancillary rooms. This rule ensures that a fresh face mask is fitted in the scrub room before every further operation.

Going to the toilet. The guidelines for hospital hygiene and preventing infection [2] recommend going through the complete operating suite sluice procedure after going to the toilet (▶ above). Adam & Daschner [1] do not find any scientific indication that the genital region of the surgeon or any other member of staff in the operating suite would constitute a special risk for postoperative wound infection. This presumes that the clothing is not soiled and that the operating staff wash their hands after going to the toilet and also disinfect them before every operation.

UCH-MHH: access to the toilets is only possible through the staff sluice, i.e. outside the actual operating suite. This means that the staff have to go through the complete operating suite sluice procedure again after going to the toilet.

Sterile surgical clothing. The surgical team enters the actual operating theatre through the scrub room where the surgical hand disinfection procedure takes place (▶ there). On entering the operating theatre, the sterile ankle-length operating gown is fitted. It is important that the gown fits closely around the neck and that the sleeves are long enough and also fit tightly around the wrists. The requirements for sterile surgical clothing depend essentially on the liquid levels. For high-moisture procedures, linen and cotton quickly lose their function as germ barrier. In such cases, the surgical clothing must be impervious to liquid at least in the sleeves and front of the body [12].

Sterile operating gloves are generally accepted as protection for patient and staff alike. It goes without saying that defective gloves must be replaced. The use of double gloves does not protect from punctures or cut injuries but does reduce the risk of contaminating the hands with blood. Everyone should be advised to use two pairs of gloves.

UCH-MHH: two pairs of gloves are not obligatory.

2.3.2 Cleaning and disinfecting the hands

Most infections in hospitals are transferred with the hands. Washing and disinfecting the hands are therefore the simplest, safest, most effective and cheapest means of controlling infection [1]. Jewellery worn on the hands and lower arms make the measures less effective. Surgeons should ensure that their hands are not impaired by stubborn dirt and soiling from work performed in their free time, e.g. from oil, grease and lubricants.

Washing hands. Washing hands with detergents cleans the hands and reduces the germ count by a factor of 100. One millilitre of pus contains about 100,000,000 germs, which can be reduced to about 1,000,000 germs by washing.

The rule for washing hands is: first disinfect, then wash. This should prevent the spread of germs by the actual washing procedure. But no one can be expected to treat for example hands contaminated with sputum by rubbing with disinfectant first. In the case of coarse soiling, the hands can be cleaned first with a disposable wet-wipe soaked in disinfectant.

Disinfecting hands. The word disinfection refers to the actual disinfection process, which always consists of the actual disinfectant, a reaction time and the means in which the disinfectant is applied. When disinfecting hands, it is necessary to distinguish between *hygienic* and *surgical* (preoperative) disinfection. Hygienic hand disinfection (3 ml alcoholic solution rubbed in for 30 s) kills off the transient skin flora and reduces the germ count by a factor of 10,000 (i.e. in the example given above, reduction to approx. 10,000 germs). Surgical hand disinfection aims at achieving an essential reduction in skin flora to rule out the risk of the hands being a source of infection.

In Germany, the main disinfectants used are based on alcohol. These are usually combinations of ethanol, 1-propanol and 2-propanol at a level of 80% by volume, to which skin care components are added. The disinfectant »bible« is the so-called DGHM list in which the German Society for Hygiene and Microbiology features all products and assesses them with regard to the corresponding application (available through mhp-Verlag, Wiesbaden).

Together with preoperative skin disinfection (▶ patient preparation), surgical hand disinfection is the most important antiseptic measure for surgical procedures. The hands are washed initially to remove any coarse soiling. The former practice of washing the hands thoroughly with soap and a scrubbing brush is considered obsolete today. Dirt should always be removed immediately and not only in the scrub room before operations. When the skin is scrubbed with a brush, deeper skin layers are opened resulting in a higher germ count on the skin. Frequent hand washing also encourages eczematization [7]. The pertinent guideline for hospital hygiene and prevention of infection [2] dated 1991 still requires fingernails and the edges of the nails to be cleaned with a nailbrush. The washing procedure should not take more than 1 min.

After washing, any remaining soap is rinsed off thoroughly and the hands dried gently. Many hypersensitive reactions are caused by mixing remaining soap and disinfectants. Low-germ towels (textile) can be used to dry the hands. Paper towels are rejected by some authors because of possible spore contamination. It is very important for a suitable disinfectant (DGHM list) to be applied to the *dry skin*. (This is easily explained: damp hands carry approx. 3 ml water; together with 3 ml 80% disinfectant, the water reduces the alcohol concentration to 40%, thus making it ineffective).

During the reaction time, the hands and lower arms should be coated with the disinfectant all the time. The disinfectant should be rubbed in, devoting particular attention to the nails and between the fingers. Approx. 12–15 ml disinfectant are required, depending on the reaction time and size of the hands. Experts fail to agree on the time that should be taken to disinfect the hands. Whereas Hingst et al. [15] fundamentally demand 5 min, Adam & Daschner [1] draw attention to the fact that surgeons abroad are already operating while their German colleagues are still disinfecting their hands in the scrub room. These authors recommend 3 min before the first operation and another 1–2 min before further operations.

UCH-MHH: hands are washed before the first operation and immediately after coarse soiling, soft brush for the fingernails, total time: 1 min. Soaked well with alcoholic disinfectant, rubbed in, not waved around, time: 3 min. Subsequent operations without significant interim contamination: no washing, but disinfection for 2 min.

2.4 Preoperative patient preparation

Body flora in the patient's nose and throat, intestinal passage and skin can be the starting point for wound infection.

Day before the operation. The length of stay in hospital before the operation is closely related to the wound infection rate. One reason could be contamination of the patient with problematical hospital germs. The aim should therefore be to reduce the length of stay in hospital before the operation. A multi-centre study in various European countries has revealed that bathing in an antiseptic agent (chlorhexidine) on the evening before the operation has no influence on the infection rate [17].

But the procedure of shaving the site of the operation before surgery has a verified effect on the incidence of wound infections. Seropian & Reynolds [19] showed that the use of a depilatory cream without mechanical hair removal resulted in a far lower infection rate than after shaving (0.6% compared to 5.7%). But depilatory agents frequently cause skin irritations. Studies by Cruse & Foord [5] showed the wound infection rate to be 0.9% when no measures were taken, 1.7% when cutting the hair with scissors and 2.3% in shaved patients. The cause of the increased infection rate after shaving the patient on the evening before is presumed to come from germ settlement and infection of tiny skin injuries. Today the operating site is only shaved immediately before the operation (in the preparation room) if thick hair is expected to interfere with the operation and simply shortening the hair is not sufficient. A strip of approx. 2 cm along the incision should be sufficient. The skin should be shaved as gently as possible, i.e. with a disinfected, sharp razor blade and using shaving soap or cream to prevent any injuries to the skin as far as possible.

UCH-MHH: patients are not bathed or shaved on the evening before the operation. Surgical preparation room: fine down and short hair is left; interfering long hair in the immediate operating site is cut with scissors; gentle shaving is only carried out in a 2-cm strip in the case of thick hair.

Skin disinfection. The disinfectants used include alcohol, iodine preparations and more rarely, phenolic preparations (see also DGHM list, 1991). Alcohol disinfectants start to act very quickly and are ideal for wound infections caused by key germ types [8]. Iodine preparations start to react more slowly and are used more for disinfection of the mucous membranes. The operating site must be intensively coated with disinfectant for the complete reaction time. Wiping disinfection is more effective than simply spraying. The disinfected area must extend well beyond the actual operating site. An area of 20 cm is recommended all around the operating site. In addition, all areas must be disinfected which are touched during the operation when changing the patient's position. For example, for a knee operation, it can be necessary to disinfect the whole leg. The reaction time depends on the areas of the body being cleaned and must be longer (5–10 min) for parts of the skin with many sebaceous glands, e.g. forehead or back or other parts of the body with a high initial germ count. For normal cases, Gundermann [8] recommends a minimum of 2 min for alcoholic preparations and a minimum of 5 min for iodine preparations. Adam & Daschner [1] stipulate 3 min.

UCH-MHH: dyed alcoholic disinfectant, generously applied with wiping disinfection, for 3 min.

Covers. The use of covers during the operation aims to prevent the penetration of germs into the wound. The material must withstand liquids and mechanical loads throughout the duration of the operation. Textile materials in damp condition are not effective germ barriers. More modern textile materials show excellent characteristics such as hydrophobic properties or consist of several textile layers. On the other hand, there are also disposable covers (plastic-coated fleece). From the point of view of preventing infections, the more modern textiles and also the disposable covers can be recommended [11, 21]. In most cases, the decision is based on economic aspects.

UCH-MHH: only disposable materials are used.

Correct awareness of hygiene at work requires knowledge and ongoing training of everyone involved. When it comes to operating hygiene, it is extremely important for every single person involved to take on his/her share of responsibility. There are many situations where appropriate knowledge, commitment and willingness help more than rules and regulations.

References

1. Adam D, Daschner F (1993) Infektionsverhütung bei operativen Eingriffen. Wissenschaftliche Verlagsgesellschaft, Stuttgart
2. Bekanntmachung des Bundesgesundheitsamtes, Kommission für Krankenhaushygiene und Infektionsprävention. Anforderung der Krankenhaushygiene in der operativen Medizin. Anlage 5.1 Bundesgesundheitsblatt 5/1991: 232–235
3. Bennett JV, Brachman PS (eds) (1993) Hospital Infections, 3rd edn. Little, Brown, Boston
4. Bühler M (1992) Hygienepläne. Bibliomed, Medizinische Verlags-Gesellschaft, Melsungen
5. Cruse PJE, Foord R (1973) A five-year prospective study of 23.649 surgical wounds. Arch Surg 107: 206–210
6. Daschner F (Hrsg) (1992) Praktische Krankenhaushygiene und Umweltschutz. Springer, Berlin Heidelberg New York Tokyo
7. Empfehlungen der Deutschen Gesellschaft für Krankenhaushygiene. Antiseptische Maßnahmen vor, während und nach Operationen. (1994) HygMed 19: 205–211
8. Gundermann KO (1990) Beitrag zur Hygiene: Hautdesinfektion vor Operationen und Punktion. Operat Orthop Traumatol 2: 145–147
9. Gundermann KO (1990) Beitrag zur Hygiene: Schutzkleidung und Händedesinfektion des Operationsteams. Operat Orthop Traumatol 2: 223–226
10. Hansis ML (Hrsg) (1994) Perioperative Infektionsprophylaxe in der Unfallchirurgie. Traumatologie aktuell, Bd 12. Thieme, Stuttgart
11. Hansis ML (1994) Perioperative Infektionsprophylaxe – Eine kritische Bestandsaufnahme. HygMed 19: 268–277
12. Heeg P (1994) Infektionsprophylaxe – Aus der Sicht des Hygienikers. In: Hansis ML (Hrsg) Perioperative Infektionsprophylaxe in der Unfallchirurgie. Traumatologie aktuell, Bd 12. Thieme, Stuttgart, S 31–38
13. Heeg P (1995) Beitrag zur Hygiene: Gesichtsmasken. Operat -Orthop Traumato 7: 141–142
14. Hierholzer G, Hierholzer S (Hrsg) (1990) Hygieneanforderungen an operative Einheiten – Aus traumatologischer Sicht. Springer, Berlin Heidelberg New York Tokyo
15. Hingst V, Juditzki P, Heeg P, Sonntag HG (1992) Evaluation of the efficacy of surgical hand disinfection following a reduced application time of 3 instead of 5 min. J Hosp Infect 20: 79–86
16. Riese J (1936) Stummes Operieren und seine Bedeutung im Vergleich zu anderen Faktoren der Aseptik. Zbl Chir 32: 1874–1890 und 33: 1922–1939
17. Rotter ML., Larsen SO, Cooke EM et al. (1988) A comparison of the effects of preoperative whole-body bathing with detergent alone and with detergent containing chlorhexidine gluconate in the frequency of wound infections after clean surgery. The European Working Party on Control of Hospital Infections. J Hosp Infect 11: 310–320
18. Sander J, Sander U (Hrsg) (1992) Praxis der Krankenhaushygiene – Umsetzungen von Gesetzen, Verordnungen und Empfehlungen. Schliehe, Osnabrück
19. Seropian R, Reynolds BM (1971) Wound infections after preoperative depilatory versus razor preparation. Am J Surg 121: 251–254
20. van Hagen C (1994) Infektionsprophylaxe – Aus der Sicht der Verhaltenstheorie. In: Hansis ML (Hrsg) Perioperative Infektionsprophylaxe in der Unfallchirurgie. Traumatologie aktuell, Bd 12. Thieme, Stuttgart, S 49–62
21. Wille B, Heeg P (1991) Beitrag zur Hygiene: Auswahl von Abdeckmaterialien unter infektionsprophylaktischen Gesichtspunkten. Operat Orthop Traumatol 3: 144–146
22. Windorfer A (1992) Gesetzliche Regelungen zur Umsetzung der Krankenhaushygiene in den Ländern der Bundesrepublik. In: Sander J, Sander U (Hrsg) Praxis der Krankenhaushygiene – Umsetzungen von Gesetzen, Verordnungen und Empfehlungen. Schliehe, Osnabrück, S 13–26

3 Legal aspects

B. Debong

3.1 Legal principles – 14

3.2 Interdisciplinary cooperation in positioning the patient – 14
3.2.1 Preoperative phase – 14
3.2.2 Positioning for the operation – 15
3.2.3 Positioning on the operating table – 15
3.2.4 Changes in position – 15
3.2.5 The postoperative phase – 15

3.3 Cooperation between doctors and nurses in positioning the patient – 15

3.4 Burden of proof – 16

3.5 Documentation of patient positioning – 16

3.1 Legal principles

A patient is to be positioned before, during and after an operation in such a way as to avoid any position-related injuries as far as possible. The doctors performing a surgical procedure and the nursing staff under their instruction share a legal obligation to ensure that the patient is positioned correctly (as explicitly stated by Cologne Intermediate Court of Appeals in the judgement pronounced on 2.4.1990 – 27 U 140/88 – AHRS 0920/33).

If a patient suffers injuries because of incorrect positioning (for the kind of positioning injuries cf. for example Vinz, Behandlungsfehler im Zusammenhang mit der Operationslagerung, Niedersächsisches Ärzteblatt 4/2000, 20), he can demand compensation from the doctor responsible for positioning and the nursing staff entrusted with positioning the patient under the doctor's instruction. In the case of hospital patients, the hospital authority is also liable for possible positioning injuries as the regular patient's contract partner. In legal terms, correct positioning of the patient constitutes a subsidiary obligation arising from the treatment contract. The hospital authority and/or doctor are liable to the patient for compensation of damages incurred as a result of the violation of such subsidiary obligation. According to § 278 of the German Civil Code, liability is also assumed by contract for so-called vicarious assistants, in this case the nursing staff entrusted with or included in positioning the patient. They are also directly liable for their own culpable mistakes made in positioning the patient in accordance with §§ 823 ff. of the German Civil Code. All those responsible for correct positioning of the patient are jointly and severally liable to the patient, i.e. the patient can demand full compensation for the damage suffered as a result of his incorrect positioning from each of the liable parties and leave any corresponding settlement to the internal relationship between the liable parties.

If a patient is injured because of culpable, i.e. wilfully or negligently incorrect positioning, the doctors and nursing staff responsible can also be prosecuted under criminal law for causing negligent bodily harm according to § 229 of the German Penal Code.

If there is a specific risk involved with a certain positioning method, e.g. the knee-elbow position (so-called »rabbit position«) such as permanent injuries to nerves compressed by the position, the patient must be *informed* about this specific risk before the operation (according to the Federal Supreme Court in its judgement pronounced on 26.2.1985 – VI ZR 124/83 – ArztRecht 1985, 214).

3.2 Interdisciplinary cooperation in positioning the patient

In positioning a patient for an operation, doctors in various disciplines work together without being accountable to each other, in particular the surgeon and the anaesthetist. This is the area of the so-called *horizontal division of labour*. Here court decisions by the Federal Supreme Court in terms of civil liability law are dominated by the thought that the risks of procedures based on the division of labour must not be to the detriment of the patient (according to the Federal Supreme Court in its judgement pronounced on 26.1.1999 – VI ZR 367/97 – ArztRecht 1999, 317 ff.).

In order to distinguish the areas of responsibility of the doctors working on an interdisciplinary basis, legal practice refers in particular to the content of the treatment contracts, the disciplinary boundaries indicated in the Code of Practice set out by the General Medical Council, the concrete distribution of roles in the specific case and on agreements between the various professions involved, which apply particularly to the aspect of patient positioning being dealt with here. Mention should be given in particular to the agreement concluded back on 28 August 1982 between the Professional Federation of German Anaesthetists and the Professional Federation of German Surgeons on cooperation in operative patient care (ArztRecht 1983, 43 ff.). This agreement has meanwhile been amended with regard to positioning the patient on the operating table (Anästhesiologie und Intensivmedizin [1987], 28: 65).

Comparable agreements also exist between other scientific societies and/or professional federations, including for example the agreement on cooperation in surgical gynaecology and in obstetrics between the German Society for Anaesthesiology and Intensive Medicine and the Professional Federation of German Anaesthetists with the German Society for Gynaecology and Obstetrics and the Professional Federation of Gynaecologists (Anästhesiologie und Intensivmedizin [1996], 37: 414 ff.).

While such agreements between professional medical federations are not binding in law, if in any doubt, as mentioned above courts refer to these agreements to distinguish the areas of responsibility so that such agreements assume great practical significance, particularly with regard to the responsibility for positioning a patient before, during and after an operation.

3.2.1 Preoperative phase

Responsibility for positioning the patient to induce the anaesthetic and for monitoring the patient's condition lies with the anaesthetist (as stated concurrently by the agreements between the professional organisations; cf. agreement between the Professional Federation of German Anaesthetists and the Professional Federation of German Surgeons, Anästhesiologie und Intensivmedizin 28 [1987], 65). This is also appropriate. During this period, where necessary the surgeon can consult his team about the operation itself and the corresponding instruments.

3.2.2 Positioning for the operation

The decision as how to position the patient for the operation is always taken by the surgeon according to the requirements of the specific procedure, with consideration of the anaesthesia risk (loc. cit. p. 65). If the anaesthetist has reservations about the positioning required by the surgeon because it impairs monitoring and sustaining the patient's vital functions or because of the risk of positioning injuries, he shall inform the surgeon accordingly. The surgeon's decision regarding positioning is part of his medical and legal responsibility for the operative procedure itself justifying the increased risk of the stipulated operative procedure (loc. cit. p. 65).

3.2.3 Positioning on the operating table

Responsibility for positioning the patient on the operating table is fundamentally part of the surgeon's task. Nursing staff who position the patient on the operating table act according to the surgeon's instructions and responsibility, regardless of which specific department they belong to. The surgeon shall give the necessary instructions; he shall check the patient's positioning before starting to operate. However, the anaesthetist is expected to draw his attention to any obvious positioning mistakes. The anaesthetist is responsible for positioning the extremities required for monitoring the anaesthetic and for administering the anaesthetic and infusions. The anaesthetist shall proceed with all specific safeguarding measures required to monitor the patient and sustain his vital functions as a result of the positioning of the patient (loc. cit. p. 65).

It is normal and correct for the anaesthetist to observe the patient's position during the operation and to inform the operating team of any changes in position (according to the Federal Supreme Court in its judgement pronounced on 24.1.1984 – VI ZR 203/82 – ArztRecht 1984, 238).

3.2.4 Changes in position

The principles stated above about the division of labour in positioning the patient also apply unchanged to any decisions for scheduled changes in positioning the patient during the operation and in implementing such decisions.

If the position of the patient is changed unintentionally as a result of the operation itself in such a way as to increase the positioning risk, the surgeon and his staff are responsible for checking the situation to the extent that the changes in position and other effects on the patient's body originate from the surgeon. If the anaesthetist notices an unintentional change in position or any other effects which are associated with risks for the patient, he must inform the surgeon accordingly (op. cit. p. 65).

In the agreement mentioned above on cooperation in surgical gynaecology and obstetrics (Anästhesiologie und Intensivmedizin [1996], 37: 414 ff., 416), explicit reference is made of the fact that during the operation, the anaesthetist is expected to check the extremities for whose positioning he is responsible.

3.2.5 The postoperative phase

Responsibility for positioning including changing the position of the patient after the end of the operation through to the end of post-anaesthetic monitoring lies with the anaesthetist, unless special circumstances require the involvement of the surgeon during repositioning (as in the agreement on cooperation in surgical gynaecology and obstetrics, op. cit. p. 416).

3.3 Cooperation between doctors and nurses in positioning the patient

Nursing staff helping to position the patient act on the instructions of the corresponding doctor. He is legally responsible for his instructions being correct (so-called *instruction responsibility*). Already the lack of general instructions about the positioning of the patient on the operating table and the lack of corresponding controls is considered to be an organisational error by legal practice (according to the Federal Supreme Court in its judgement pronounced on 24.1.1984 – VI ZR 203/82 – op. cit.). The (senior) doctor must also check that his instructions have been implemented correctly (according to the Federal Supreme Court in its judgement pronounced on 8.3.1960 – VI ZR 45/59 – legal decision on doctor liability 0500/4 regarding monitoring a nurse who is responsible for the positioning of a patient during surgery with an electric knife).

The nursing staff responsible for positioning the patient according to the doctor's instructions are liable for correct implementation of the positioning tasks entrusted to them (so-called *implementation responsibility*).

The doctor entrusting a nurse with the positioning of a patient must convince himself that the nurse is adequately experienced in the technique to be used for positioning the patient. As part of the so-called vertical division of labour, »liability is attributed from the bottom upwards«. In contractual terms, the hospital authority and doctor are liable for any positioning mistakes made by nursing staff in accordance with § 278 of the German Civil Code. When it comes to statutory tortious liability, while on the one hand § 831 of the German Civil Code offers exculpatory possibilities if evidence is provided that due care was taken in the selection and supervision of the nursing staff, on the other hand, high demands are made in this context according to the court decisions taken by the Federal Supreme Court: at least occasional controls by the doctors are necessary (judgement pronounced on 8.3.1960 – VI ZR 45/59 – loc. cit.).

A nurse who positions a patient on a doctor's orders is tied to the doctor's instructions. If the nurse performs the instructions correctly, she is only liable for any possible positioning injuries if she omits to perform a required demonstration in breach of her duties or if she can be accused of assumed fault (cf. judgement pronounced by the Palatinate Intermediate Court of Appeals Zweibrücken dated 20.10.1998–5 U 50/97 – MedR 1999, 419).

3.4 Burden of proof

The possibilities for the courts to come to a decision are also limited. For this reason, it is not always possible for civil liability proceedings to ascertain the material truth. Frequently the outcome of such proceedings depends rather on whether the party bearing the burden of proof can really provide the proof expected of it. As a basic rule, the patient as claimant has to demonstrate and prove all facts justifying his claim. But technically correct positioning of the patient on the operating table and compliance with all medical rules to be observed in order to protect the patient from any positioning injuries are measures falling within the risk area of the hospital and the medical staff. The nursing staff and responsible doctors are capable of coping fully with these measures. In contrast to the patient, the nursing staff and doctors are in a position to clarify the facts of the matter in this respect. According to the Federal Supreme Court, this justifies shifting the burden of proof to the hospital and to the doctors to prove that the patient has been correctly positioned on the operating table and that this has been checked correctly by the doctors (according to the Federal Supreme Court in its judgement pronounced on 24.1.1984 – VI ZR 203/82 – ArztRecht 1984, 238). The nursing and medical staff can, for example, provide the necessary evidence of correct positioning by virtue of the fact that the patient was brought into the correct position on the operating table by an experienced member of the nursing staff, without there being any signs of deviations from what is required from a medical point of view (cf. Eberhardt, Ärztliche Haftpflicht bei intra-operativen Lagerungsschäden, MedR 1986, 117 ff., 121).

Given that the nursing and medical staff have to provide the proof for correct positioning in any legal dispute, great significance is accorded in practical terms to documentation of the patient's positioning, because the nursing and medical staff will have to answer for any documentary omissions. In the case of documentary omissions in civil liability proceedings, it is presumed that the documented measure was not performed. It is then up to the nursing and medical staff to provide other evidence, such as evidence by witnesses that the measure had indeed been performed, that the patient for example had been correctly positioned on the operating table although there is no corresponding documentation. In this context, it is advisable for hospital authorities, surgeons and anaesthetists to issue written procedural instructions for positioning the patient, in accordance with the specific type of operating table being used, technical equipment, coverings, disinfectants, etc. (as rightly stated by Vinz in Behandlungsfehler im Zusammenhang mit der Operationslagerung, Niedersächsisches Ärzteblatt 4/2000 S. 20 f.).

3.5 Documentation of patient positioning

The documentation of the surgical procedure includes all essential diagnostically and therapeutically relevant documents, circumstances and measures, in a form which is adequately clear for the experts, i.e. not so that a lay person can understand them straight away (as in Laufs, Arztrecht, 5th edition 1993, margin number 455, p. 257).

This means that it is not necessary to draw up a detailed report about how the patient was positioned in concrete terms. On the contrary, it is sufficient for the positioning to be described in technical keywords or illustrated by symbols to make it clear for an expert which method was used for positioning and operating on the patient (as pronounced explicitly by the Federal Supreme Court in its judgement on 24.1.1984 – VI ZR 203/82 – ArztRecht 1984, 238). In the case of an operation for a slipped disk in which the patient was positioned on the operating table in the so-called knee-elbow position (»rabbit position«), the Federal Supreme Court considered it to be sufficient that this kind of positioning was documented. If the type of positioning during the operation is generally accepted, then the technical procedure for positioning the patient transpires from generally accepted medical rules which must be observed in this case. This does not have to be recorded in writing each time. This would only be necessary if in isolated cases the positioning deviated from the standard procedure or if not insignificant corrections took place during the operation. On the other hand, if an

3.5 Documentation of patient positioning

operation proceeds without anything special happening, there is no need to make any records about the unchanged position of the patient (according to the Federal Supreme Court in its judgement pronounced on 24.1.1984 – VI ZR 203/82 – ArztRecht 1984, 238).

The routine measures which do not require documentation also include actually controlling the correct position of the arm before and during the operation (adjusting the abduction angle and observing the infusion arm) (according to the Federal Supreme Court in its judgement pronounced on 24.1.1995 – VI ZR 60/94 – ArztRecht 1996, 62). By contrast, it is advisable to make corresponding reference to any risk factors in the operating report, documenting how these were taken into account, for example including any effects on the positioning of the patient (as stated by Vinz, loc. cit. p. 21). Such risk factors can include severe emaciation, neurological disorders, joint contractures, atrophic skin diseases, abnormal perspiration, excessively extended positioning of the operating table because of blameless, intraoperative surgical or anaesthesia complications, long-term blameless cardiovascular depression or allergies to skin.

4 Use of X-rays in the operating suite

General aspects and X-ray Ordinance, radiation generation and radiation protection

H. Kreienfeld, H. Klimpel, V. Böttcher

4.1	Radiation protection in the operating suite	– 20
4.1.1	Introduction – 20	
4.1.2	Legal principles for the use of X-rays in medicine – 21	
4.1.2.1	X-ray Ordinance, Atomic Energy Law, Euratom Directives, ICRP recommendations – 21	
4.1.2.2	Use of X-rays on people – 22	
4.1.2.3	Radiation protection manager, radiation protection officer – 24	
4.1.2.4	Obligations when operating an X-ray machine – 24	
4.1.2.5	Occupational exposure to radiation, personal dosimetry – 25	
4.1.2.6	Helpers – 27	
4.1.2.7	Information and instruction procedures – 27	
4.1.2.8	Records – 29	
4.1.2.9	Quality assurance according to the X-ray Ordinance – 29	
4.1.3	Generating X-rays – 30	
4.1.4	The image receiver system for surgical image intensifiers – 32	
4.1.5	The main components in surgical image intensifiers – 32	
4.1.6	Technical minimum requirements for examination with surgical image intensifiers – 32	
4.1.7	Application-related radiation protection in the operating suite – 32	
4.1.8	Correct positioning of the image receiver system – 34	
4.1.9	Correct use of the automatic dose control (ADR) – 34	
4.2	Surgical image intensifier systems	– 35
4.2.1	Expert inspection – 36	
4.2.2	X-ray radiation – 36	
4.2.3	Radiation protection – 36	
4.2.4	Structure and technique of a surgical image intensifier – 37	
4.2.5	Application – 38	
4.2.6	Use of the surgical image intensifier – 38	
4.2.7	Tips and tricks for daily routine – 38	

References – 39

4.1 Radiation protection in the operating suite

H. Kreienfeld, H. Klimpel

4.1.1 Introduction

In 1895, the physicist Wilhelm Conrad Röntgen in Würzburg discovered a »new type of ray« which was later called X-ray or »Röntgen« in Germany in recognition of his pioneering discovery (Fig. 4.1).

In physical terms, X-rays are attributed to ionising radiation (Fig. 4.2).

The possibility of using this radiation successfully in human medicine for diagnostic purposes or also for therapy in certain diseases led to a dramatic development in the following decades, both in examination techniques and also in the corresponding equipment required for this purpose. X-rays could be used for both *short-term exposure* for X-ray pictures, and also for so-called radiography for *continuous exposure*. During the 1950's, the development of X-ray image intensifiers had progressed to such an extent that radiography was also possible in the operating theatre for support or documentation of surgical procedures, without the room having to be darkened accordingly for this purpose. This technical development – initially the pictures were viewed through a monocular or binoculars – and the subsequent addition of television cameras and monitors paved the way for the versatile applications of mobile surgical image intensifiers (»mobile C-arm units and C-arm units on the ceiling mount in the operating theatre«).

The principle of these X-ray scanning machines has remained the same through to today, even though technical refinements have been introduced with developments in microelectronics in newly developed machines. These include for example the CCD camera (charge-coupled device – light-sensitive chip camera) *together with digital image storing and processing.*

Mobile C-arm X-ray machines are not shielded from leakage radiation in the design of the machine because of the special aspects of their use, so that the user has to pay special attention to radiation protection. But it is also possible for radiation protection for the patient to be impaired quite considerably, for example by unacceptable positioning and use of the emitter/image receiver system. As a result, it is absolutely mandatory for all users of surgical image intensifiers to be well instructed in correct use of the equipment (▶ § 18 of the X-ray Ordinance [RöV]) and in addition, they also have to possess the qualification »*special knowledge* in radiation protection« according to the regulation »*special knowledge according to the X-ray Ordinance/Medicine*« which is anchored in the X-ray Ordinance [1]. The assistants working under the medical staff must have »*knowledge* of radiation protection« if they are expected to trigger X-rays under the instruction of a doctor with special knowledge in radiation protection (specialised doctor) or to assume the »technical execution« of the radiation application.

Although the application techniques for X-ray examinations and surgical image intensifiers have undergone further development, X-ray diagnosis in the operating theatre still differs in character from »classical X-ray diagnosis« in the X-ray department of hospitals, which is geared to differentiated »X-ray diagnosis«. »Surgical X-ray diagnosis« differs on account of the following features:

– In the operating theatre, the X-ray examination is an indispensable aid for supporting and documenting surgical procedures.

Fig. 4.1. First handwritten message from Röntgen about his discovery

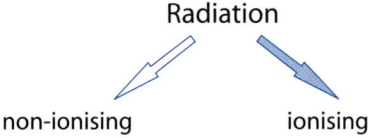

Fig. 4.2. Attributing X-rays to ionising radiation

Radiation

non-ionising
- radio and microwaves
- electromagnetic fields
- optical radiation

ionising
- X-rays
- gamma rays
- particle radiation of radioactive substances

- Surgeons, anaesthetists, surgical nurses and assistants are also present during perioperative radiation application in the operating theatre and thus also within the stipulated *control zone*.
- Given the necessary wide range of applications of surgical image intensifiers, it is not possible to fix any radiation protection shielding for the operating staff to the C-arm machines, which have to be able to turn and swivel to all sides, in contrast for example to the close-control scanning machines used in the X-ray diagnosis department.
- The room brightness required for the operation can possibly impair viewing and evaluation of the monitor picture.
- The necessary presence of several doctors and assistants in the operating theatre can make it more difficult for the individual to stay for any length of time in places with low local dose or local dose rate.
- Operations under sterile conditions and special positioning of the patient, particularly for procedures to the trunk, can considerably impair or even prevent optimum radiation protection precautions.
- For simple issues and pictures for documentation purposes, e.g. after the removal of implants, it is possible to accept less than optimum image quality in the interests of low radiation exposure.

4.1.2 Legal principles for the use of X-rays in medicine

4.1.2.1 X-ray Ordinance, Atomic Energy Law, Euratom Directives, ICRP recommendations

In Germany, the medical use of X-rays has been regulated since 1973 in the *X-ray Ordinance* (RöV). This legal provision was issued as an ordinance on account of the *authorisation provisions in the Atomic Energy Law* (AtG). The X-ray Ordinance was amended in 2002 [2] because of the stipulations in the directive 96/29/EURATOM »laying down basic safety standards for the protection of the health of workers and the general public against the dangers of ionising radiation« [3] and in the patient protection directive 97/43/EURATOM »on health protection of individuals against the dangers of ionising radiation in relation to medical exposure« [4] and came into effect on 1 July 2002.

The new X-ray Ordinance gives special priority to the *radiation protection principles*
- justification,
- dose limitation,
- prevention of unnecessary radiation exposure and
- dose reduction

together with the newly worded Radiation Protection Directive (StrlSchV).

To this end, the new X-ray Ordinance contains clearer regulations of the medical and technical requirements for the use of X-rays on people than before. These regulations include in particular new definitions:
- »use of X-rays« (for X-ray examinations with a differentiation between »technical implementation« and »evaluation«),
- »image quality« (»diagnostic image quality« and »physical image quality«),
- »diagnostic reference values« (DRW),
- »justifying indication«.

The sub-section »use of X-rays on people« in the new X-ray Ordinance contains above all specifications for »justifying indication«, on the »authorised persons« and »application principles« together with »documentation obligations«.

The new X-ray Ordinance also includes two important, updated implementing regulations (Fig. 4.3):
- the »ordinance on expert inspections according to the X-ray Ordinance (SV-RL)« dated 27 August 2003 [5] and
- the »ordinance for performing quality assurance with X-ray equipment according to §§ 16 and 17 of the X-ray Ordinance (QS-RL)« dated 20 November 2003 [6].

Both ordinances stipulate the technical radiation protection requirements and the corresponding tests and the requirements for »physical image quality« with the corresponding intended quality assurance (quality tests) for the various medical X-ray diagnosis equipment, also for surgical image intensifiers.

For surgical image intensifiers, i.e. for »mobile C-arm units (including C-arm units on the ceiling mount in the operating theatre), these requirements for radiation protection and for quality control are featured essentially in the test positions according to section 2.2.4 of the SV-RL.

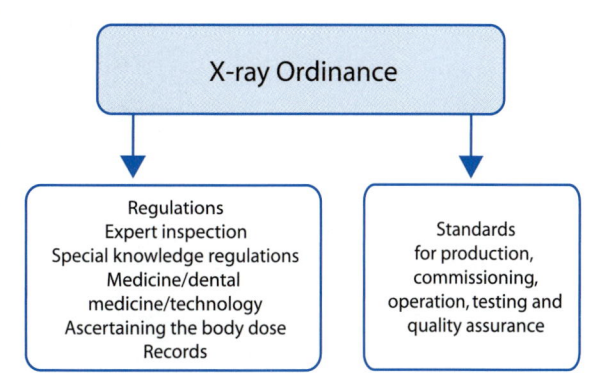

```
                    ┌─────────────────┐
                    │ X-ray Ordinance │
                    └─────────────────┘
                      ↙             ↘
    ┌──────────────────────┐   ┌──────────────────────┐
    │ Regulations          │   │ Standards            │
    │ Expert inspection    │   │ for production,      │
    │ Special knowledge    │   │ commissioning,       │
    │ regulations          │   │ operation, testing   │
    │ Medicine/dental      │   │ and quality          │
    │ medicine/technology  │   │ assurance            │
    │ Ascertaining the     │   │                      │
    │ body dose            │   │                      │
    │ Records              │   │                      │
    └──────────────────────┘   └──────────────────────┘
```

Fig. 4.3. X-ray Ordinance and corresponding regulations and standards

According to the X-ray Ordinance, when operating X-ray diagnosis equipment it must be guaranteed that
- the regulations of the Medical Product Law (MPG) are fulfilled for putting the equipment into circulation for the first time and commissioning the equipment,
- all state-of-the-art equipment is present and measures taken as required to ensure that the protection regulations are heeded and
- given the intended type of examination, it is guaranteed that the necessary image quality is achieved with the lowest possible radiation exposure.

The guarantee of the »necessary (physical) image quality« is a prime prerequisite in order to achieve the necessary »diagnostic image quality« in medical X-ray examinations (▶ definitions in § 2 No. 5 RöV). Diagnostic image quality for the various X-ray examinations is described in the »medical quality requirements« according to the »Guidelines for quality assurance in X-ray diagnosis« [7]. These guidelines must fundamentally also be applied when using surgical image intensifiers. The wide range of applications of these X-ray diagnosis machines is also indicated in the *know-how* recommendations for the application area »emergency diagnosis« in the above mentioned special knowledge ordinance (▶ Sect. 4.1.2.2). Given that when surgical image intensifiers are used it is also frequently necessary to perform treatment and progress checks, for example, and take documentation pictures, the corresponding »medical quality requirements« according to the stated guidelines can be considered and used in individual cases with clear differentiation to the requirements for »classical projection radiography (▶ Sect. 4.1.1).

One essential aim of the amended X-ray Ordinance consists of minimising the radiation exposure of patients resulting from medical X-ray diagnosis as far as possible while complying with a defined image quality and use-related radiation exposure standards (»diagnostic reference values« – DRW). The measures mentioned above for radiation protection and quality assurance and the requirements made of the special qualifications of the doctors and their assistants apply to this specific end.

In addition, the amended X-ray Ordinance also implements the clearly reduced dose limit values for »persons with occupational exposure to radiation« and for the general public in national law (◘ Table 4.1).

The amended version of the X-ray Ordinance applies to X-ray radiation generated by accelerated electrons in the energy range between 5 kilo-electron-volt and 1 mega-electron-volt. All equipment for generating ionising radiation with higher energy, as used for example in radiotherapy, are subject to the provisions of the Radiation Protection Ordinance (StrlSchV). The basic aim of optimising radiation protection applies to both the Radiation Protection Ordinance and to the X-ray Ordinance and is also described by the so-called ALARA principle (»as low as reasonably achievable) in corresponding recommendations of the »International Commission on Radiological Protection« (ICRP), which comes into effect in interpreting radiation protection precautions.

4.1.2.2 Use of X-rays on people

According to the *application principles* of § 25 of the X-ray Ordinance, X-rays can be used »on people only in medical healing or dental healing, in medical research, in other cases intended or permitted by law or for examination according to the specifications of general occupational safety«.

◘ **Table 4.1.** The new dose limit values [mSv]

Body dose	Limit values of the body dose for		
	persons with occupational radiation exposure in		individuals in the population
	Cat. A	Cat. B	
1. Effective dose	20/50	6	1
2. Organ dose: iris	150	50	15
3. Organ dose: skin[a], unless stated under 4	500	150	50
4. Organ dose: hands, lower arms, feet and ankles including corresponding skin[b]	500	150	

[a] The limit values apply regardless of the exposed surface for a mean dose on every surface of 1 cm^2.
[b] The effective dose for persons with radiation exposure in Cat. A may amount to up to 50 mSv in one single calendar year if the total dose of 100 mSv is not exceeded in the 5 successive calendar years.

According to § 23 Para. 1 No. 1 of the X-ray Ordinance, X-rays may »only be used directly on people in medical or dental healing if a person has made a *justifying indication* according to § 24 Para. 1 No. 1 or 2«.

Furthermore, when a justifying indication has been made, X-rays may always only be used on people under the responsibility of doctors who possess *specialised knowledge in radiation protection,* i.e. have acquired specialist know-how in radiation protection and can verify corresponding training (»justified persons« according to § 24 of the X-ray Ordinance). Here it must be noted that doctors are not considered to be specialists in accordance with radiation protection just on the basis of completing their medical training. The acquisition of the specialist knowledge and radiation protection know-how is stipulated as an implementing regulation to the X-ray Ordinance in the above mentioned specialist ordinance in the version dated 1991 [1] (This ordinance will probably come into effect in an updated version during 2005 on the basis of the amended X-ray Ordinance dated 2002). According to the currently valid ordinance dated 1991, specialist knowledge in radiation protection consists of the »*technical knowledge*« and successful attendance of »*courses in radiation protection*«. The technical knowledge »contains theoretical knowledge and practical experience in using X-ray radiation in the specific area of application«. The courses in radiation protection »convey a knowledge of the laws, other theory and practical exercises in radiation protection in the specific area of application«.

Technical knowledge »includes the practical implementation and assessment of X-ray examinations under the special aspects of radiation protection.« For surgeons at the moment as a rule, a minimum 12-month period is required for acquiring the technical knowledge in the area of »emergency diagnosis (extremities, skull, vertebral column, thorax, abdomen)«.

To this end, the specialist knowledge ordinance explains among others:
- Emergency diagnosis: simple X-ray diagnosis as part of initial care and emergency treatment and
- Emergency diagnosis of the abdomen: digestive, urinary and biliary tracts, reproductive organs.

If the technical knowledge has been verified in the corresponding application area with successful attendance of radiation protection courses – when using surgical image intensifiers after an initial 8-h »Instruction … in radiation protection…«, a »basic course in radiation protection« and a »special course in X-ray diagnosis«, the responsible state Medical Council issues a corresponding specialist certificate. This specialist certificate is a prerequisite for the operation of surgical imaging intensifiers under their own responsibility by surgeons working in general practice.

A doctor *without* specialist knowledge in radiation protection, even a surgeon, may only use X-rays according to the X-ray Ordinance if he has the necessary »know-how in radiation protection« according to § 24 of the X-ray Ordinance and works »under constant supervision and responsibility« of a doctor »with specialist knowledge in radiation protection«. Know-how in radiation protection refers to an applied method of X-ray examination and the corresponding necessary radiation protection rules and is conveyed according to the specialist knowledge ordinance of 1991 as »instruction for doctors about radiation protection in diagnosis with X-ray radiation« in the 8-h special courses mentioned above.

For the use of surgical image intensifiers, it is stipulated that also those persons working as assistants only in the operating suite and using or switching on X-ray equipment under the direct instruction of the immediately present specialist doctor (technical execution) must have *know-how in radiation protection.* According to the above mentioned specialist knowledge ordinance, the necessary *know-how in radiation protection* is acquired in special courses which currently last 24 h.

With regard to transitional rulings, the amended X-ray Ordinance prescribes that *specialist knowledge* and *know-how* in radiation protection must be updated for the corresponding group of people at least every 5 years by attending corresponding radiation protection courses or other acknowledged training courses.

4.1.2.3 Radiation protection manager, radiation protection officer

The radiation protection manager requires a permit or notification according to the X-ray Ordinance (owner). Where necessary for safe operation, the radiation protection manager shall appoint in writing the required number of radiation protection officers to run or supervise the facility. The radiation protection manager is still responsible for compliance with the protection regulations even after he has appointed radiation protection officers (▶ § 13 Para. 2 of the X-ray Ordinance).

In a university clinic or hospital with several independent departments with X-ray equipment, as a rule, the radiation protection manager (e.g. dean of the university or administrator of the city or district hospital) appoints the senior physician or medical director in writing as the radiation protection officer. »Required number of radiation protection officers to run or supervise the facility« means that a deputy must be appointed also in the event of the absence of a radiation protection officer while on holiday or incapacitated. A radiation protection officer must also be appointed to cover the eventuality that the use of X-ray radiation is planned on days being worked in several shifts, during night shifts, at the weekends or on public bank holidays.

Fig. 4.4. Important dose definitions in radiation protection

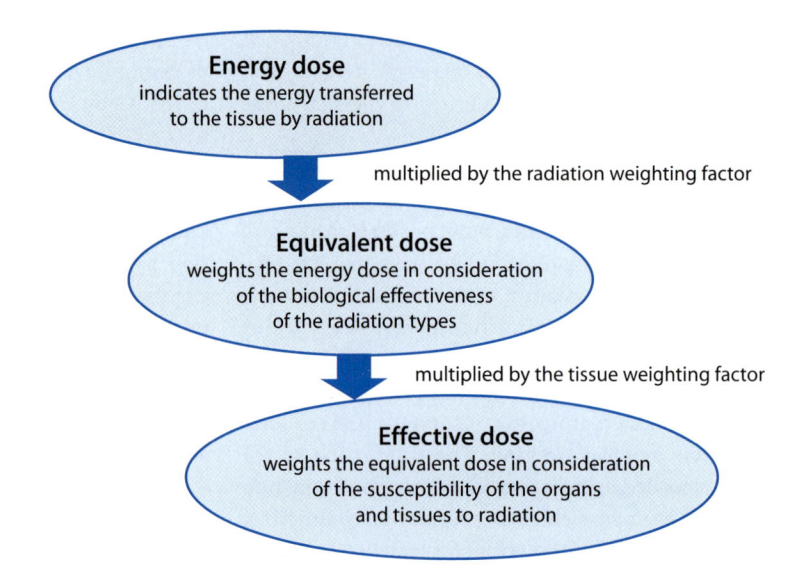

Energy dose
indicates the energy transferred to the tissue by radiation

multiplied by the radiation weighting factor

Equivalent dose
weights the energy dose in consideration of the biological effectiveness of the radiation types

multiplied by the tissue weighting factor

Effective dose
weights the equivalent dose in consideration of the susceptibility of the organs and tissues to radiation

The basic rule applies that medical staff in the possession of only »know-how in radiation protection« is only allowed to work in the application of radiation »under the constant supervision and responsibility« of a specialist doctor. This rule has meanwhile been interpreted by the responsible authorities in such a way that following a justifying indication (in other words, »order for radiation application«) by a doctor with »specialist knowledge in radiation protection«, this doctor (or another specialist doctor) does not necessarily have to be personally present during the radiation application; however, he must be capable of arriving (back) in the place where radiation is being used within 15 min.

4.1.2.4 Obligations when operating an X-ray machine

Instruction of the staff. Given the special use of radiation with surgical image intensifiers in the operating theatre and the necessary presence of the doctors and assistants while using the radiation within the control area, the »instruction« in the correct handling of this equipment required in § 18 Para. 1 No. 1 of the X-ray Ordinance is of very special significance. This instruction, which must be arranged by the owner on the basis of an operating manual in the German language provided by expert staff of the machine manufacturer or supplier, is only required »at initial commissioning«, but should be repeated at appropriate intervals by the radiation protection officer in view of the special potential for danger involved in using the equipment, together with the frequently high fluctuation rate among staff in surgical departments. Records must be kept about holding such instruction sessions for the staff.

Radiation protection areas – control area. According to the X-ray Ordinance (§ 19), areas where persons can receive a higher effective dose than 6 mSv per calendar year (Sv, Sievert: dose unit for the effective equivalent dose) are to be marked off and identified as control areas. Given standard use of surgical image intensifiers, the control area depends not only on the radiation exposure times but also on the size of the maximum possible effective radiation field; in standard applications it ends between 2.5 m and 3.5 m from the region of the patient's body where the radiation was used. When using surgical image intensifiers for long procedures with long radiation exposure times, under certain circumstances the whole operating theatre is to be declared as control area. The control area identification must be clearly visible, containing at least the words »No entry – X-rays«. It can also be affixed to the (mobile) image intensifier in a clearly visible form stating the stipulated distance. But given the meanwhile wide range of applications of surgical image intensifiers, it is advisable to consider the whole operating theatre as control area in each case, and to apply the protection regulations of the X-ray Ordinance to all persons present there.

Monitoring areas. Monitoring areas are areas not belonging to the control area where persons can receive an annual effective dose higher than 1 mSv. These areas are to be set up as monitoring areas and given a permitted presence time of 40 h/week and 50 weeks/ calendar year, as in the control areas, unless other details apply to the actual presence time (§ 19 of the X-ray Ordinance).

The »effective dose« stated in § 2 No. 6 Letter b of the X-ray Ordinance is a dimension for the total damage or total risk from stochastic radiation effects which can occur with the comparatively low radiation exposure of persons with occupational radiation exposure in X-ray diagnosis. The effective dose is the sum of the weighted mean equivalent doses in the individual organs and tissues,

Fig. 4.5. Official personal dosimeter (film badge)

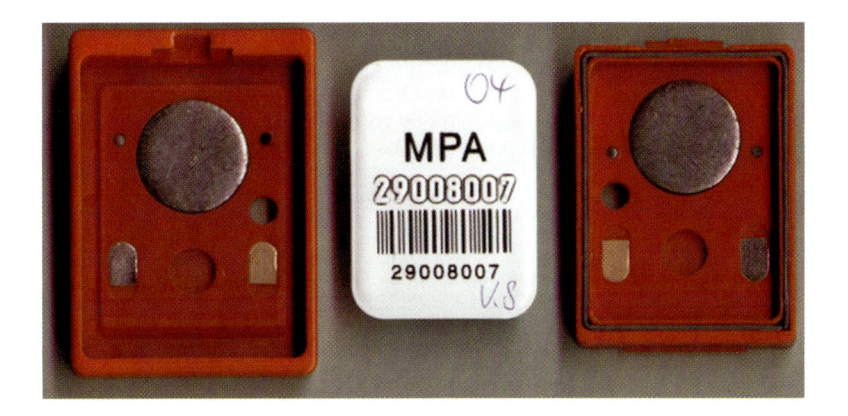

which are possibly exposed to differing amounts of radiation (Fig. 4.4). The unit of measurement for the effective dose is the sievert (Sv). The effective dose allows for a better comparison of the risks with regard to cancer or genetic damage for whole body exposure or exposure of just individual parts of the body. Stochastic radiation effects are random biological effects whose probability increases with radiation exposure, but for which no limit dose is presumed. As far as the stochastic effects are concerned, it is presumed that these are mono-cellular processes, i.e. the malignant transformation of one single cell is sufficient to trigger this kind of effect. It is only with considerably higher radiation exposure, such as that used for example in radiotherapy, that random (stochastic) effects reliably no longer occur; the effects here are deterministic (non-stochastic) radiation effects where the severity increases with increasing radiation exposure according to the number of damaged cells; here a limit dose is presumed. These effects come about as a result of multi-cellular processes, i.e. many cells have to be damaged before these effects are manifested. These radiation effects include all acute radiation effects, e.g. cataract or fibrotic processes in various tissues.

4.1.2.5 Occupational exposure to radiation, personal dosimetry

When surgical image intensifiers are being used in the operating theatre, the medical and nursing staff can receive a body dose as effective dose or part body dose of more than 1 mSv/a in certain organs. This group of persons is thus considered as having »occupational exposure to radiation«, and their radiation exposure, i.e. their body dose, must be monitored by measuring the personal dose. So-called personal dosimeters (film badges) are used for this purpose; they are usually replaced once a month and evaluated by the authority responsible according to state law (Fig. 4.5).

The result of this evaluation is the amount of the received body dose. The radiation protection manager, radiation protection officer or person supervised by them can stipulate the use of a second dosimeter in addition to the official dosimeter, which can be read off at any time, e.g. a rod dosimeter (Fig. 4.6).

The details of the type and scope of personal dosimetry for occupational exposure to radiation are stipulated in the amended »Guideline for physical radiation protection control for ascertaining body doses« dated 8 December 2003 [9]. Given the significance of occupational exposure to radiation when »using X-rays in the operating theatre«, Figure 4.7 shows the suggestions made by these guidelines for personal dosimetry in the operating theatre and in interventional radiology.

The intensity of radiation used in the operating theatre is very unevenly distributed. In the case of unhindered, free dissipation, radiation from a punctiform origin will decrease in intensity according to the distance square law. Although these perquisites usually do not apply when using radiation in the operating theatre, enlarging the distance to the patient volume being exposed to radiation always considerably reduces the

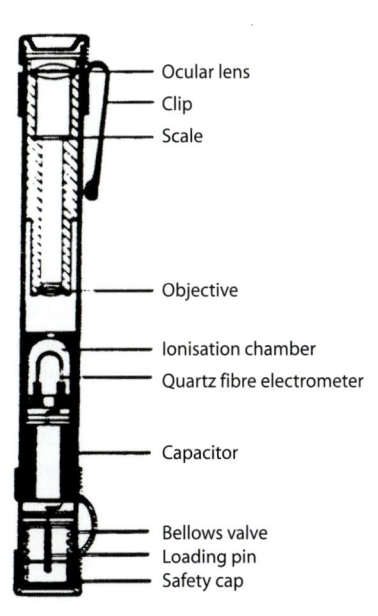

Fig. 4.6. Rod dosimeter which can be read off at any time

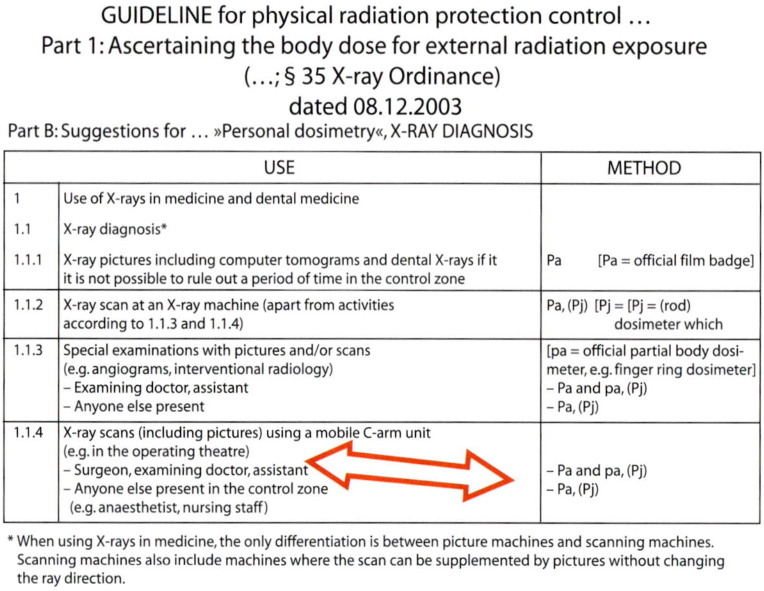

Fig. 4.7. Suggestions for personal dosimetry

GUIDELINE for physical radiation protection control …
Part 1: Ascertaining the body dose for external radiation exposure
(…; § 35 X-ray Ordinance)
dated 08.12.2003
Part B: Suggestions for … »Personal dosimetry«, X-RAY DIAGNOSIS

	USE	METHOD
1	Use of X-rays in medicine and dental medicine	
1.1	X-ray diagnosis*	
1.1.1	X-ray pictures including computer tomograms and dental X-rays if it is not possible to rule out a period of time in the control zone	Pa [Pa = official film badge]
1.1.2	X-ray scan at an X-ray machine (apart from activities according to 1.1.3 and 1.1.4)	Pa, (Pj) [Pj = [Pj = (rod) dosimeter which
1.1.3	Special examinations with pictures and/or scans (e.g. angiograms, interventional radiology) – Examining doctor, assistant – Anyone else present	[pa = official partial body dosimeter, e.g. finger ring dosimeter] – Pa and pa, (Pj) – Pa, (Pj)
1.1.4	X-ray scans (including pictures) using a mobile C-arm unit (e.g. in the operating theatre) – Surgeon, examining doctor, assistant – Anyone else present in the control zone (e.g. anaesthetist, nursing staff)	– Pa and pa, (Pj) – Pa, (Pj)

* When using X-rays in medicine, the only differentiation is between picture machines and scanning machines. Scanning machines also include machines where the scan can be supplemented by pictures without changing the ray direction.

radiation exposure for the persons present in the control area (Fig. 4.8).

In this context it is worth mentioning that together with the tolerable annual limit value for the effective dose, limit values have also been stipulated for persons with occupational exposure to radiation for organs or areas of the body »iris, skin, hands, lower arms, feet and ankles«, and compliance with these limit values must be safeguarded by corresponding protection measures. In addition, § 31b of the X-ray Ordinance stipulates a limit value for the effective dose measured in all calendar years (occupational life dose) for persons with occupational exposure to radiation as 400 mSv. If this limit value is exceeded, the supervisory authorities can permit that the effective dose in subsequent years does not exceed 10 mSv per calendar year.

Persons with occupational exposure to radiation are allocated to category A or B depending on the expected radiation exposure. Persons in category A must undergo a check-up by an »authorised doctor« (occupational health check-up) within 1 year before starting to work in the control area. The doctor must ascertain whether there are any health concerns against working in the control area. For persons in category B, the supervisory authorities *can* stipulate that this kind of check-up takes place before starting to work in the control area. If the check-up shows that there are no health concerns to working in the control area, the »authorised doctor« issues a corresponding certificate which has to be submitted to the radiation protection manager.

The main difference between the two categories consists in the fact that persons with occupational radiation exposure in category A have to be examined by an »authorised doctor« *regularly every year*. Such regular check-ups are not prescribed for persons with occupational radiation exposure in category B.

If the information from the official personal dosimeter evaluated every month shows that the limit value of 6 mSv for the annual effective dose has been exceeded in a person with occupational radiation exposure in category B, then this person must be allocated to category A of persons with occupational radiation exposure, and then has to undergo regular yearly check-ups by an »authorised doctor«, as described above. Persons subject to monitoring by an »authorised doctor« must tolerate the necessary medical check-ups.

In the case of female operating staff, it must be noted that
— in women capable of bearing children, the body dose at the womb accumulated over 1 month must not exceed 2 mSv (§ 31a of the X-ray Ordinance) and
— the working conditions for pregnant women must be organised in such a way that the equivalent dose to which the unborn child is exposed is kept as low as reasonably possible and the dose probably does not exceed 1 mSv during the remainder of the pregnancy. In compliance with these marginal conditions, pregnant women are not prohibited from working in the control area.

Outside staff. The new X-ray Ordinance now also contains occupational safety regulations for employees working for example as *anaesthetist* in *another hospital* or in doctor's surgeries when using surgical image intensifiers in the operating suite, without belonging to the regular staff there. The supervisory authorities must be informed of the activities of these persons according to § 6 Para. 1 No. 3

4.1 · Radiation protection in the operating suite

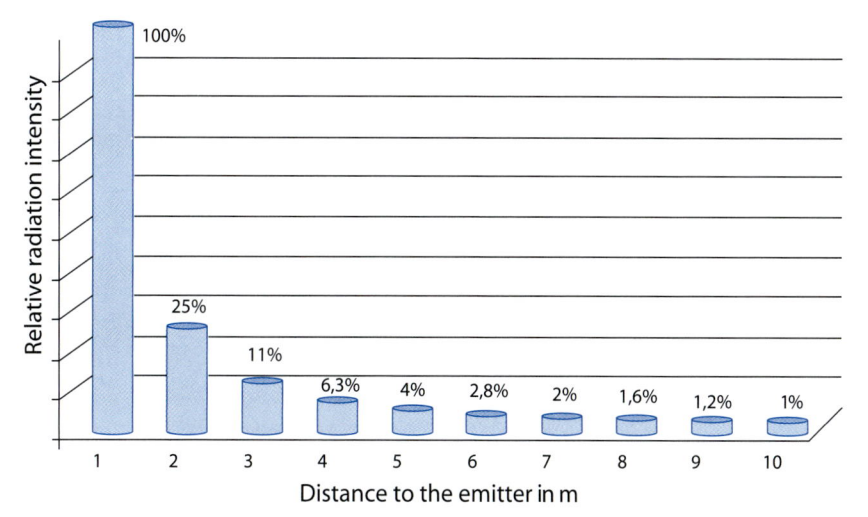

Fig. 4.8. Distance square law. Decrease in radiation intensity by the distance to the emitter for punctiform free dissipation

of the X-ray Ordinance, and they must hold a radiation card (▶ see § 35 Para 2 and 3 of the X-ray Ordinance).

Immediate measure to be taken on exceeding the limit values. If it is possible for the dose limit value for persons with occupational radiation exposure to be exceeded for one or several persons when operating an X-ray machine as a result of »extraordinary events or circumstances« (§ 42 of the X-ray Directive), this »event«, which the old X-ray Ordinance referred to as accident, must be reported immediately to the supervisory authorities. In addition, the affected persons must consult an »authorised doctor« immediately. As a rule, the authorities will check the event or circumstances resulting in this »accident« on the spot and order further measures to guarantee compliance with the dose limit values for persons with occupational radiation exposure. Given the fact that such incidents, which also have to be reported to the responsible Professional Association, are extremely rare when operating surgical image intensifiers, they will not be given any further attention here.

4.1.2.6 Helpers

§ 2 of the amended X-ray Ordinance contains a definition for »helpers« based on the rulings in the directive 97/43/Euratom. Accordingly, helpers, e.g. members of the patient's family (previously called »accompanying persons«) are persons who support and look after the patient »voluntarily outside their occupational activity« where X-rays are being used as part of medical treatment. No dose limit values apply to helpers, because their exposure always depends on the exposure of the person being helped or cared for. The demand for protective measures to restrict the radiation exposure of helpers indicates that their dose should not exceed a few millisievert.

In addition, the regulations of »physical radiation protection control« do not apply to helpers, i.e. the use of »official dosimeters« (film badges) is not necessary when present in the control area. The body dose can be ascertained by measuring the personal dose, e.g. with dosimeters which can be read off at any time, by multiplying the period of presence with the local dose measured at the place where the helper is, or »by other suitable means«.

4.1.2.7 Information and instruction procedures

The *annual* instruction of persons using X-rays or permitted to enter the control area as employees, »helpers« or trainees stipulated in the X-ray Ordinance is of great significance for the radiation protection of staff and patient when using radiation in surgical image intensifiers. This instruction according to § 36 of the X-ray Ordinance essentially deals with

— the intended working methods,
— the possible risks,
— the safety and protection measures being used,
— the essential contents of the X-ray Ordinance referring to the activity or presence and
— the radiation protection instruction.

Together with persons with authorised access to the control area, instruction must also be given to those who *use* X-rays or are involved in the *technical aspects* of using radiation, without having to be present in the control area. As far as the instructions are concerned, § 36 of the X-ray Ordinance says: »Records are to be kept about the contents and time of the instructions and must be signed by the person receiving the instructions. The records are to be kept for five years (one year for helpers) and submitted to the supervisory authorities on request.«

The instructions do not have to be provided by the radiation protection manager or radiation protection officer: they can be delegated to another person, e.g. well qualified doctors of the department or an external expert. The radiation protection manager still remains responsible for the contents and delivery of the instructions. From the requirement to provide instruction »about the safety and protective measures to be used«, it can be deduced that »general« or »sweeping« instructions e.g. just about the radiation protection regulations in the X-ray Ordinance, are inadequate. The particular special type of radiation application and the activities of the persons being instructed must always be taken into account in the instructions. On the other hand, together with verbal instruction it is also possible to use specially elaborated instruction texts, together with including film or video recordings during the instructions.

Patient protection. Radiation protection of the patient is featured in the X-ray Ordinance in the application principles of § 25 as already mentioned above. According to these principles, X-rays must only be used on persons if
— this is advisable resulting from a medical indication and a person with the necessary expertise has made the »justifying indication«,
— the health benefits from using radiation on the individual outweigh the radiation risk,
— other procedures with similar health benefit which entail no or lesser radiation exposure have already been considered,
— it is certain that the radiation exposure can be limited to an extent which is compatible with the requirements of modern medical science.

Together with these principles, § 16 of the X-ray Ordinance demands compliance with so-called diagnostic reference values (DRW) which are published by the Federal Department for Radiation Protection, in order to guarantee good practice when performing medical and dental X-ray examinations. The diagnostic reference values do not constitute limit values for patients and do not apply to individual examinations. But the use of radiation in the various examinations should be organised and optimised so that the diagnostic reference values are not exceeded in average for an adequate number of examinations of one specific examination type.

Personal radiation protection of the patient also includes the requirement in § 25 of the X-ray Ordinance that parts of the body, which do not have to be affected by the effective radiation in the intended use of X-rays, must be protected as far as possible from radiation exposure. Here is it necessary to keep available and use suitable radiation protection accessories, such as patient protection aprons, gonadal shields and other lead rubber covers. Up to now according to the meanwhile withdrawn standard DIN 6813 issue July 1980 [10], patient protection aprons had to have a lead equivalent value of min. 0.4 mm and gonadal shields

Table 4.2. Radiation protection accessories

For the **radiation user** (doctor and assistant) with the necessary lead values in mm Pb according to DIN 6813, issue July 1980	
Radiation protection apron, front	0.35
Radiation protection apron, back	0.25
Radiation protection surgical apron	0.25
Gloves	0.25
For the **patient** as per DIN 6813, issue July 1980	
Patient protection apron, gonadal protection apron	0.4
Gonadal shield	1.0

a lead equivalent value of min. 1.0 mm. The new DIN EN 61331-3, issue May 2002 [11] stipulates for »gonadal protection aprons« an attenuation equivalent of min. 0.55 mm Pb according to standard sizes (for children and adults). In addition, this new standard also recommends »*light* testicle protection« with min. 0.5 mm Pb and »*heavy* testicle protection« and »ovary protection« each with an attenuation equivalent of min. 1.0 mm Pb. It goes without saying that existing patient protection devices according to the old DIN 6813 can still be used. The specialist doctor decides about using the existing radiation protection accessories from case to case.

Annex III of the Expert Guidelines [5] lists the *necessary* patient protection devices for X-ray diagnosis machines depending on the various areas of application. For surgical and orthopaedic applications, the devices are as follows:
— gonadal protection aprons in several sizes,
— testicle capsule (enclosing) in several sizes,
— ovary shields,
— patient protection aprons,
— lead rubber covers in several sizes.

Together with these *necessary* patient protection devices as per DIN 6813 [10], the *recommendations for use* of the accessories in the (old) standard must also be heeded. The radiation protection accessories as per DIN 6813 must have at least the lead equivalents shown in Table 4.2.

The effectiveness of the shields decreases out of all proportion in the face of higher energy radiation, i.e. generated with higher tube voltage. But the radiation protection accessories are still ideally effective for the tube voltage range of about 70 kV required in surgery. So consistent use of the radiation protection accessories constitutes a very effective radiation protection measure.

Radiation protection of the patient should also be mentioned by the responsible surgeon in his personal information session with the patient. This is part of his duty to inform as required in the *professional code of conduct* of the state Medical Councils in order to obtain the patient's consent for the intended medical procedures.

4.1.2.8 Records

According to § 28 of the X-ray Ordinance, suitable records are to be produced about using X-rays on persons, which must also contain

- information about earlier medical use of ionising radiation, insofar as this is significant for the intended application and
- in the case of female persons of an age capable of bearing children, information about whether they are pregnant or not.

In the case of X-ray examinations, X-ray cards are to be kept available and offered to the patient (§ 28 Para. 2 of the X-ray Ordinance).

The records in the X-ray card should help to avoid unnecessary X-ray pictures or examinations in individual cases. But the patient is not obliged to keep such an X-ray card on him.

Together with the information obtained by asking the patient about past X-rays, records must also be kept of every use of X-rays. These records must contain all information required to reconstitute the radiation exposure in each individual case, even months and years after the radiation application. Since the amended X-ray Ordinance came into effect in 2002, all newly commissioned X-ray radiography equipment including surgical image intensifiers must be equipped with devices for registering the exposed radiation, for example a dose surface product measuring device or a device which calculates and displays the exposed radiation from the operating parameters. Correct recording of the dose surface product (DFP) is therefore particularly important – also including the unit of measurement, for example in »µG*m²« or »cGy*cm²«. The dose surface product can be used to reliably ascertain the effective dose for a patient for a defined application. All surgical image intensifiers already in use must be retrofitted with a device to register the radiation exposed during operation within an interim period. Furthermore, since 2003 standard DIN 6868 Part 7 [12] has been available to all users, which allows for reliable estimation of the radiation exposure for the patient on the basis of the application parameters for the patient.

The records of X-ray examinations, i.e. also about radiation applications with surgical image intensifiers, must be kept for 10 years. The records must be organised in such a way that they indicate

- the point in time,
- the type of application,
- the parts of the body being examined,
- information about justifying the use and
- the obtained findings.

The records about the point in time of the application, the parts of the body being examined and the details of the doctor performing the examination are to be entered in the X-ray card if submitted by a patient.

4.1.2.9 Quality assurance according to the X-ray Ordinance

According to § 16 of the X-ray Ordinance, the rules for quality assurance also apply to surgical image intensifiers, as described in detail in the above mentioned guidelines for quality assurance [6]. This includes in particular the acceptance test and possibly also partial acceptance tests in accordance with the X-ray Ordinance by the manufacturer or supplier of the X-ray machine, regular constancy tests to be carried out by the owner, and advice from the Medical Department of the corresponding federal state. The overall concept of quality assurance and radiation protection for X-ray diagnostic equipment is shown in Fig. 4.9 in a simplified manner in relation to the operating time of an X-ray diagnosis machine.

Advice from the Medical Department (▶ § 17a of the X-ray Ordinance) suggesting measures to reduce radiation exposure of patients and optimise image quality is based on the new guidelines »Medical and Dental Departments« dated 5 November 2003 [13] and consists essentially in evaluation and assessment of

- the documents required for acceptance tests or partial acceptance tests, for radiation protection inspection by an officially appointed expert and the regular constancy tests by the owner, together with the
- required patient X-ray pictures (direct or indirect X-ray pictures either from the X-ray image intensifier output or from another downstream imaging system).

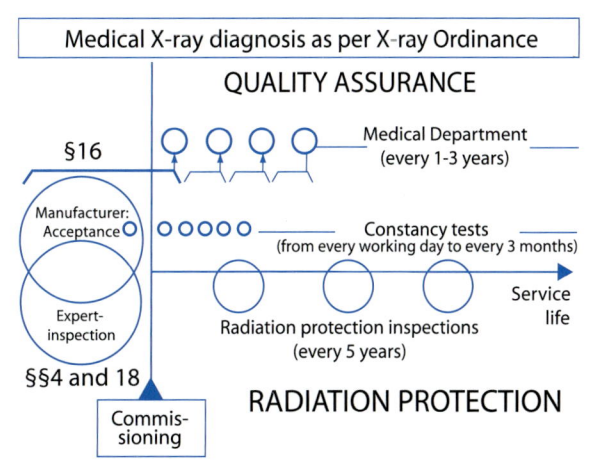

Fig. 4.9. Regulations for quality assurance in X-ray diagnosis

The records of constancy tests for X-ray imaging equipment also include X-ray film pictures of a special technical test body. These test body pictures are compared with the reference pictures taken during the acceptance test by the manufacturer or supplier. Such objective picture documents must be produced during constancy tests of radiography equipment with image intensifier TV chains, i.e. also with surgical image intensifiers, if these units are used to produce X-ray pictures e.g. for documentation purposes. The constancy tests of these units also assesses the monitor picture of the test body by the owner or doctor in visual terms in reference to certain parameters for »physical picture quality«. This assessment cannot be based without doubt on the comparison monitor picture assessed during the acceptance test by the manufacturer or supplier. In order to ascertain gradual changes in the monitor picture over time, the Medical Department rightly insists that the owner's records about the constancy tests on these radiography machines are confirmed on an annual basis by the manufacturer, e.g. as part of regular maintenance, or by an officially appointed expert.

The new X-ray Ordinance and its implementing regulations also contain stricter rules and standards for the requirements made of the reproduction systems for X-ray examinations, i.e. at the end of each complete imaging system, also with regard to the increasing digitisation of X-ray diagnosis and its integration in medical IT systems in hospitals and general medical practices.

The quality assurance guidelines therefore also state technical requirements for film viewing equipment (film viewers) for image documentation systems (e.g. hardcopy cameras, hardcopy printers) and for image reproduction units. Insofar as this equipment is also used as part of surgical image intensifiers, it has to fulfil the corresponding requirements. Quality tests (acceptance test and constancy test) are to be performed in particular for image reproduction systems for C-arm units. Section 8 of the quality assurance guideline describes the requirements for image reproduction systems from a medical point of view and defines the terms *evaluation* and *viewing*. *Evaluation* refers to the diagnostic image quality as defined in the X-ray Ordinance. By contrast, *viewing* (only) refers to the image features and contents of images which have already been evaluated as part of doctor information, demonstration and control. According to the quality assurance guideline, image reproduction units (monitors, VDUs, displays) and film viewers must be marked by the radiation protection manager according to their purpose for *evaluation* or *viewing*.

Image reproduction units which were already commissioned when the new quality assurance guideline came into effect (old units) are to be tested along the lines of the acceptance test according to DIN V 6868–57 [8]. This additional acceptance test of old units is to be completed by *31 December 2005 at the latest* with verification sent to the supervisory authorities. Following the acceptance test,

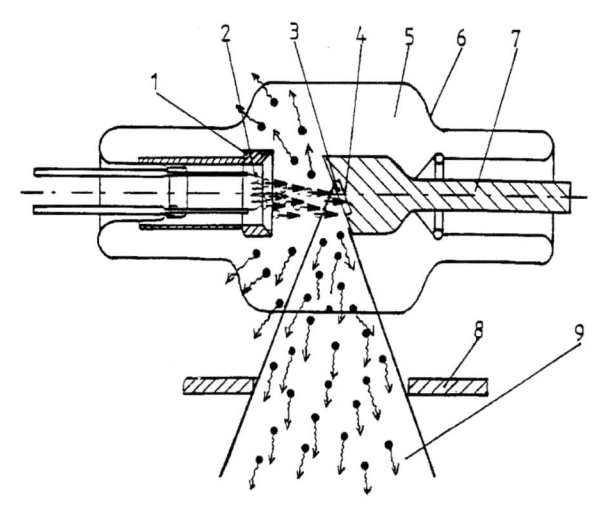

Cut through a standing anode X-ray tube
1 Cathode
2 Filament (electron source)
3 (Thermal) focal spot
4 Tungsten diaphragm
5 Vacuum chamber
6 Hard glass piston
7 Anode (copper shaft)
8 Primary ray diaphragm
9 Effective ray cone (shaded)
∿ X-ray quantum
o— Electron

Fig. 4.10. Diagram to show the generation of X-rays

constancy tests are to be carried out for these units on a daily, quarterly or 6-monthly basis, depending on the characteristics of the image reproduction unit.

Quality tests are also prescribed for film viewers and image documentation systems.

4.1.3 Generating X-rays

Since the almost coincidental discovery of X-rays in 1895 by Wilhelm Conrad Röntgen in his physical laboratory at the University of Würzburg, X-rays have been used for many medical and technical purposes. The key role in their discovery was played by the so-called luminescence effect. The light emitted by a barium platinum cyanide screen, which was accidentally hit by X-rays during experiments with cathode ray tubes, prompted Röntgen to pursue these phenomena and to examine the newly discovered rays and how to generate them in greater depth.

X-rays are produced among other things by the interaction of accelerated electrons, i.e. negative charge carriers, with a metallic anode (positive pole), e.g. a heat-resistant tungsten anode. This interaction of the electrons with the atomic shell of the tungsten atoms produces the so-called X-ray Bremsstrahlung (or braking radiation), which plays the major role in X-ray diagnosis. This interaction process is triggered in a high vacuum glass vessel, the so-called X-ray tube. High electric voltage applied between the cathode and anode accelerates the electrons emitted by

4.1 · Radiation protection in the operating suite

Table 4.3. Measurable effects of the interaction between X-ray radiation and material

Effects	X-ray radiation capability
Attenuation effect	to penetrate material while being attenuated
Luminescence effect	to make certain substances luminant
Ionisation effect	to ionise certain substances, i.e. make them electrically conductive
Photographic effect	to make photographic films black
Semiconductor effect	to change the electrical conductivity of semiconductors
Biological effect	to cause changes to the tissue of living creatures

the heated cathode (electron current or also called tube current defined in the physical unit amperes [A] or milliamperes [mA]) within the X-ray tube to such an extent that this is stopped at high speed at the atomic shell of the anode material and generates X-rays in this process (◘ Fig. 4.10).

The higher the electric voltage – between 25 kV and 150 kV (*kV*, kilovolt; *1 kV*, 1000 V) depending on the application – the higher the speed of the electrons on their way to the anode and the higher the energy in the resulting X-rays. When the tube high voltage is switched off, the electron bombardment of the anode is interrupted so that no more radiation can be generated.

The efficiency of this conversion of electrical energy into radiation energy amounts to about 1%, i.e. about 99% of the electrical energy is converted into heat energy. This efficiency balance illustrates the huge thermal load on X-ray tubes and their anodes. The heat problems have also resulted in the use of X-ray tubes with rotating anodes for X-ray emitters in surgical image intensifiers.

During the interaction between X-ray and material, the effects featured in ◘ Table 4.3 can be observed and measured in technical terms.

Technically constrained bundling of the electrons on their way to the anode means that X-rays are generated in a punctiform part of the anode, the so-called focal spot, from where they spread as a divergent radiation field strictly limited by the emitter diaphragm, so that the decrease in radiation intensity depends on the distance from the focal spot in accordance with the *distance square law* (◘ Fig. 4.8): »The intensity of the radiation from a divergent radiation field of punctiform origin decreases with the square of increasing distance from its point of origin.« This law is also important for practical radiation protection in terms of image generation.

Tube protective housing with X-ray tube. For several reasons, the X-ray tube is installed in a *tube protection housing* (◘ Fig. 4.11) which offers protection from

- tube high voltage (contact protection and insulation protection),
- thermal loads (heat dissipation by laying the tubes for example in insulating oil),
- emitted X-ray radiation outside the effective radiation bundle and
- mechanical loads.

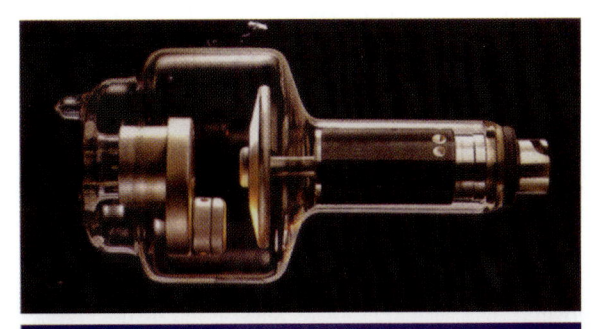

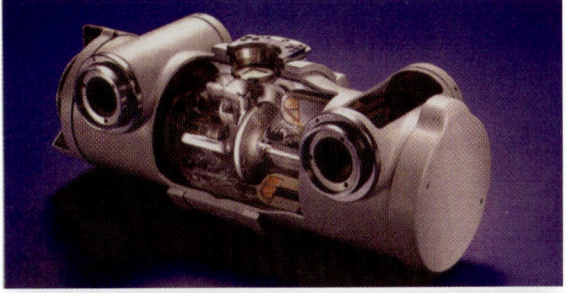

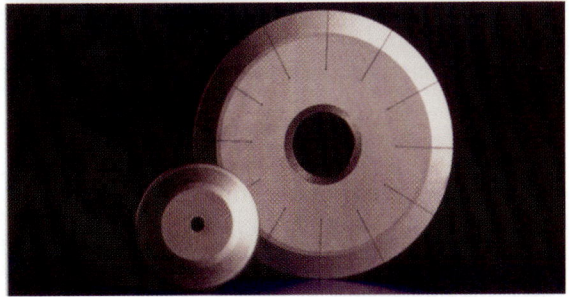

◘ **Fig. 4.11.** Tube protection housing and X-ray tube

Fig. 4.12. Diagram to show image receiver system in scanning units

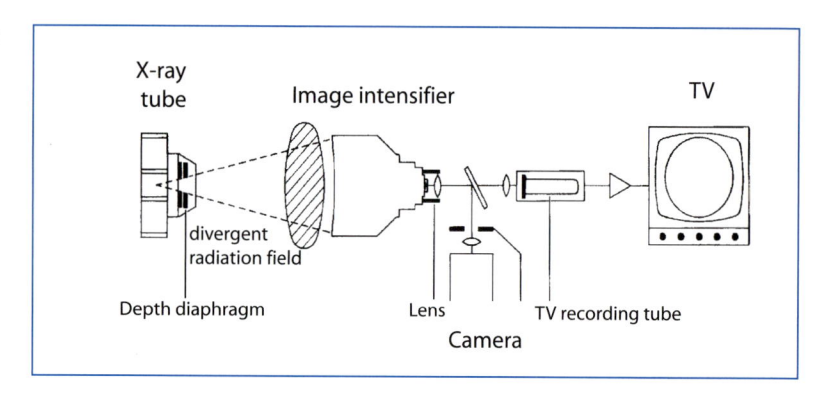

In addition, the tube protective housing also offers structural possibilities for fitting *diaphragms* to limit or variably restrict the effective radiation field.

4.1.4 The image receiver system for surgical image intensifiers

The image receiver system for surgical image intensifiers consists of the *X-ray image intensifier (RBV)*, a downstream TV camera and a monitor (Fig. 4.12).

This system is also referred to as image intensifier/TV chain. Together with the TV camera and a monitor, other recording and image storing cameras are also used, such as a film camera (e.g. 35 mm camera for »cinema films«, 100 mm camera for single pictures of the image intensifier output screen), storing on magnetic tape, digital image storing and image processing together with video imager technology, i.e. photographing the stored monitor picture from a special monitor. The rapid development and production of high-performance electronic storage media has resulted in digital image generation, image storage and image reworking possibilities substituting the conventional imaging procedures. This development is also considered in the amended X-ray Ordinance from 2002 in § 28, which states that digitally documented records and X-ray pictures must be made available in a suitable form to a doctor sharing in the treatment or responsible for follow-up treatment, together with the Medical Departments. The records and X-ray pictures must coincide in terms of images and contents with the original data records and be suitable for evaluation of the findings. When data are transmitted by electronic means, it must be certain that no information will be lost during remote data transfer.

4.1.5 The main components in surgical image intensifiers

The main components in surgical image intensifiers are:

— the radiation emitting system with its components high voltage generator and controller, together with tube protection housing with X-ray tube and radiation apertures,
— the image receiver system or depiction system with the X-ray image intensifier (RBV), TV camera, monitor and the downstream digital image storage devices.

4.1.6 Technical minimum requirements for examinations with surgical image intensifiers

According to the above mentioned »Guideline for the technical testing of X-ray equipment and interference emitters subject to permission« (expert test guideline – SV-RL) [5], certain technical minimum requirements have to be fulfilled for examinations with image intensifiers (Table 4.4).

The technical minimum requirements for the application must be used as the basic appraisal standards for tests during initial commissioning (§ 3 and § 4 of the X-ray Ordinance) and for repeat tests according to § 187 of the X-ray Ordinance.

4.1.7 Application-related radiation protection in the operating suite

The effective radiation hits the patient's body and penetrates it in part, so that it then arrives as a so-called radiation relief at the input of the image receiver system where it is used for imaging. Another part of the effective radiation is absorbed by the patient's body and therefore cannot contribute to imaging.

Yet another part of the effective radiation is scattered in the patient's body (»Compton scattering«) and leaves the patient's body again on all sides as so-called scattered lower energy radiation. *Radiation protection for the user refers essentially to protection from this scattered radiation.* The share of scattered radiation is far lower for radio-

4.1 · Radiation protection in the operating suite

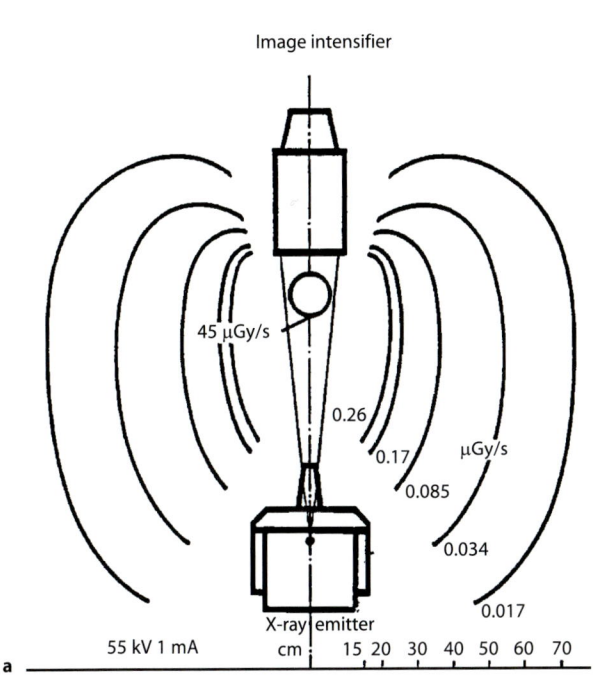

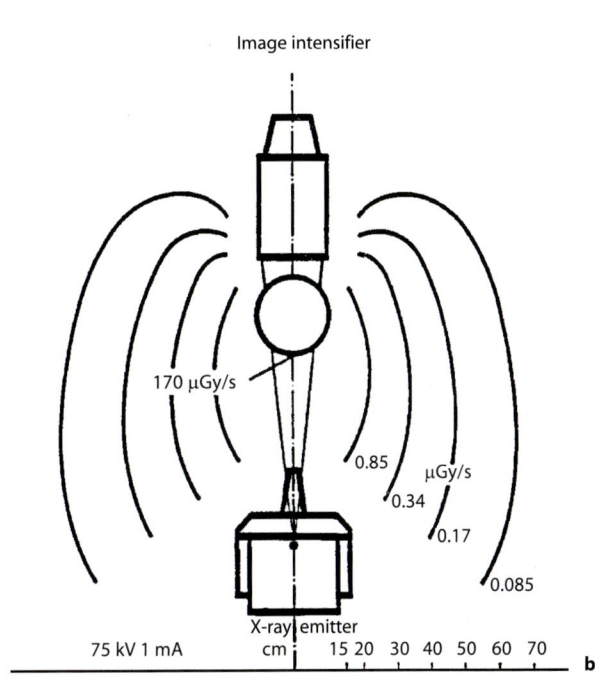

Fig. 4.13 a, b. Leakage radiation in surgical image intensifiers with small and larger scanned patient volume, shown using *isodoses*, i.e. curves with the same dose

graphy of smaller patient volumes than in the case of larger volumes (Fig. 4.13).

Together with scattered radiation from the patient volume, notable radiation exposure can also be caused by leakage radiation through the housing of the X-ray emitter, if the medical activities which the users have to perform entails them staying close to the X-ray emitter (e.g. at a distance of less than 20 cm).

When using surgical image intensifiers in the operating theatre, it is apparently not possible to rule out the risk of the hands and lower arms of the users being in the effective radiation bundle or in the area of intensive interference radiation during their surgical activities, at least occasionally and usually only for a short period. To protect the hands and lower arms during such activities, DIN EN 61331–3 [11] recommends radiation protection gloves (five finger gloves) and surgical radiation protection gloves (mittens with open hand surface) with an attenuation equivalent of at least 0.25 mm Pb.

An important rule for practical radiation protection for patient and user can be derived from all this:

Gate the effective radiation field well!

A well gated effective radiation field improves not only radiation protection for patient and user but also the »physical image quality« of the monitor image and the image documentation systems downstream from the imaging process.

Depending on the situation, the effective radiation field can be gated using the iris diaphragm or the parallel diaphragm from the control desk. The diaphragms then appear in the monitor picture and stay in position even after the scan has been briefly interrupted so that repeated gating will not be necessary. In some new machines, the position of the effective radiation diaphragms is also illustrated for the user on the monitor when there is no radiation exposure, so that the effective radiation diaphragms can be brought into a suitable, favourable position for the application, already during the preparatory phase. Many new machines offer enlargement possibilities for special situations (sector enlargement or zoom formats) for the specific part of the body by changing over to a smaller image intensifier input format. The effective radiation diaphragms on the X-ray emitter then automatically adjust to a smaller image intensifier input format when the system changes over.

Another important aspect of radiation protection, which unfortunately is still not given sufficient attention, is:

Keeping radiation times as short as possible!

All newer machines today offer technical support to help implement this radiation protection aspect in the form of an *interrupt setting*: with compulsory interruption of scanning after a certain interval, which can be preset in some cases. The user then has to trigger a further scanning interval again.

A similar possibility for reducing the radiation times consists of pulsed, intermittent scanning when the ON-switch is held down. In this case, the X-rays are emitted in adjustable time intervals (pulse frequency) for an adjustable period of time, with considerable reductions in radiation exposure for patient and user.

All new surgical image intensifiers are equipped with digital image memories as another contribution to reducing scanning times. After only a short scanning time, the user has a saved monitor image which allows him to evaluate the current situation. For documentation purposes, as far as possible indirect scanning (video imager technology or multi-format camera) should be used, or digital image documentation. Interim results can be produced with video printers, but this is no substitute for documentation on an X-ray picture generated by direct and indirect scanning.

4.1.8 Correct positioning of the image receiver system

Another radiation protection measure resulting from equipment handling consists of positioning the image receiver part of the surgical image intensifier as close as possible to the patient's body. This not only improves the physical image quality but also considerably reduces radiation exposure for the patient. Misalignment of the emitter/image receiver system becomes apparent to the user when during the scan, the examined part of the body or organs are extremely enlarged on the monitor.

■ Figure 4.14 shows the normal patient incident dose (main dose) for various focus/object distances when using surgical image intensifiers. For very small focus/object distances, the patient incident dose increases out of all proportion. The figure also shows the object enlargements resulting from misalignment for the listed focus/object distances.

4.1.9 Correct use of the automatic dose control (ADR)

According to the X-ray Ordinance, all scanning equipment for examining the human body and therefore also all surgical image intensifiers must be equipped with *automatic dose control (ADR)* or at least an equivalent device and a device for electronic image intensifying with TV chain. In

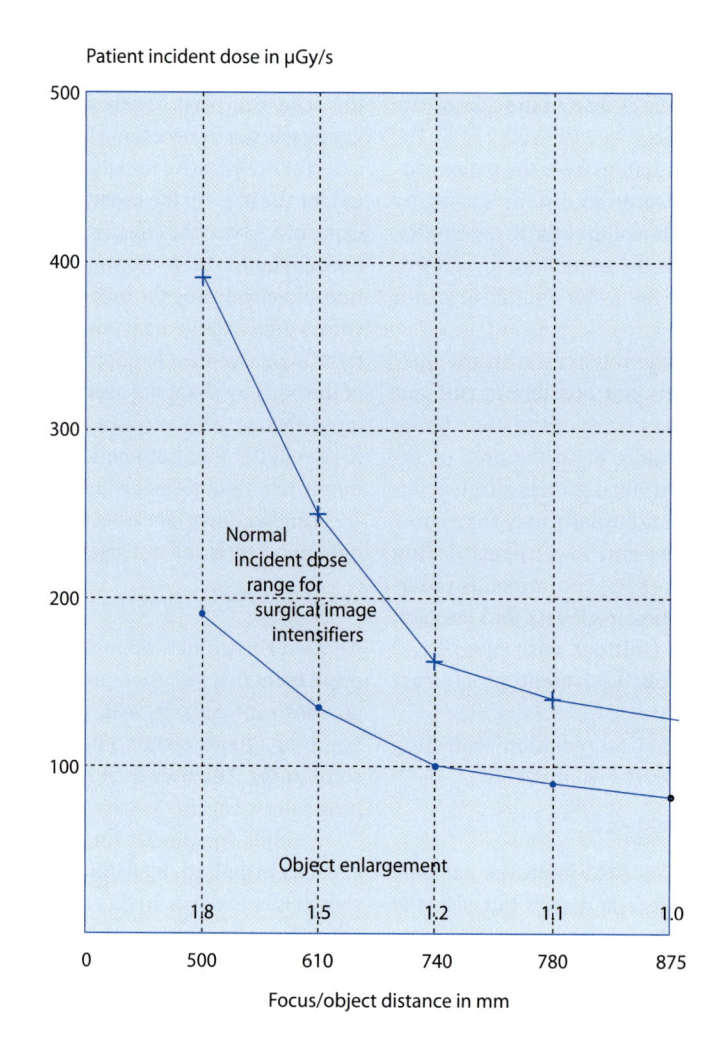

■ **Fig. 4.14.** Influence of the focus/object distance on the incident dose and object enlargement

addition, all devices have the possibility of interrupting this control for certain situations (*automatic stop*) before continuing to work either with the last controlled operating values (kV and mA) or in manual mode. In the so-called manual mode, tube voltage can be adjusted by the user.

The techniques involved in *automatic dose control*, *automatic stop* and *manual mode* are highly significant for situations where instruments or implants of low radiation transparency, e.g. metallic materials, are placed in the effective ray path. In these cases, the automatic function adjusts the voltage and current values in such a way that sufficient radiation passes through these objects, because the *automatic dose control* does not differentiate between body tissue and foreign bodies or other materials. As a result, the radiation passes over the parts of the body which are more transparent to radiation so that the picture on the monitor is too bright with insufficient contrast for the body regions. In these situations, use must be made of the *automatic stop* or *manual setting* just before such materials are introduced into the effective ray path. In the *manual setting*, the operating values for tube voltage can then be varied by the user at the controller so that the tissues or parts of the body concerned are shown with an optimum picture on the monitor.

In the case of surgical procedures where the parts of the body concerned are scanned initially for guidance without any implants or metallic instruments, the user should use the *automatic stop* button already during this initial step so that the operating parameters adjusted for an optimum X-ray picture can then remain unchanged for all further stages of the operation.

The following list summarises the most important radiation protection rules when using surgical image intensifiers:
- reduce the radiation times as far as possible,
- gate the effective radiation field well,
- keep the greatest possible distance between staff and the effective radiation field and the patient's body,
- use optimum radiation protection clothing for the users (doctors and assistants),
- when using radiation for the head and extremities, cover the patient's trunk with radiation protection aprons,
- position the image receiver system as close as possible to the patient's body,
- do not start the scanning equipment until the emitter and image receiver system are correctly positioned,
- use the interrupt switch and perhaps the possibility of intermittent scanning (pulsed scanning),
- use the high-level mode carefully and for the shortest possible time (with an incident dose of >0.087 Gy/min at a distance of 30 cm to the image intensifier input side of the C-arm unit)
- use the parts of the body being examined when repositioning emitter and image receiver system, not the image on the monitor,
- use the *automatic stop* button or *manual setting* when metallic instruments or implants have to be brought into the radiation path,
- keep records about the X-ray times, exposed parts of the body and the value of the dose surface product (or in machines without this feature, the operating parameters image intensifier input format, automatic dose control curve type or level) together with tube voltage (kV), the mAs product or current (mA), shutter times and the radiation field size and position for X-ray pictures produced in the direct method in the operating suite for documentation purposes; these records are then kept with the patient's records.

4.2 Surgical image intensifier systems

Volker Böttcher

After the discovery of the X-ray by Wilhelm Conrad Röntgen in 1895, another 50 years passed before this technique for supporting surgical procedures made an impact on the operating theatre.

During the 1950s, the development from luminescent screen to image intensifier tube and the rapid progress in camera and monitor technology made it possible to work without having to darken the room. The generator was a 1- or 2-pulse generator, the image intensifier had a lens coverage of 15 cm diameter, and the picture taken by the camera was only visible on the monitor during radiation.

The key components of surgical image intensifier (also called C-arm because of its shape) were therefore already present:
- generator (usually single-tyke generator, X-ray tube and high-voltage generator in one housing),
- image intensifier,
- camera,
- monitor.

Together with their diagnostic use, X-rays also have a harmful effect so that rules and laws for radiation protection were issued at a very early stage. The most important set of regulations on this topic is the X-ray Ordinance. The aim of this ordinance is to reduce the dose for patient and medical staff as far as possible. To this end, technical minimum requirements were stipulated for the equipment which were regularly adjusted to technical progress.

These minimum requirements (◘ Table 4.4) and competition between manufacturers of surgical image inten-

Table 4.4. Minimum requirements for surgical image intensifiers (SV-RL dated 27 August 2003)	
Focal spot rating	≤ 1.8 mm
Rating of the shortest cycle time	≤ 100 ms
Limit dose for direct radiography	≤ 5 µGy
Limit dose for digital radiography (with 23 cm image intensifier BV)	≤ 2 µGy
Limit dose for X-ray radiation (with 23 cm image intensifier)	≤ 0.6 µGy/s
Limit resolution (including memory image with 23 cm image intensifier 23 cm BV)	≤ 1.0 Lp/mm

sifiers resulted in huge progress in technology and above all in radiation protection over the next few years.

The generator. It was developed into a high-frequency generator (almost direct current) with a clear increase in radiation hygiene.

The image intensifier. The luminous layers at input and output and the intensification were considerably improved. The diameter of the lens coverage was increased to 23 and 31 cm, removing the need for elaborate positioning.

The camera. Highly sensitive, non-ageing CCD cameras with high photosensitivity have replaced the tube camera.

Image memory. Image memories brought an essential reduction in radiation dose. Following a short radiation pulse, the picture is »frozen« on the monitor. The surgeon can now assess the picture without any time pressure.

The monitor. High-resolution, high-contrast monitors make it easier to assess the picture. Introduction of a second monitor allows for the direct comparison of two pictures.

Automatic dose control (ADR). This automatically adjusts the optimum dose for the corresponding object.

Image processing. Filter techniques have improved the image quality in spite of a lower dose. Subsequent picture processing allows for visual improvement of the picture. Cinema memories make it possible to access and repeat dynamic procedures from the image memory without having to repeat the radiation.

Documentation. Direct radiography has been extensively replaced by digital radiography and indirect systems such as video printers.

4.2.1 Expert inspection

A system of inspection and monitoring was developed for compliance with these regulations. After completion, every surgical image intensifier undergoes acceptance testing by the manufacturer. A corresponding report must be drawn up. During initial commissioning, the acceptance is checked by an independent expert. The owner of the machine must perform constancy tests at regular intervals. An independent expert checks the machine again every 5 years. This guarantees that all machines comply with the statutory regulations at all times.

4.2.2 X-ray radiation

When using X-rays on a patient, a differentiation is made between effective radiation and scattered radiation. The effective radiation passes through the patient and is absorbed to a differing extent by the body, depending on the density of the organs. The radiation leaving the patient's body thus forms a so-called radiation relief on the image receiver input screen which is used to produce the pictures.

Part of the effective radiation is scattered by the patient's body and leaves the body as lower-energy scatter radiation in all directions. The user is essentially exposed to this scattered radiation.

4.2.3 Radiation protection

The first commandment is to protect the user and the parts of the patient's body not being examined from this scattered radiation. The following rules should be observed:
- *Prevention of scattered radiation*
    - Keep the radiation times as short as possible. Memorising technology today makes it possible to »freeze« a top quality picture on the monitor after a short X-ray pulse.
    - Use pulse techniques for procedures with movement.
    - As far as possible, always work with the program with the lowest dose (half-dose program).
    - Use the slot or iris diaphragm for gating because the amount of scattered radiation is directly related to the patient volume through which radiation has passed.

4.2 · Surgical image intensifier systems

- If possible, change over to a smaller image intensifier format (magnifier). An additional advantage here is the enlargement of the object.
- Use a saved radiation picture for documentation (indirect radiography).
- *Protection from scattered radiation*
  - Distance is the best radiation protection, because radiation decreases by the square of the distance.
  - Use radiation protection clothing.
  - Cover those parts of the patient's body which are not being examined.

4.2.4 Structure and technique of a surgical image intensifier

A modern surgical image intensifier consists of a mobile stand which can be moved with great precision millimetre by millimetre with very little effort. Cable deflectors are needed at all wheels. It must be possible to push it parallel to the operating table. The C-arm with the radiation source (generator) and the image receiver (image intensifier with camera) is positioned on this mobile stand in such a way that it can be moved and turned to all sides (▶ Figs. 4.15–4.19). The C-arm has the largest possible inner width and penetration depth to make it easier to position it at the operating table. A laser light visor makes it easier to position the machine without radiation and helps during the locking nailing procedure. All functions required during the operation can be controlled from the control desk. A dose-optimised automatic function makes it easy to control the machine, improves image quality and reduces scattered radiation. The dose measuring system provides information about the applied patient dose.

The second component is the monitor trolley. This can also be moved with very little effort. It contains the image memory unit, image processing unit, both monitors and the documentation unit. Today the image memory unit and image processing unit consist of one single device and should be capable of storing at least 100 images. Image

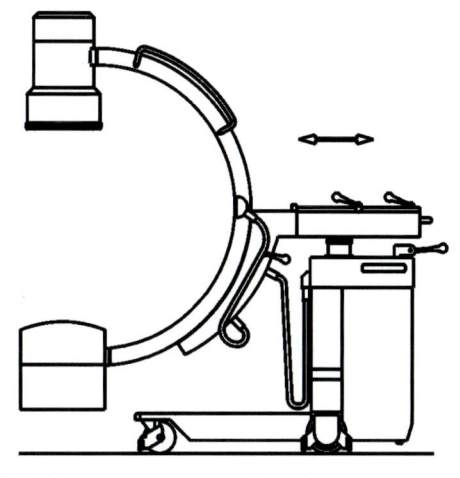

Fig. 4.16. Movement transverse to the patient

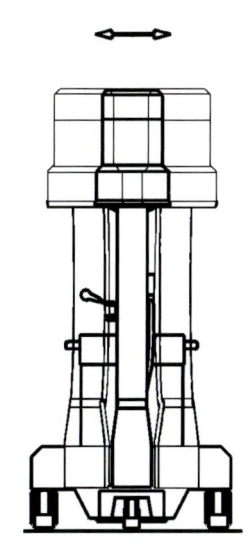

Fig. 4.17. Movement longitudinal to the patient, also possible by parallel displacement of the complete unit

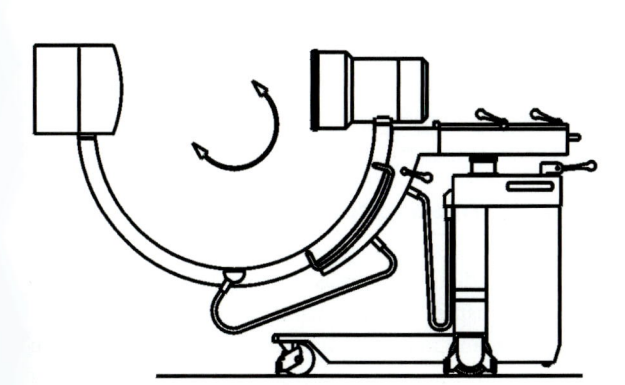

Fig. 4.15. Orbital movement around the patient

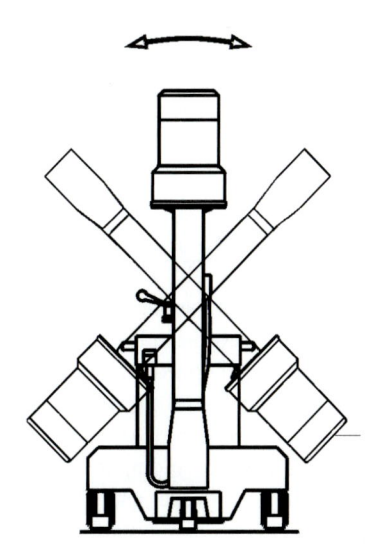

Fig. 4.18. Rotation of the C-arm

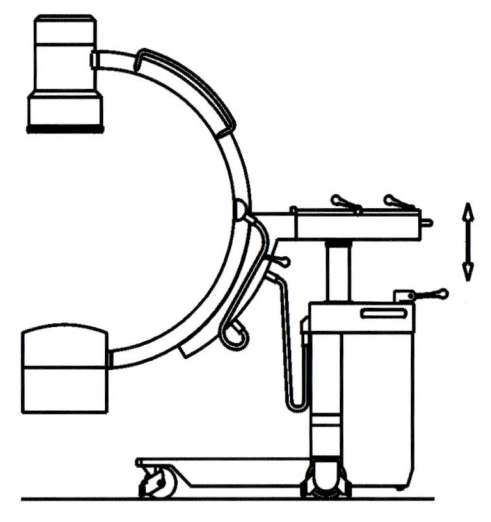

Fig. 4.19. Adjusting the height

processing uses various filter techniques to produce high-contrast pictures at a low dose; these are then visually improved by subsequent image processing (e.g. electronic magnifier, Windows technology). When used in vascular surgery, image processing must be capable of performing subtraction procedures. A cinema function is available to assess these dynamic procedures which it records in the memory at differing recording speeds. The memory capacity should be at least 1000 pictures. For documentation purposes, integrated video printers can be used with thermal paper or foil, together with video recorders. State-of-the-art systems today are capable of transferring image data via a digital interface (DICOM) to a laser printer or digital archive (PACS). It should always be possible to transfer images to a digital data carrier (e.g. floppy disk, MO disk, CD-ROM) so that they can be processed in a conventional PC.

Today, two monitors are mandatory for surgical machines. For special applications (e.g. outpatients) where two monitors are not necessary, machines are available with just one monitor on the mobile stand. The complete image processing and memory functions are integrated in the mobile stand.

4.2.5 Application

Surgical image intensifiers are used today in all surgical disciplines. They have become indispensable in the outpatients department, in orthopaedics, traumatology, neurosurgery, general surgery, hand surgery, vascular surgery, for radiotherapy and endoscopy. An ongoing flow of new technology is constantly expanding the range of applications. Increasing possibilities for using the machines also make increasing demands on the staff who operate them. Some manufacturers have recognised this fact and offer

special machines developed for certain applications, e.g. in the emergency room, on the intensive care unit or for gastroenterology.

Even the new navigation systems currently penetrating the market which used to need pictures produced with a CT can now produce comparable results when coupled with a C-arm.

4.2.6 Use of the surgical image intensifier

Before every operation, it is important to check that the machine is fully functional. After the patient has been positioned, in the case of difficult operations the machine should be positioned at the patient first without radiation. This is the only way to guarantee trouble-free use during the operation. The patient should be washed and covered only after this has been completed. An example for special positioning techniques is shown in Fig. 4.20 and Fig. 4.21.

As soon as the surgeon needs an X-ray picture, the machine should be brought into position, ensuring that the distance between image intensifier input and the patient is as short as possible. This not only improves image quality but also makes a contribution to radiation protection. The larger focal spot/skin distance reduces the radiation burden on the patient. Positioning without radiation is made easier in modern machines with a laser light visor. The X-ray program (organ automatic mode) is chosen. Everyone in the room must wear protective clothing. After the first X-ray has been taken, the position of the image on the monitor can be adjusted by reflecting and/or turning the picture. Modern machines rotate the image directly on the monitor. Rotation takes place by digital means in the image memory so that no additional radiation is required for position control. The object is then gated using the iris or slot diaphragm.

Automatic dose control usually ensures that there is a perfect image. The optimum dose is adjusted depending on the object. But metal implants or instruments in the ray path prevent the automatic dose control from working properly. In this case, it is advisable to press the automatic stop button and adjust the image manually. Some machines have a program which is capable of ignoring metal in the ray path during the control phase. This prevents radiating over the organs.

4.2.7 Tips and tricks for daily routine

Keep the radiation times as short as possible. A smaller image intensifier format (magnifier) reduces the radiation burden and makes it easier to recognise details. Store images with important interim results so that they are available later on for documentation. Whenever an image

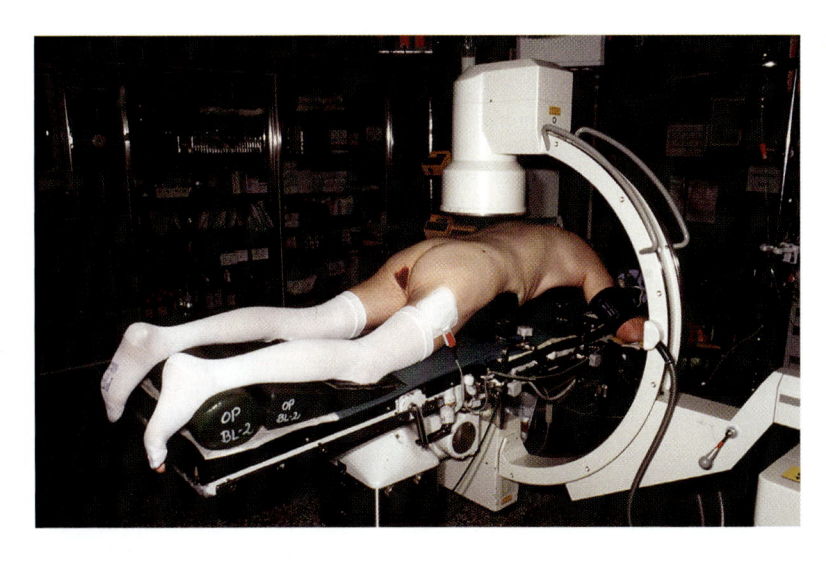

Fig. 4.20. Spinal column anteroposterior.

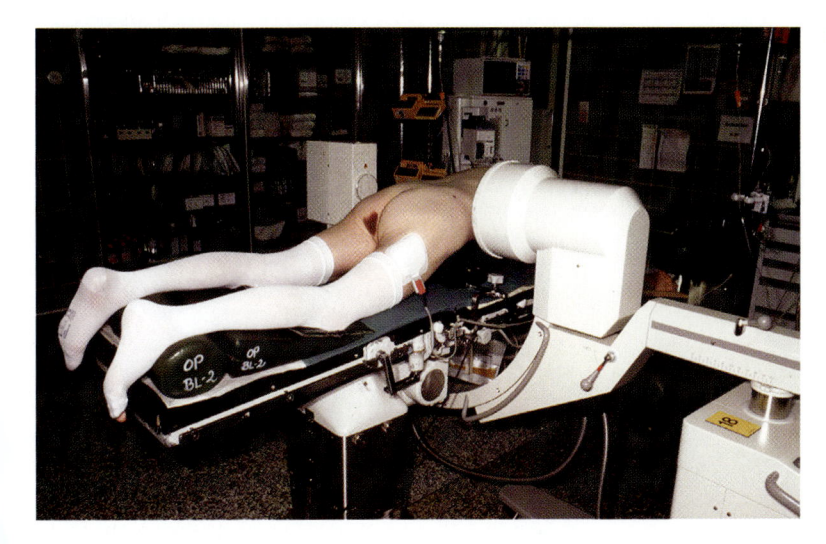

Fig. 4.21. Spinal column, from the side

has to be compared with another one (e.g. in two-level operation), transfer one image to the auxiliary monitor with the image change button. If the machine has to be re-positioned, never continue with radiation during the movement but use the laser light visor for re-positioning. After the operation, save the results in all necessary levels. If top quality is required for documentation, use digital radiography (snap shot) for the final images.

After the operation, document the necessary images. A video printer with thermal paper or foil can be used for this purpose; modern machines have a DICOM interface to produce the images directly on a laser printer or store them in a digital archiving system (PACS). Modern machines can also save the images on digital memories (e.g. floppy or MO disk or CD) so that they can be processed on any PC.

References

1. Richtlinie Fachkunde und Kenntnisse im Strahlenschutz für den Betrieb von Röntgeneinrichtungen in der Medizin, Zahnmedizin und bei der Anwendung von Röntgenstrahlen auf Tiere (Fachkunde nach Röntgenverordnung/Medizin) BArbBl. 9/90, S, 67 und BArbBl. 9/91, S. 88
2. Verordnung über den Schutz vor Schäden durch Röntgenstrahlen (Röntgenverordnung – RöV) vom 7. Januar 1987 in der Fassung der Bekanntmachung vom 30. April 2003 (BGBl. I S. 604)
3. Richtlinie 96/29/EURATOM des Rates vom 13. Mai 1996 (»EURATOM-Grundnormen«) zur Festlegung der grundlegenden Sicherheitsnormen für den Schutz der Gesundheit der Arbeitskräfte und der Bevölkerung gegen die Gefahren durch ionisierende Strahlungen, Amtsblatt der Europäischen Gemeinschaften DE Nr. L 159 vom 29 Juni 1996, S. 1
4. Richtlinie 97/43/EURATOM des Rates vom 30. Juni 1997 (»EURATOM-Patientenschutz-Richtlinie«) über den Gesundheitsschutz von Personen gegen die Gefahren ionisierender Strahlung bei medizinischer Exposition und zur Aufhebung der Richtlinie 84/466 EURATOM, Amtsblatt der Europäischen Gemeinschaften DE Nr. L 180 vom 9. Juli 1997, S. 22

5. Richtlinie für die technische Prüfung von Röntgeneinrichtungen und genehmigungsbedürftigen Störstrahlern – Richtlinie für Sachverständigenprüfungen nach der Röntgenverordnung (SV-RL) – vom 27. August 2003
6. Richtlinie zur Durchführung der Qualitätssicherung bei Röntgeneinrichtungen zur Untersuchung oder Behandlung von Menschen nach den §§ 16 und 17 der Röntgenverordnung – Qualitätssicherungs-Richtlinie (QS-RL) – vom 20. November 2003
7. Leitlinien der Bundesärztekammer zur Qualitätssicherung in der Röntgendiagnostik, Qualitätskriterien röntgendiagnostischer Untersuchungen (Überarbeitete und ergänzte Fassung), Deutsches Ärzteblatt 92, Heft 34/35, 28. August 1995 A 2272 – A 2285
8. DIN V 6868-57 Sicherung der Bildqualität in röntgensdiagnostischen Betrieben, Teil 57: Abnahmeprüfung an Bildwiedergabegeräten
9. Richtlinie für die physikalische Strahlenschutzkontrolle zur Ermittlung der Körperdosen, Teil 1: Ermittlung der Körperdosis bei äußerer Strahlenexposition (§§ 40, 41, 42 StrlSchV; § 35 RöV) vom 08.12.2003
10. DIN 6813: 1980–07, Strahlenschutzzubehör bei medizinischer Anwendung von Röntgenstrahlen bis 300 kV; Regeln für die Herstellung und Benutzung
11. DIN EN 61331–3 Strahlenschutz in der medizinischen Röntgendiagnostik, Teil 3: Schutzkleidung und Gonadenschutz, Ausgabe Mai 2002
12. DIN 6809-7 Klinische Dosimetrie – Teil 7: Verfahren zur Dosisermittlung in der Röntgendiagnostik, Ausgabe Oktober 2003
13. Richtlinie »Ärztliche und zahnärztliche Stellen« (Richtlinie zur Strahlenschutzverordnung (StrlSchV) und Röntgenverordnung (RöV) vom 05.11.2003 (Anwendung ab dem 1. März 2004)

5 High-frequency surgery

V. Hausmann

5.1 General aspects – 42
5.1.1 How it works/Definition – 42
5.1.2 Incision – 43
5.1.3 Coagulation – 44
5.1.4 Influences on the surgical effect – 45

5.2 Neutral electrode – 46
5.2.1 Task – 46
5.2.2 Safety systems – 46
5.2.3 The neutral electrode – which, where, how? – 46
5.2.4 Burns under the neutral electrode? – 47

5.3 Rules for safe use – 48
5.3.1 General – 48
5.3.2 Use of high-frequency surgery in minimally invasive surgery – 48
5.3.3 Other information – 49

Glossary – 50

References – 54

5.1 General aspects

5.1.1 How it works/Definition

What is electrosurgery?

High-frequency surgery or electrosurgery today is an established feature in every operation. Its advantages compared to other techniques are as follows:
- Tissue dissection possibly with simultaneous haemostatic effect (stops bleeding).
- Combinations with other techniques, e.g. argon gas surgery or ultrasonic dissection (e.g. CUSA) result in further simplification in surgery.

In addition, electrosurgery is used in both open surgery and also in minimal invasive surgery (MIS).

The user's know-how about handling high-frequency surgical devices is based on what he has been told and also on his own experience. But training literature contains little information about how high-frequency surgery works and its risks.

Basic idea: heat

The basic idea behind electrosurgery is to generate heat. This principle was already known in the past. It was known that glowing metal or hot stones would have a haemostatic or coagulating effect on a wound. Later, technological developments provided other sources of energy, namely electricity (◘ Fig. 5.1).

Cauterisation

One simple means of generating heat by electricity is to reduce the diameter of an electrical conductor to increase the electrical resistance. Heat is produced at the point of reduced diameter by the greater current density (◘ Fig. 5.2).

Using normal mains power (230 V, 50 Hz), a corresponding transformer could be used to make a generator which lets a thin wire glow red hot for use for local haemostasis. This technique is called cauterisation. But the drawback is that more tissue is damaged by radiant heat than is actually wanted. In addition, this technique cannot be used for cutting.

Cautering or cauterisation are frequently incorrectly confused with high-frequency surgery.

High-frequency surgery

Another possibility is to consider the tissue as resistance between two electrical conductors. In order to generate a surgical effect at the specific site, a small contact surface is required (active electrode), generating a very high current density at the metal/tissue interface. This causes the required heat in the corresponding tissue.

A far larger, conductive area is provided on the other side of the tissue (neutral electrode) which ensures that the current leaves the tissue with a very low density without developing any heat (◘ Fig. 5.3).

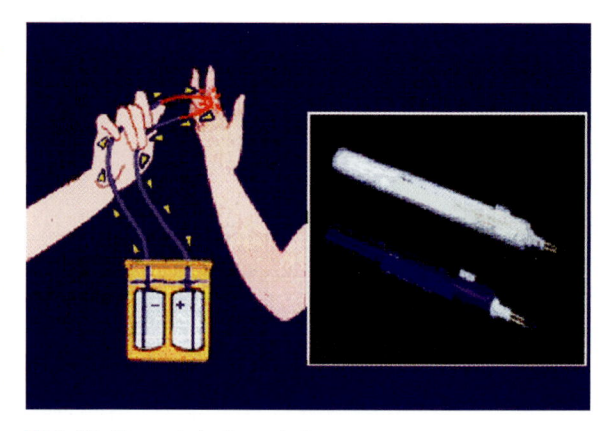

◘ **Fig. 5.2.** The cauterisation technique

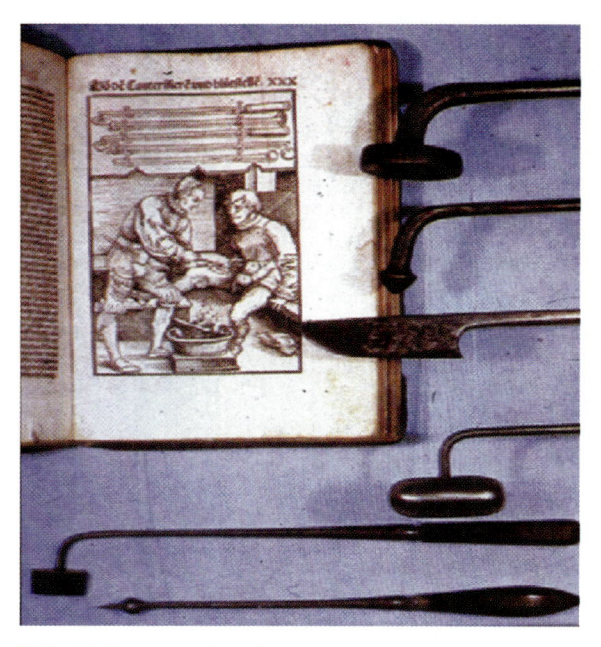

◘ **Fig. 5.1.** Instruments from the past

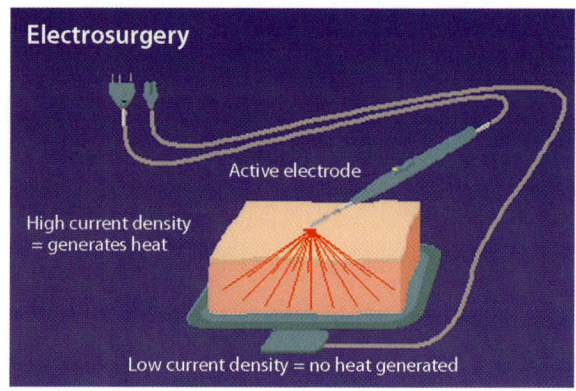

◘ **Fig. 5.3.** High and low current density

5.1 · General aspects

The human body sends conduction pulses as little electrical currents to the muscles to make them contract. To ensure that electrosurgery does not stimulate the whole body to uncontrolled muscular contractions, alternating current is used with a frequency above the stimulus threshold of the human body. This threshold is at about 10 kHz, i.e. about 10,000 changes of current direction per second. The human body is too inert to react to electrical current above this frequency. This also applies to the heart muscle, so that a high-frequency current through the heart does not cause any damage.

Most high-frequency surgical devices today work with a frequency in a range of about 450–550 kHz (Fig. 5.4).

Electrosurgical techniques

Surgical effects can be divided into two main groups, depending on the application:

Incision and coagulation. Incision separates the tissue and coagulation dries the tissue out (Fig. 5.5).

These two surgical effects are in turn broken down into two sub-groups each (Fig. 5.6):
- pure or smooth incision with as little lateral haemostatic effect as possible
- incision with lateral haemostasis by including coagulation shares (mixed current, »blend«, mixing)
- and contact coagulation (desiccation) and
- non-contact coagulation (fulguration and spray).

Many users are not familiar with the difference between desiccation and fulguration. But there is a fundamental difference between the two, because if these techniques are used incorrectly, the surgeons can suffer from painful discharges through their gloves.

5.1.2 Incision

Pure cut

During the pure cut, the main aspect is to heat only the tissue at the point of contact very quickly with the active electrode. This is achieved best using an electrode with a small contact surface (e.g. needle electrode) which produces a high current density. This in turn causes »cell explosions« in the tissue. A »micro spark rain« is produced between the electrode and the tissue at high temperatures of more than 100°C. The continuous supply of energy heats the tissue cells so quickly that they explode. This causes the tissue to separate (incision) (Fig. 5.7). The supplied heat is dissipated again mainly by means of the evaporated cell liquid. No heat is transferred to the surrounding tissue, producing a smooth cut with a minimum coagulation zone.

Cutting is not possible without micro-sparking.

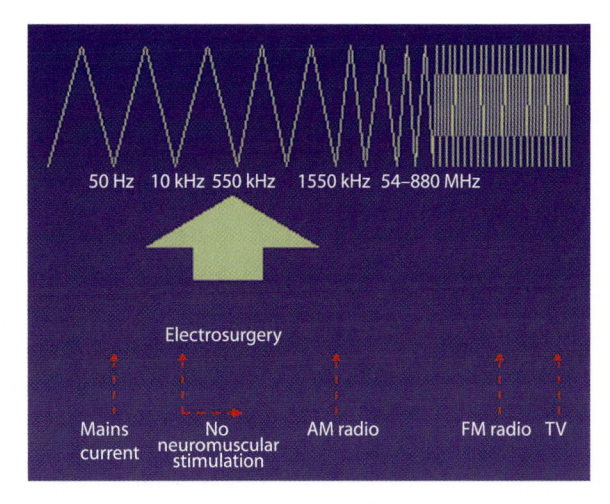

Fig. 5.4. Frequency range for most high-frequency surgical devices

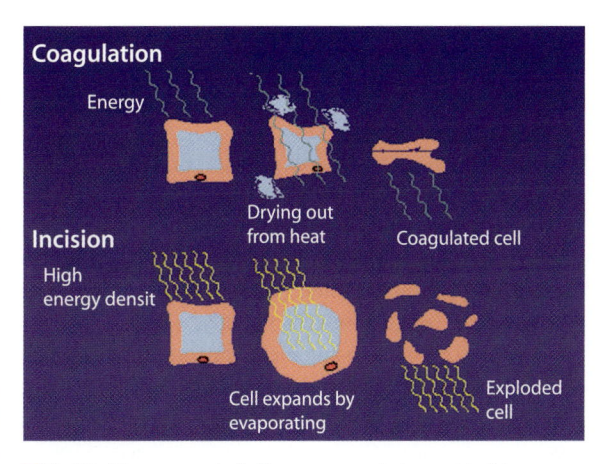

Fig. 5.5. The two surgical effects are coagulation and incision

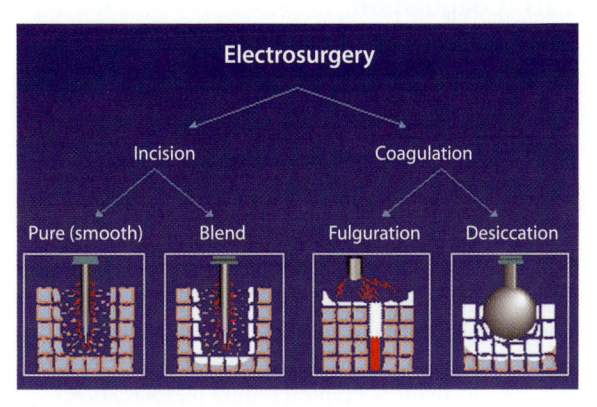

Fig. 5.6. The surgical effects and their subgroups

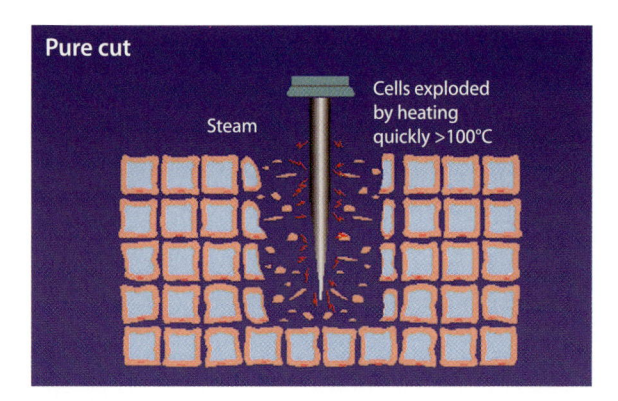

Fig. 5.7. Pure cut

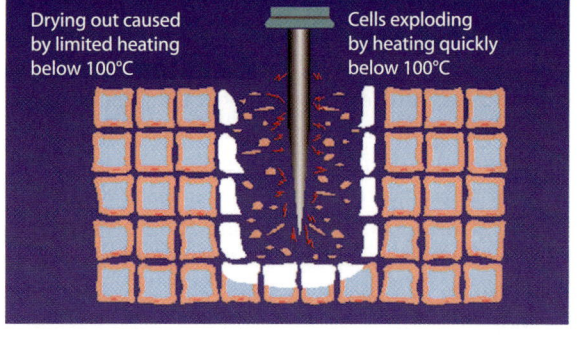

Fig. 5.8. Blend cut

Blend cutting
(Incision with coagulation)

For certain incisions, e.g. through parenchymal or capillary tissue, a haemostatic effect is wanted together with the cut. This haemostasis can be produced in various ways:
- by a cut at low speed,
- by a cutting electrode with a larger surface
- and finally by modulating the cutting signal.

This method causes energy and thus warmth to penetrate deeper into the surrounding tissue during the incision, producing the coagulating effect (Figs. 5.8 and 5.9).

One indication for using blend cutting is an incision through subcutaneous tissue; coagulation is then usually required for only a few vessels so that time is saved in this way.

5.1.3 Coagulation

Desiccation or contact coagulation

The difference between incision and coagulation lies in the large current density, resulting in rapid, local heating of the cell tissue, triggering a cell explosion and causing separation of the tissue.

By contrast, in coagulation the current density is decreased so that the developed heat diffuses through the cell wall into the cell liquid, transforming the protein (visible in the white colouring). This procedure dries the cell out and the cell wall stays intact (Fig. 5.10). Direct contact with the tissue is a typical feature of desiccation.

At a lower current density, heat penetrates deeper into the tissue so that the tissue dries out to the side of the electrode. The time factor plays a major role: 100 W applied for 0.1 s has a more superficial heating effect on the tissue, whereas 10 W applied for 1 s has a deeper effect and is more likely to produce the required coagulation effect. So a higher power setting does not necessarily result in better or deeper coagulation. On the contrary, if the power

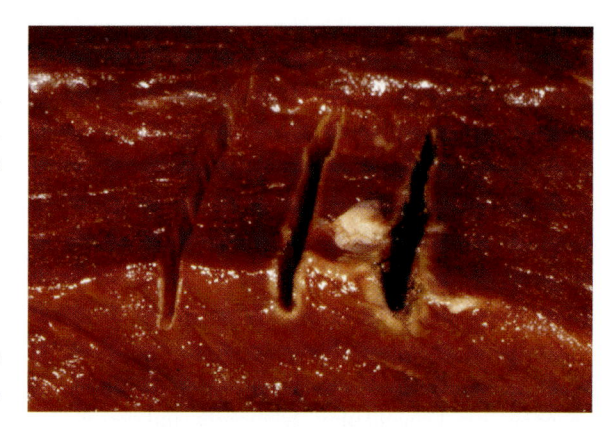

Fig. 5.9. Cutting with coagulation shares

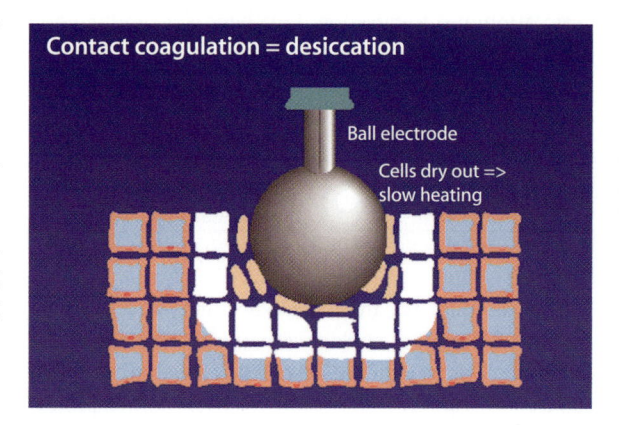

Fig. 5.10. Desiccation

setting is too high, the tissue then carbonises and sticks to the electrode (Fig. 5.11).

Non-contact coagulation – fulguration and spray coagulation

Fulguration. The second form of coagulation is fulguration (fulgur, lat.: the spark, spray coagulation). The main difference to desiccation is that no contact is necessary

5.1 · General aspects

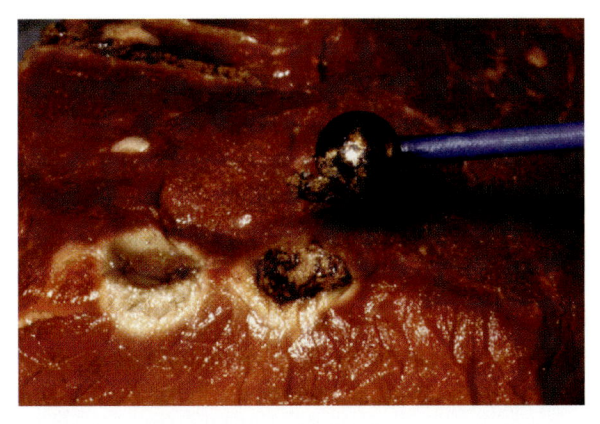

Fig. 5.11. Sticking to the electrode when the output is too high

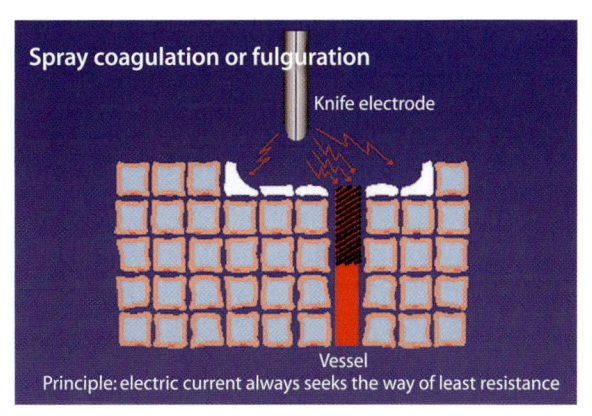

Fig. 5.12. Fulguration

with the electrode. This effect is preferably used when sealing tissue over a large surface. In order to generate the necessary sparking effect, high momentary voltage peaks are required.

The advantage of fulguration is that the sparks are sprayed or »jump« to the tissue. Current seeks the way of least resistance (physical principle) so that it is easy to imagine how these sparks »seek« bleeding vessels and coagulate them because they have better conductive properties (Fig. 5.12).

This naturally also happens in situations in which blood vessels are not visible. Suitable areas of application therefore include for example surgery to the liver, coagulation of the sternum, coagulation of not visibly open veins during transurethral resection and generally widespread, diffuse bleeding.

Fulguration always causes a flat, flexible necrosis at the sparking point. These points are then also less conductive for heat, so that deep coagulation is not possible.

Spray coagulation. Spray coagulation is high-intensity fulguration. This means that a spark jumps already at a very early stage so that widespread coagulation can be performed more easily and faster.

5.1.4 Influences on the surgical effect

It is not only the power setting and mode which influence the effect on the tissue: the surgical effect is in fact the sum of the following factors.
- Power setting:
  A high power setting causes more tissue damage than a lower power setting
- Type:
  Incision has a different effect on the tissue from coagulation
- Mode:
  A smooth cut (pure cut) generates less lateral haemostasis than a blend cut. Contact coagulation generates deeper protein denaturation than fulguration or spray coagulation which is more superficial.
- Shape of the electrode:
  A needle electrode concentrates the power on a small contact surface, producing higher power density for an easier cut. A ball electrode or forceps generate larger contact to the tissue: the power density decreases and with it the temperature generated in the tissue, resulting in coagulation.
- Incision speed:
  With the incision speed through the tissue, the user has a direct influence on the degree of haemostasis to the side of the cut: more energy can be emitted laterally at a lower speed, generating more haemostasis than at a fast incision speed.
- Kind of tissue:
  Fat or glandular tissue has higher electrical resistance than muscular tissue, for example. The user therefore feels higher mechanical resistance during the incision at the interface between muscular and fat tissue. The power setting of the HF surgical device is then usually increased.
- Distance between active electrode and neutral electrode
  The distance between the site and the positioned neutral electrode also influences the quality of the surgical result. The reason for this is that the electrical resistance increases with the distance of the neutral electrode to the site. This means that part of the power emitted by the HF surgical device can be lost by higher body resistance (▶ see also Sect. 5.2).

5.2 Neutral electrode

5.2.1 Task

The root »neutral« in the word »neutral electrode« implies a certain safety. But this impression is false in view of the fact that the same power which passes through the electrode handle also penetrates the neutral electrode and corresponding connection cable.

The function of the neutral electrode is to close the alternating current circuit from the high-frequency surgery device – electrode handle – patient – neutral electrode – high-frequency surgery device with the lowest possible current density at the contact surface. Which is quite the reverse of the »active« electrode, where a high current density is required for the surgical effect.

As far as the contact surface and size of the neutral electrode are concerned, the physical rule applies: the larger the contact surface of the neutral electrode, the better for the patient because the current density is smaller.

But if this contact surface is too small, the neutral electrode comes loose or was not applied completely, this can result in serious burns because of the high current density, with the »neutral electrode« also becoming an »active electrode« (▶ see also Sect. 5.2.4).

5.2.2 Safety systems

Current high-frequency surgery devices come with monitoring systems which notice a decrease in the contact surface (when the neutral electrode works loose) and draw the user's attention to the situation with an alarm and by stopping the power, before the patient can be harmed.

This function is best illustrated by the example of the monitoring system make Valleylab.

The »Return Electrode Monitoring« (REM) system was developed to avoid burns under the neutral electrode. This neutral electrode monitoring measures the quality of the contact surface between the neutral electrode and the patient all the time, also while the device is activated, and registers every change during the entire surgical procedure.

A visible and audible alarm is generated when the quality of the contact surface is inadequate and the power is switched off immediately to prevent any dangerous situation.

The REM system consists of an electronic monitoring system, a divided neutral electrode and a two-wire connection cable.

The electronic control unit in the generator emits high-frequency alternating current as measuring current; this flows across one-half of the neutral electrode through the patient's tissue and back across the other half of the neutral electrode: the generated electrical resis-

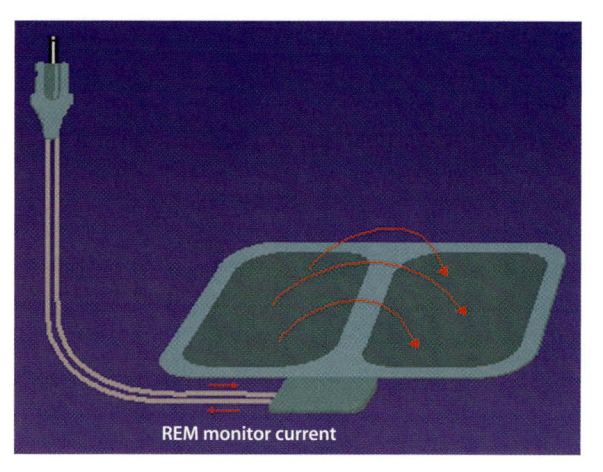

Fig. 5.13. Measuring current at the divided neutral electrode

tance is a dimension of the contact quality of the neutral electrode (◘ Fig. 5.13).

So the neutral electrode and thus the patient are *always* integrated in the monitoring of the REM system. The properties of the skin (hair growth, circulation, fat, temperature) differ in every patient, the personal limit value is ascertained individually for each patient and monitored during the entire operation (adaptive REM system).

The alignment of the neutral electrode to the site is irrelevant with this system, because an electronic feature ensures that the high-frequency current always flows symmetrically across the divided neutral electrode

The effectiveness of this safety system depends crucially on how the characteristics of its components interact. These are the inert resistance of the used neutral electrode and the used connection cable, and the resistance value of the patient's skin.

The electronic control unit of the REM system is ideally adapted to the corresponding neutral electrodes and connection cables.

5.2.3 The neutral electrode – Which, where, how?

In spite of all technical possibilities and different versions, there are a few general rules for using the neutral electrode.

Positioning
- Positioning as close as possible to the site:
  This ensures that the procedure can be carried out with the lowest possible power setting, reducing the risk of alternative currents in the body.
- Positioning on tissue with good circulation:
  Tissue with good circulation has lower transition resistance, making it easier to close the current circuit: and lower power settings are required.

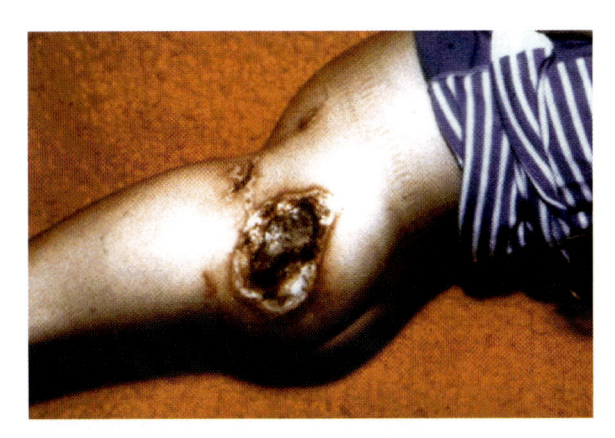

Fig. 5.14. Burns under the neutral electrode

Unsuitable application points

The following application points or an application leading the current through these points should be avoided:
- Bony structures:
  They have a high electrical resistance. This could result in a higher power setting in the device.
- Scar tissue:
  This is also dry tissue with high resistance and therefore not suitable as an application point
- Metal implants:
  Metal implants in the body can be artificial hip joints, pacemakers or other conductive implants. Electric current has the physical property of seeking the way of least resistance, so it will prefer to flow across these particularly good conductors. There is then a risk that the current density and therefore energy density at the entrance or exit point is so high that internal burning is caused.
- ECG electrodes, monitor leads, etc:
  If a neutral electrode is placed on these similarly conductive materials, high-frequency current can overcome any existing insulation and couple into these conductors. Here again there is a risk that the current density and therefore energy density at the entrance or exit point is so high that internal burning is caused.

Considerations when choosing the neutral electrode

The following considerations should be included when selecting the individual neutral electrodes:
- Gel or adhesive electrodes?
  A gel electrode adapts to uneven parts of the skin and hair growth better than an adhesive electrode. Shaving is not usually necessary in top quality gel electrodes, thus avoiding the risk of micro-lesions.
- Neutral electrode with small or large contact surface
  The task of the neutral electrode is to achieve the smallest current concentration possible, which means the larger the neutral electrode, the smaller the current density.
- Prescribed application arrangement?
  A prescribed application arrangement can restrict the possibilities of fixing the electrode.
- Neutral electrodes with integrated connection cable or clip-on connection lead?
  A clip-on solution is usually less expensive, but in some indications (heart surgery, paediatric surgery) a clip should be avoided so as not to harm the patient through pressure necrosis

5.2.4 Burns under the neutral electrode?

Burns from high-frequency current under the neutral electrode: how do such burns occur, how can they be detected, and how can they be avoided?

A burn from high-frequency current is always generated when the current density is very large in a small point. The same electrosurgical effect is then caused at this point as at the »active« electrode, resulting in a tissue lesion in the form of a 3rd degree burn. In the case of intensive activation, the tissue continues to burn and the lesion spreads (Fig. 5.14).

Possible causes for concentration of current under the neutral electrode

- Contact surface is too small:
  The neutral electrode has not been adhered completely or has worked partly loose during the operation. When reusable rubber neutral electrodes are being used, the contact surfaces can very quickly become inadequate or too small (tent formation, placed on body recesses or uneven areas of skin).
- Good contact over a small area:
  The neutral electrode is in contact across its complete surface, but parts of this contact surface have far better contact. This can happen if liquids flow under the neutral electrode, or when adhesive electrodes are applied with the fingertips and not pressed on with the full surface of the hand.

Today damage of this kind is caused only rarely because of the safety features integrated in high-frequency surgical devices. But in many cases, skin lesions are incorrectly said to be damage caused by high-frequency current (Figs. 5.15 and 5.16):

These are changes to the skin consisting of reddening, blisters and flaky skin caused by the following factors:
- Heat: e.g. warming mats, warming cushions, warm surroundings …
- Pressure, e.g. from the patient's own weight, poor positioning, the surgeon leaning on the patient …

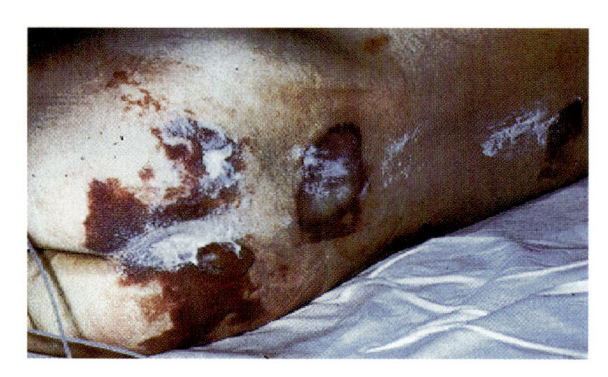

Fig. 15. Skin lesions

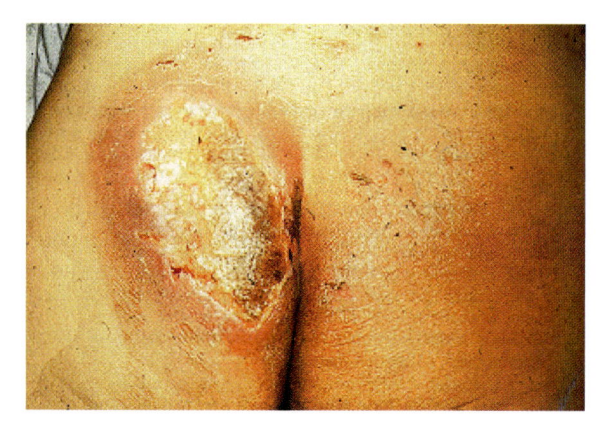

Fig. 5.16. Skin lesions

— Time: the entire time for the operation, also including the time for transporting and preparing the patient
— Chemicals, e.g. alcoholic cleaning and disinfectant, urine …
— Moisture, e.g. sweat, water, amniotic fluid …

Not all the above factors have to be present to cause such changes to the skin. Such skin lesions are *not* caused by the influence of high-frequency current.

It is important for the user to recognise which cause is involved in order to take the necessary measures.

5.3 Rules for safe use

5.3.1 General

According to the regulations of the Medical Product Law (MPG), high-frequency surgical devices are classified in class IIb. The classification is based on a risk analysis, and the risk potential posed by the use of high-frequency surgery is set on equal terms with the risks from radiotherapy equipment, lasers, anaesthetic equipment and respirators.

It is therefore vital for every user to know the rules for safe use of high-frequency surgery, to minimise the risk of danger for the user, the patient and all staff working in the operating theatre.

User know-how. Most manufacturers of products for high-frequency surgery provide information on how the equipment functions and its correct use (e.g. courses, instructions, manuals, etc.). Every user (doctors, operating staff, medical technicians) should make himself familiar with the handling and possibilities of the HF surgery device being used; this is a mandatory requirement according to the Medical Product Owner Ordinance (MPBetreibV) §§ 2.2, 2.4, 2.5 and § 5. In addition, offers for advanced training should be taken up in order to acquire basic knowledge about the procedures and techniques involved as well as operating the devices.

Power settings. High-frequency devices are often adjusted to very high power settings. These high power settings can then cause problems such as ECG artefacts or faults in the monitor. Apart from that, usually excessive amounts of tissue undergo necrosis with an unnecessary burden on the patient. The same effect can be produced at a lower power setting simply by the choice of electrode (change from knife electrode to needle electrode). The aim should always be to choose the lowest possible power setting to minimise the potential risks.

Choice of the right system. Which is the right system which will cause the least harm to the patient? The bipolar system has only a locally limited effect, but the high power setting required for some indications causes extensive damage to the tissue, which can be avoided when using the monopolar system with less power and a fine needle electrode.

Choice of the right mode. Not every mode is ideally suited for every indication; the choice should depend on the indication. There is no point in choosing a fulguration or spray mode, i.e. non-contact coagulation, when working with the forceps coagulation system (contact coagulation). This can cause injuries to the surgeon from discharges through the gloves (▶ see also: »Glove discharges«).

5.3.2 Use of high-frequency surgery in minimally invasive surgery

As far as minimally invasive surgery is concerned, the same rules naturally apply as for open use of HF surgery. But there are additional dangers involved because of the limited vision, the usually confined space available and the special instruments.

Insulation faults. Defect insulation of the active electrode can cause unwanted burns. Even only slightly damaged instrument insulation (scratches, blisters, cracks ...) can puncture during an operation and cause serious injuries (Fig. 5.17).

Direct coupling. Direct coupling refers to the contact of an active instrument with another conductive instrument, e.g. forceps, needle holder etc. Tissue contact by this instrument then inevitably causes unwanted damage (Fig. 5.18).

Capacitive coupling. Two electrical conductors separated by insulation have the property of saving energy in an alternating current circuit. This kind of electrical element is called »capacitor«. A monopolar instrument (conductor), its insulation and a metal trocar (conductor) constitute this kind of energy accumulator. As long as the metal trocar has widespread contact with the abdominal wall, no energy can gather. But as soon as it becomes insulated from the patient by a plastic fixator (grip), this energy accumulator becomes charged and discharges its energy on contact with conductive structures (colon, mesenterium etc.), causing burns (Fig. 5.19).

The following recommendations should be observed to reduce the risks for minimal invasive surgery.
- Check the insulation of monopolar instruments thoroughly.
  Replace instruments as soon as any signs of scratches, scores etc. can be seen or felt. Use disposable instruments.
- Use low power settings.
  The risk of injuring the patient decreases with lower power settings.
- Avoid high-voltage modes as far as possible.
  The high-voltage modes fulguration and spray should only be used specifically and deliberately, e.g. for fulguration of the liver bed during a cholecystectomy.
- Only activate the instruments when in contact with the tissue.
  This avoids charging any energy accumulators and unwanted »hot« contacts with other instruments.
- Avoid bringing the active electrode into contact with or into the vicinity of other metal instruments.
  Alternative current paths via these instruments can be avoided in this way.
- Use purely metal or purely plastic trocars.
  No capacity is generated.

5.3.3 Other information

Use of high-frequency surgery for pacemaker patients

The heart is a muscle which is not impaired in its functions or damaged by the flow of high-frequency current.

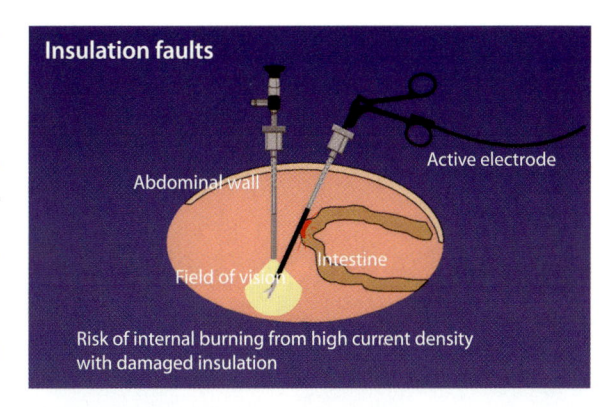

Fig. 5.17. Insulation faults

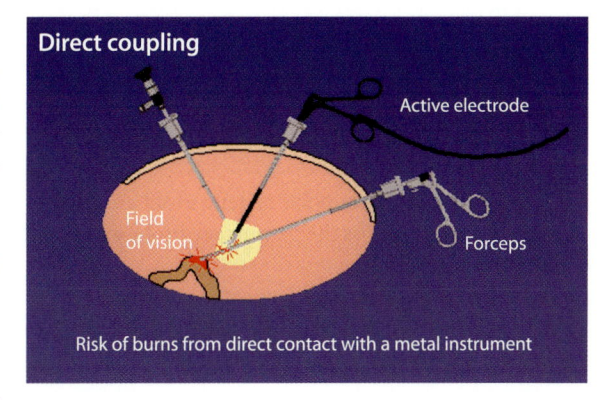

Fig. 5.18. Direct coupling

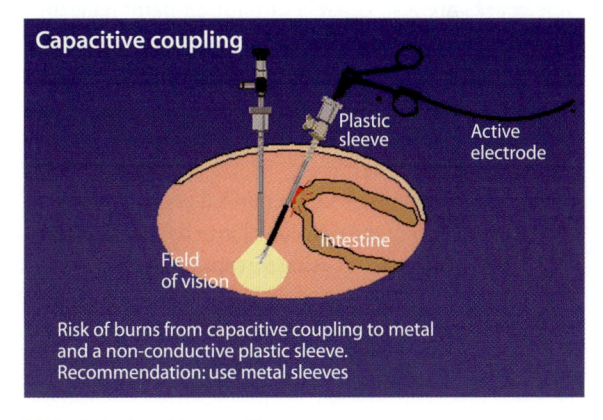

Fig. 5.19. Capacitive coupling

However, if a pacemaker probe is implanted in the heart, a current can easily couple into this conductive probe. A burn can then be caused at the exit point in the heart muscle as a result of the high current density at the tip of the probe (small surface). The pacemaker is not hindered in its internal settings and functions, but the necrotised tissue in the heart cannot stimulate an emitted pulse.

The recommendations for using high-frequency surgery in pacemaker patients are as follows:

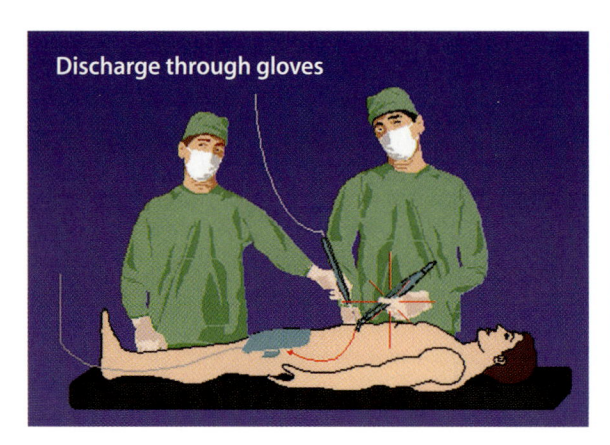

Fig. 5.20. Glove discharge

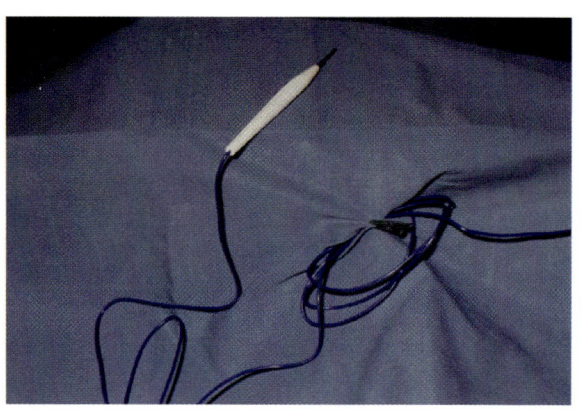

Fig. 5.21. Winding the cable generates an electromagnetic coil

- The safest solution is not to use electrosurgery at all, but this is not always practicable.
- The current flow is limited locally in the bipolar system.
- When using the monopolar system, avoid an obvious flow of current across the pacemaker, probe and heart muscle.
- Use a low power setting.
- Consult the recommendations issued by the pacemaker manufacturer.

Use with inflammable gases and substances

The use of high-frequency surgery generates sparks. But these sparks are also capable of igniting flammable and explosive gases and vapours. Care is required when opening hollow organs (e.g. colon, oesophagus) and in the presence of alcoholic disinfectants.

Glove discharges

The glove discharge is usually a painful effect. This refers to the destruction of the surgeon's glove by a high-energy spark during coagulation using forceps (contact coagulation (Fig. 5.20).

There are several reasons for this discharge:

On the one hand, if the power setting is too high, this can cause discharge through the glove. On the other hand, the quality of the glove always plays a role.

But the cause is normally to be found in using the wrong technique.

If the fulguration or spray mode has been selected on a high-powered high-frequency surgery device but the user then proceeds with contact coagulation using forceps, the tissue around the forceps dries out and forms a high electrical resistance. The high-frequency current then looks for an alternative path by using the lower resistance of the glove and closes the circuit across the surgeon who is in contact with the patient and thus with the neutral electrode. This effect is provoked all the more if the electrode handle was already activated before contact with the forceps or the forceps are already carbonised.

The remedy is to reduce the power, adjust the desiccation mode, not to use carbonised instruments and not to activate the electrode handle until the first contact with the forceps.

Wiring

A wound up cable gives a tidy impression, but also constitutes a risk. Winding the cable creates an electromagnetic coil – a transformer – which generates a magnetic field and another current circuit. If the wound cable is then fixed with a metal clip (towel clip) this reinforces the effect even further (Fig. 5.21).

If the towel clip touches the patient, this can cause burns. The cable should therefore be laid out on the floor to its full length. If cables are routed parallel to each other, electrical energy can couple into the other cable and cause interference (e.g. artefacts in the ECG monitor).

Glossary

Leakage current	Current which flows along an unwanted path, normally to the earth potential. In insulated high-frequency surgery, this is high-frequency current flowing to the earth potential.
Active electrode	HF surgical instrument or accessory which concentrates the electrical (therapeutic) current in the operating site.

Glossary

Adapter	Connection between incompatible connectors and sockets, facilitating correct connection and closure of the current circuit.
Ampere (A)	Unit of measurement for electrical current. One ampere (A) corresponds to 6.242×10^{18} electrons per second.
Tipping the vessel forceps/forceps coagulation	Surgical procedure for coagulating bleeding blood vessels, where the active electrode makes contact with the vessel forceps: the current passes through the vessel forceps to the target tissue. Typical for contact coagulation.
Output current/voltage/power	The current, voltage or power produced by an electrical device, e.g. HF surgical device (HF generator, HF device).
Auto bipolar	Mode selected by a user, allowing for automatic application and interruption of the bipolar current depending on the impedance of the tissue between the branches of the bipolar forceps.
Bipolar output	Insulated output in HF surgery where the electrical current flows between two bipolar electrodes positioned around the tissue to achieve a surgical effect in this tissue (usually desiccation).
Bipolar HF surgery	HF surgical procedure where the electrical current flows between two bipolar electrodes positioned around the tissue to achieve a surgical effect in this tissue (usually desiccation). The current flows from one electrode through the target tissue to the other, closing the circuit, without the current penetrating in any other part of the patient's body.
Bipolar instrument	HF surgical instrument or accessory in which the active and neutral electrodes are close together.
Blend	Wave mode including both incision and coagulation wave modes; current for incision with different levels of haemostasis.
Crest factor	Dimension for the capability of a coagulation form to achieve haemostasis without separating or cutting tissue. A higher crest factor indicates better coagulation with less tissue damage.
CUSA system	Cavitational ultrasonic dissector and aspirator produced by Valleylab, with selective tissue removal in contrast to ultrasonic knives. Can be used for ultrasonic high-frequency surgery.
Desiccation	HF surgical effect of hydrating the tissue and denaturising the protein, resulting from direct contact between the HF surgical electrode and the tissue.
Direct coupling	Condition occurring when an electrical conductor (the active electrode) has direct contact with another, second conductor (e.g. endoscope, forceps). The electrical current flows from the first conductor to the second and supplies it with energy.
Electrode	Conductor transferring or receiving the HF surgical current. see also active electrode, neutral electrode.
Effective voltage	Effective amount of voltage; square mean voltage (mean amount of voltage at any point in time) of a wave mode.
Electrosurgery (HF surgery)	Achieving the required surgical effect by conducting high-frequency electrical current through the tissue.
Endoscope	Fibre-optic tubular or hose-shaped instrument for examining body cavities and organs.
Earth potential	Universal conductor and joint current return point for electric circuits; earthing.
Frequency	Speed at which a cycle repeats. In HF surgery, the number of cycles per second in which the direction of current changes.
Fulguration	Use of electrical arcs (sparks) for coagulating tissue. The sparks jump from the electrode across an air gap to the tissue.
Spark	Discharge of electric current across an air gap; essential for incision and fulguration procedures in HF surgery.
Vessel forceps	Forceps for clamping a bleeding vessel to stop the flow of blood.

Generator	Device which converts low-frequency alternating current into high-frequency HF surgical current (HF surgical device, HF generator, HF device).
Haemostasis	Coagulation; in HF surgery, the use of heat generated by the HF current to stop the bleeding of a cut blood vessel.
Hertz (Hz)	Unit of measurement for frequency; one Hertz corresponds to one cycle per second.
HF surgery (electrosurgery)	Achieving the required surgical effect by conducting high-frequency electrical current through the tissue
HF surgical device	The HF surgical generator and its connection cables.
HF surgical circuit	The path taken by the therapeutic current. HF surgical device – active electrode – through the body tissue – neutral electrode – HF surgical device and in another direction (alternating current circuit).
HF surgery burns	Destruction of tissue caused by the concentration of HF current. This expression also includes the surgical effect, but usually refers to unintentional tissue damage; see also unintentional burns.
High frequency (HF)	Frequencies at which radio signals can be transferred; here the high-frequency current used for HF surgery.
Impedance	Resistance in the alternating current circuit, the ohmic resistance and the resistance generated by capacity or inductivity. The resistance of a material measured in ohms is its tendency to withstand the flow of current or, in other words, the tendency of a material not to conduct the current.
Instant Response Technology	HF device technology using a feedback circuit to scan the tissue resistance. The resistance of the target tissue can vary, so that the computer-controlled output voltage of the HF surgical device is automatically adjusted in certain modes. The result is a constant output power which achieves the same surgical effect in all tissue types.
Insufflation	Introduction or injection of gas, steam or powder into body cavities or organs (e.g. carbon dioxide in the abdominal cavity during a laparoscopy).
Insulated output	Output of an HF surgical device which has no connection to the earth potential.
Insulation	Material which does not conduct electric current.
Insulation fault	This condition occurs when the insulation around an electrical conductor is damaged. The result can be that the current flows outside the intended current circuit.
Capacity	Characteristic of a current circuit to transfer an electric charge from one conductor to another, even if these are separated by insulation.
Capacitive coupling	Transfer of energy from one conductor (the active electrode) through the intact insulation into adjacent conductive material (tissue, trocars, wires, etc.).
Coagulation	Clotting of blood or destruction of tissue without incision effect; HF surgery differentiates between desiccation and fulguration.
Coagulation mode	Intermittent high-voltage wave mode which has been optimised for HF surgical coagulation.
Coagulation across forceps/clip	Surgical procedure for coagulating bleeding blood vessels, where the active electrode makes contact with the forceps/clip: the current passes through the vessel forceps to the target tissue. This procedure is a form of contact coagulation.
Electrode holder	Insulated container for safe storage of the active HF electrode when not in use during the operation. Recommended to avoid accidents.
Cross coupling	Transfer of electric power between two neighbouring circuits.
Short circuit	Condition of a HF surgical circuit when the high-frequency surgical device is activated and the active electrode has direct contact with the neutral electrode. An electrical circuit without load (consumer).
Load	In HF surgery, the body tissue which is included in the HF surgical circuit; the electrical impedance in this circuit.

Glossary

Power	Quantity of energy produced per second, expressed in watt.
Conductor	Material which conducts electric current.
LLETZ/LEEP	HF surgical excision procedure in gynaecology, where a loop is used to remove the transformation zone of the cervix (large loop excision of the transformation zone).
Macro bipolar	HF surgical wave mode used in bipolar surgery with higher voltage and power than the normal bipolar HF surgical wave modes. It is used for bipolar incision or fast coagulation.
Micro bipolar	Bipolar wave mode with low voltage used for precise desiccation.
Monopolar HF surgery	HF surgery procedure where the active electrode is in the surgical wound. One active pole.
Monopolar output	Earthed or insulated output for a HF surgical device which conducts current through the patient to the neutral electrode.
Monopolar instrument	HF surgical instrument or accessory consisting of just one electrode; one active electrode.
Necrosis	Destruction of tissue.
Neutral electrode	Conductive surface in direct contact with the patient's skin during HF surgery. During the operation, it absorbs the HF current from the patient across a wide surface, distributes it and returns it to the HF surgical device, closing the circuit. Standard neutral electrodes today are disposable electrodes fixed with an adhesive gel.
Ohm (Ω)	Unit of measurement for electrical resistance; volt per ampere.
REM contact quality monitoring system	Special Valleylab safety system which continuously monitors the impedance level between patient and neutral electrode. If the REM system registers dangerous impedance levels as a result of poor contact between the neutral electrode and the patient, the system produces an acoustic and optical signal and the HF surgical device is switched off. To guarantee maximum safety, HF surgical devices equipped with REM must use a compatible neutral electrode. This electrode can be recognised as having two separate areas and a special connector with a middle pin.
Incision	HF surgical effect resulting from high current density in the tissue causing intracellular fluid to evaporate. This results in the cell wall bursting with destruction of the cell structure. Low voltage, high current flow.
Cut	Continuous low-current wave mode optimised for HF surgical incision.
Self-restricting power	Power feature of the HF surgical device which limits the power output at certain tissue resistances.
Voltage	Force pressed across the resistance by the electrical current; electromotor force or potential difference, expressed in volt.
Voltage from peak to peak	The voltage of a wave mode, measured from its maximum negative value to its maximum positive value.
Peak voltage	The maximum voltage of a wave mode, starting from zero (0) in a positive or negative direction to the maximum value.
Spray	Coagulation mode allowing for optimum fulguration.
Current	Number of electrons passing a given point in a second, measured in ampere (A).
Current density	Amount of current flow per surface unit; the current density is directly proportional to the heat generated in the material.
Circuit	Path along which the electric current moves.
Current division	Electrical current which leaves the intended HF surgical circuit and follows an alternative path with the least resistance to the earth potential; typically the cause for unintended burns at earthed HF surgical devices far from the operating site.
Transformer	In HF surgical devices an electrical connection circuit which changes the ratio of current to voltage and converts wave modes with low voltage and high current into wave modes with high voltage and low current.

Burns under the neutral electrode	HF surgical burns resulting from an excess concentration of current or current density under the neutral electrode.
Volt (V)	Unit of measurement for electrical potential (voltage).
Watt (W)	Unit of measurement for power.
Wave mode	Graphical representation of electrical activity; it shows how voltage varies with the change in current over time.
Resistance	Lacking conductivity of a material, measured in ohms.

References

1. Aigner, König, Wruhs (1993) Komplikation bei der Anwendung der Hochfrequenzchirurgie. Osteo, Wien, 1/1993
2. Bedienungshandbuch Force FX-A (1999) Valleylab Inc. Boulder/CO, USA, März
3. Benders D. Electrosurgery interference-minimize ist effects on ECG monitors, B.S.E.E.
4. Gendron F (1980) »Burns« occuring during lenghty surgical procedures. J Clin Eng 5(1): 19–26
5. Gesetz über Medizinprodukte (Medizinproduktegesetz – MPG) v. 2. Aug. 1994, in der Fassung vom 6. Aug. 1998
6. Pierson MA. In: Alexander's Care of the patient in surgery, 10. Aufl., S. 25 ff.
7. Tucker RD, Ferguson S (1991) Do surgical gloves protect staff during electrosurgical procedures? 110(5): 892–895
8. Verordnung über das Errichten, Betreiben und Anwenden von Medizinprodukten (Medizinprodukte-Betreiberverordnung – MP-BetreibV) v. 29. Juni 1998
9. Zap Facts, Valleylab Inc. Boulder, CO, USA, Mai 1995
10. Laparoscopy for the general surgeon
11. Fire during surgery of the head and neck area, Health Devices 9(2): 50–53

6 New technologies

D. Kendoff, L. Mahlke, T. Hüfner, C. Krettek, C. Priscoglio

6.1 Navigation – 56
6.1.1 Equipment, installation and modalities – 56
6.1.2 Iso-C3D general – 57
6.1.3 Iso-C3D navigation – 58

6.2 AWIGS/VIWAS – New systems for image-guided surgery – 60
6.2.1 Introduction – 60
6.2.2 Overview of the system components – 60
6.2.3 AWIGS – 60
6.2.3.1 Use and benefits of the system – 60
6.2.4 VIWAS – 65
6.2.4.1 VIWAS in combination with an angiography system – 65
6.2.4.2 VIWAS in combination with a sliding gantry – 66
6.2.5 Prospects – 66

References – 66

6.1 Navigation

D. Kendoff, L. Mahlke, T. Hüfner, C. Krettek

6.1.1 Equipment, installation and modalities

A complete navigation module includes the following units (Fig. 6.1):
- Computer workstation with monitor
- Camera
- Reference bases
- Navigated instruments

The reference bases (RB) are marked with LED dots or reflecting materials which are recognised by the camera. The RBs are affixed to the bone being operated in alignment with the camera. Signals are transmitted between camera, patient and navigated systems by means of infrared signals.

Before starting the operation and actual registration process, it is vital to stipulate exactly how the system is to be arranged, i.e. the exact position of all equipment in the navigation system in relation to each other. This also includes the C-arm or Iso-C-arm. The equipment should be arranged before starting or parallel to the positioning of the patient.

The attachment of the RBs must be rotationally stable during the operation to avoid relative movements; if the RBs work loose, this causes inaccuracies (Fig. 6.2). If the RBs work loose during the operation after registration of the system, this must be repeated. The alignment and side-dependency of the RBs and instruments should be kept the same to guarantee optimum communication to the camera during the navigation process. After registration of the RBs and the C-arm, the patient can be moved freely. The instruments are moved relative to the RBs on the patient.

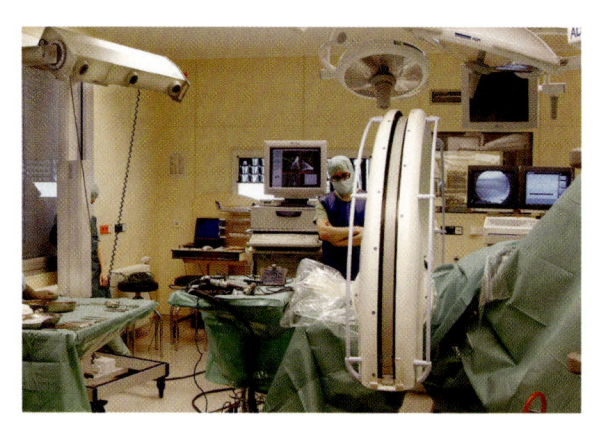

Fig. 6.1. View of the equipment

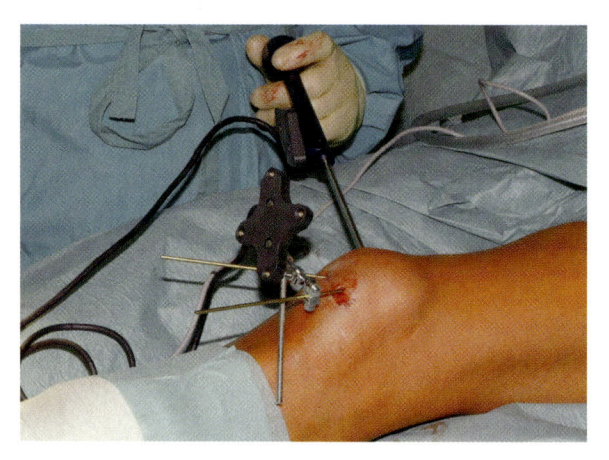

Fig. 6.2. The attachment of the RBs must be rotationally stable during the operation

At present there are various different imaging modalities in use for navigation; these are as follows:
- CT
- Fluoroscopy
- Iso-C
- Kinematic (non-imaging) navigation

In CT-based navigation, during the operation attention only has to be given to the positioning of the workstation and possibly also the camera. Pictures produced before the operation are used while the operation is taking place and as a rule, no further pictures are taken during the operation. Fluoroscopy and Iso-C navigation entails consideration of the C-arm and image intensifier monitor. The C-arm or camera must be positioned to allow for unimpaired communication for registration during the scan. In particular for Iso-C navigation, this must be guaranteed throughout the whole scanning process. Before the operation it is important to check whether troublefree scanning without artefacts will be possible in the necessary anteroposterior and lateral projections. It is sensible to put the monitor in an ergonomic position directly next to the workstation. Kinematic navigation does not require additional imaging. Various anatomic regions are depicted on the basis of non-picture data obtained during the operation. In this case, the camera and workstation are positioned together or separately depending on the system (Fig. 6.3).

Various different navigation systems are currently available; in many cases the camera is integrated directly at the workstation. The corresponding angles and settings of the camera can be changed at short notice using a handle (Fig. 6.4).

Other models have an independent mobile camera unit with correspondingly different arrangements in the operating theatre. Details can be found in the special section.

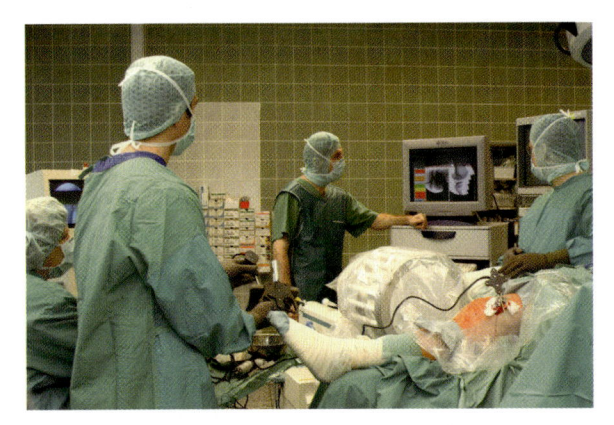

Fig. 6.3. Fluoroscopy-based navigation

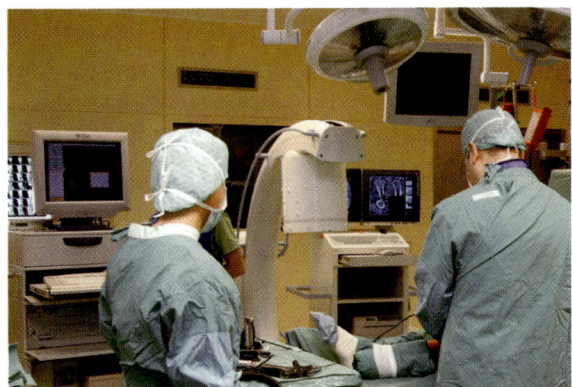

Fig. 6.5. C-arm and monitors on the side opposite the surgeon

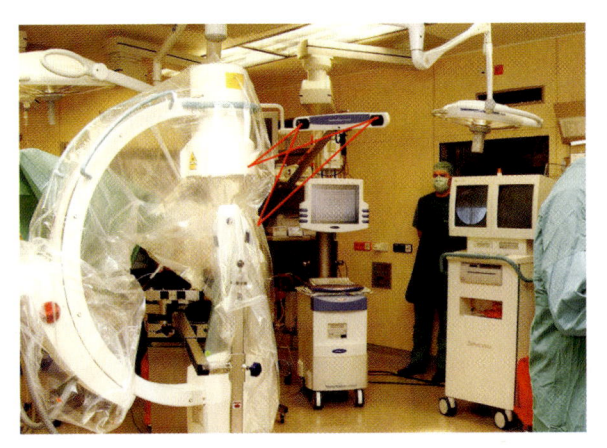

Fig. 6.4. Workstation with camera

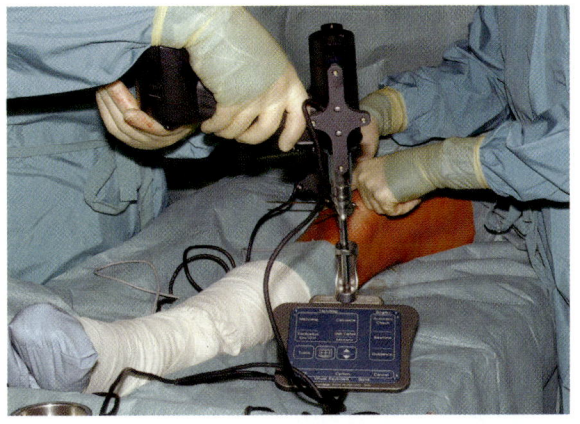

Fig. 6.6. Navigated instruments

It must be possible for the surgeon to look at the monitor easily without special effort during the whole operation. In most cases it is preferable to position it on the side opposite the surgeon. Some indications deviating from this arrangement are described in the special section. In the case of fluoroscopy or Iso-C navigated operations, the image intensifier monitor can be positioned next to the navigation module. Generally, the C-arm should also be placed on the side opposite the surgeon. In the case of necessary control scans, the position of the C-arm is defined and the control scans can be performed without complicated repositioning (Fig. 6.5).

Before the operation it is important to stipulate whether the surgeon will control the workstation himself, e.g. using a sterile touch screen or special handling instruments, or whether an assistant performs this directly in sterile/non-sterile conditions at the system (Fig. 6.3).

Basically for all fluoroscopy or Iso-C navigation, care is required to ensure that there are no X-ray aprons in the region being scanned. Consideration should also be given to partly adjoining joints, e.g. hip or knee joint when defining the navigated leg axis.

6.1.2 Iso-C3D general

A solid carbon (CRP) table should always be used. The region being scanned should be positioned centrally in the middle of the table where possible (Figs. 6.7, 6.8).

If this is not available, the region being scanned must be arranged in the middle of the table, away from all metal braces/brackets. In the case of peripheral extremities such as the hand or foot, the extremity can be hung over the end of the table.

When positioning the patient, it is important to ensure that side supports, leg holders and other supports do not interfere with the direct X-ray path or in the area of the orbital movement of the device. When the patient is positioned on the side, the side supports in particular must be moved towards the thorax. For abdominal positioning, padded cushions should be given preference over metal bolsters. In the case of deep solid carbon (CRP) tables, lateral positioning is only conditionally possible because of the restricted clearance to the C-arm. Similarly, abdominal positioning with high bolsters/cushions is difficult with obese patients.

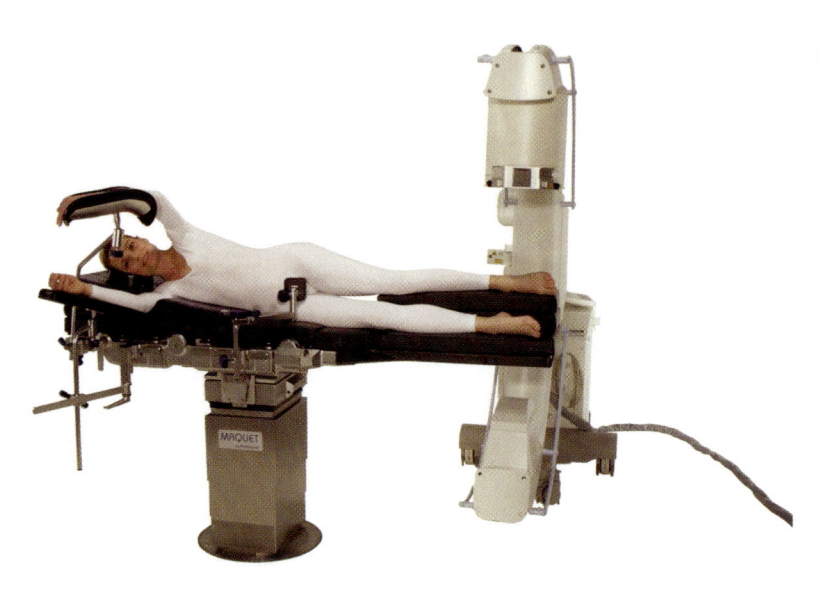

Fig. 6.7. Scanning the left foot on a carbon (CRP) leg plate

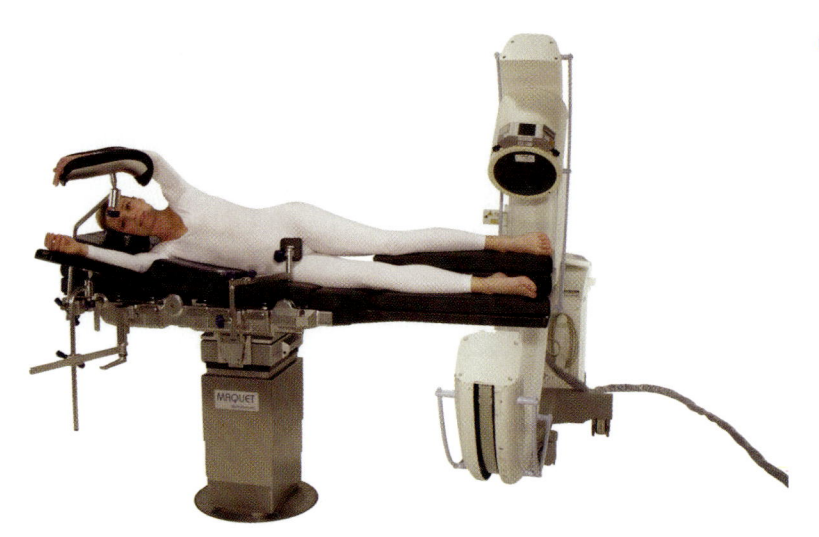

Fig. 6.8. Swivelling movement

Only exact preoperative adjustment of the Iso centre allows for complete orbital movement. Additional intraoperative covers, cloths and equipment restrict the clearance even further.

Before the operation it is important to check whether the operating site is exactly in the Iso centre in both anteroposterior and lateral projections. The possibility of performing the full orbital movement through 190° should be checked by swivelling through this angle once. Bumping against the table or the operating site causes the automatic scan to abort.

Before being brought to the operating table, the system should be protected with specific sterile covers for the Iso-C system. It is also advisable to cover the site additionally with sterile cloths for the actual scan itself. For example, here the extremities can be wrapped in stockinette.

To guarantee sterility while the system is rotating, the table can also be wrapped in a sterile cloth from below. All cloth covers used in this way can be removed again easily after the scan (Figs. 6.9, 6.10).

All instruments and cables in the X-ray path should be removed before the scan to avoid any artefacts.

For surgical procedures to the extremities, the contralateral side interferes a little in the X-ray path; the calculation and display of the multiplanar reconstructions is based on the 12×12×12 cm cube in the Iso centre (Figs. 6.11, 6.12).

6.1.3 Iso-C3D navigation

In the case of ISO-C navigation, the RBs affixed to the bones for registration must not be covered by the sheets during the scan. The monitor should be positioned next to the navigation workstation. During the scan, all operating staff should leave the immediate area of the operation to guarantee that the camera has a permanent view of the C-arm.

6.1 · Navigation

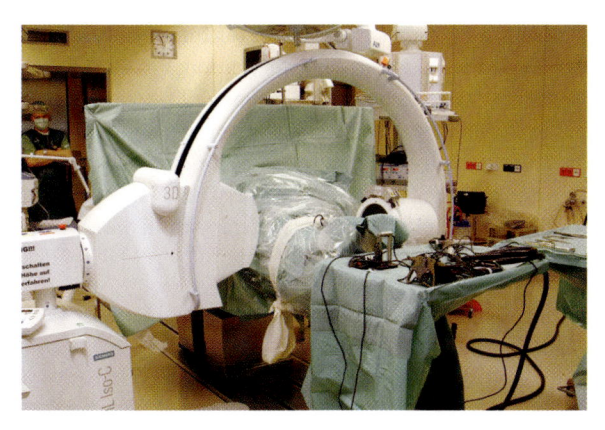

Fig. 6.9. Scanning procedure with the lower extremities in sterile covering

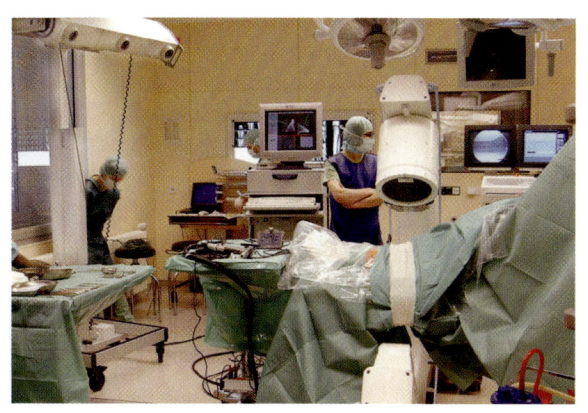

Fig. 6.10. Swivelling movement

Fig. 6.11. Supine position with knee in a middle position on the carbon (CRP) patient board

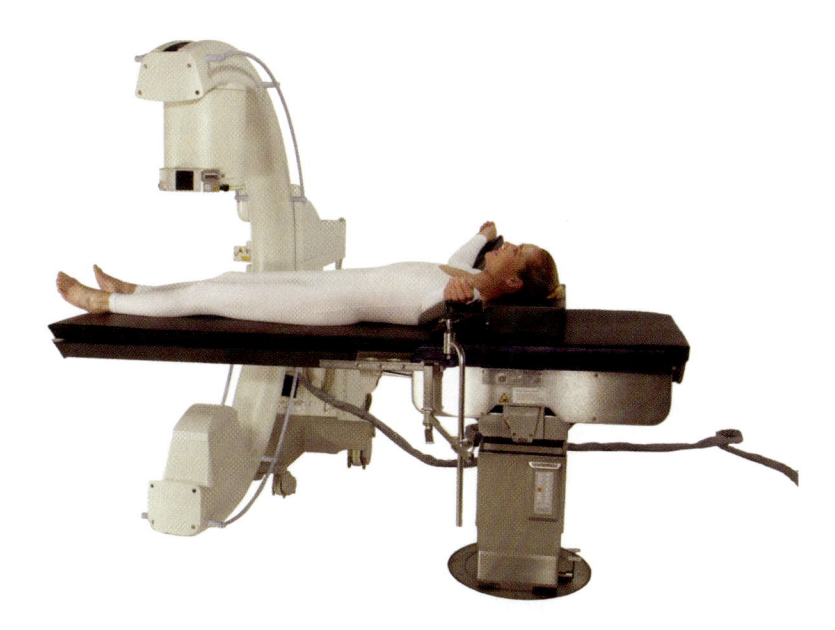

Fig. 6.12. Swivelling movement

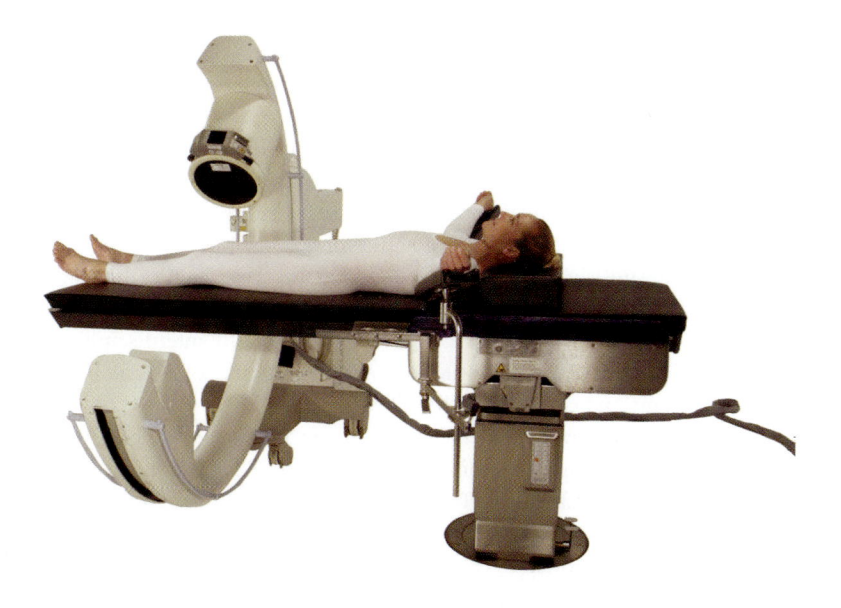

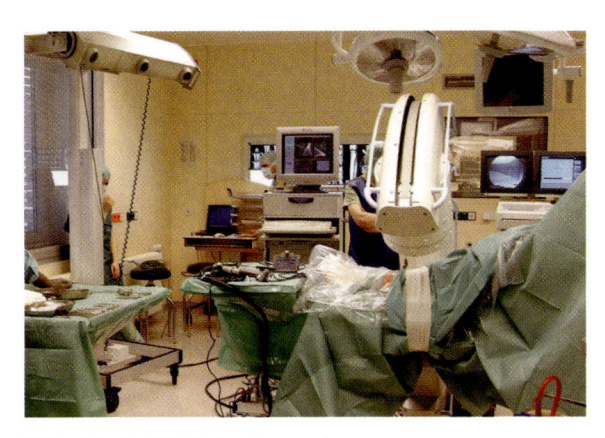

Fig. 6.13. Iso-C3D during the scanning process

Basically the Iso-C can then still be used as a normal scanning unit; if necessary, another scan can be performed as a direct control on success after the end of navigation (Fig. 6.13).

6.2 AWIGS/VIWAS – new systems for image-guided surgery

C. Priscoglio

6.2.1 Introduction

The whole field of medicine is currently witnessing a trend towards interdisciplinary centres of expertise and treatment in view of increasing complexity and the growing demand and pressure for efficiency.

For some time now, surgical disciplines have seen a growing trend to minimally invasive procedures. Alongside the surgical disciplines, originally purely diagnostic, non-invasive disciplines have developed and promoted minimally invasive methods. Such disciplines include for example cardiology, gastroenterology, angiology and, above all, radiology, which have the most efficient imaging systems and the corresponding special know-how. Imaging systems are all the more important when direct vision is not possible to reduce the invasive nature of a procedure. Minimally invasive therapy is image-guided therapy, based on special optical techniques or digital image processing.

Surgery is attaching increasing importance to modern imaging systems and computer technology. This applies to both elective surgery and emergency medicine. Interdisciplinary networking of diagnosis and therapy reveal new paths in the surgical future. The AWIGS and VIWAS systems have been developed as a concept for allowing these two disciplines, which were previously separated in physical terms as well as in time, to grow together.

AWIGS (Advanced Workplace for Image Guided Surgery) and VIWAS (Vascular Interventional Workplace for Advanced Surgery) open up new possibilities for treating patients, and form a bridge between surgery and radiology. The two high-tech systems allow for diagnosis, operation and checking results in one unit. This avoids the need for time-consuming patient transfers, with all the associated dangers (Fig. 6.14).

6.2.2 Overview of the system components

The two systems are based on two structural columns, the so-called duplex column, which offers the greatest stability. The columns can be moved along a linear guide, offering free access to all parts of the body on an operating table, for the first time in imaging diagnostics. The systems consist of various support surfaces, two patient transporters, an AWIGS transfer table specially developed for standard diagnosis and an AWIGS CT table which, in this concept, is positioned behind the computed tomography (CT) unit. It is thus possible to proceed with whole-body scans without having to re-bed or turn the patient.

The AWIGS/VIWAS system can be combined with the diagnostic components computed tomography unit (GE Medical Systems or Siemens Medical Solutions) and with an angiography system (of various makes).

The components can be linked together in different ways, depending on the application (Fig. 6.15).

6.2.3 AWIGS

The AWIGS system has been developed as a high-tech unit to integrate diagnosis, operation and control in one surgical workplace. The AWIGS system is the globally unique unit made up of the operating table and computed tomography.

6.2.3.1 Use and benefits of the system

There is an extremely wide range of possible uses. The AWIGS system can be used in traumatology, neurosurgery and orthopaedic procedures, for general surgery or oral and maxillofacial surgery. The AWIGS system is thus an interdisciplinary element in the operating theatre, in radiology and in the emergency room.

The trauma concept

It is in particular the time savings in traumatology which support the life-saving measures of the surgical team. Even if an average time of 71 min (time between the accident and arrival at hospital for polytraumas – the so-called »golden hour« [2]) sees a patient receiving relatively fast

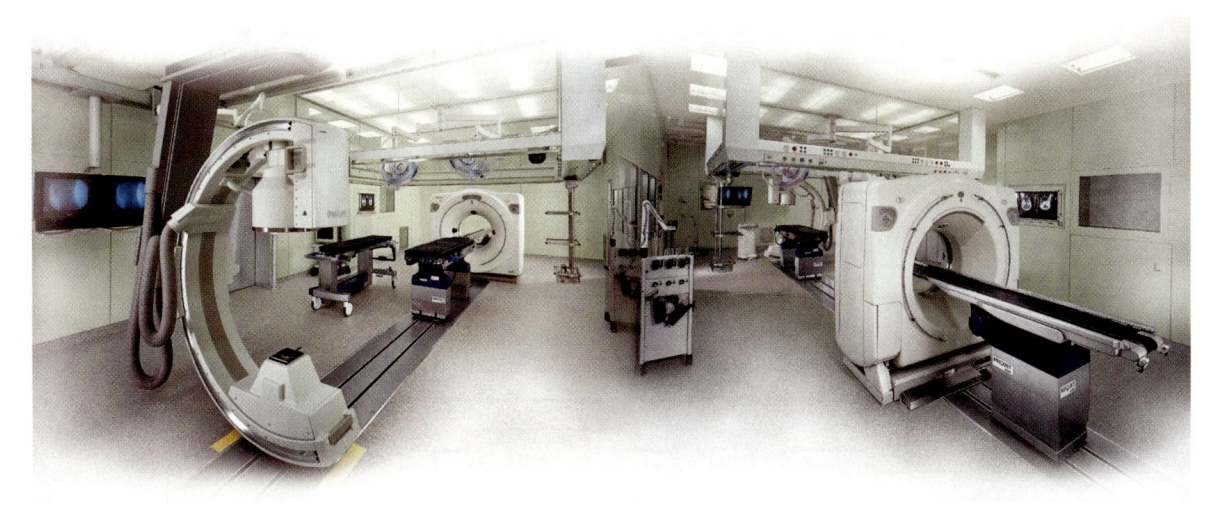

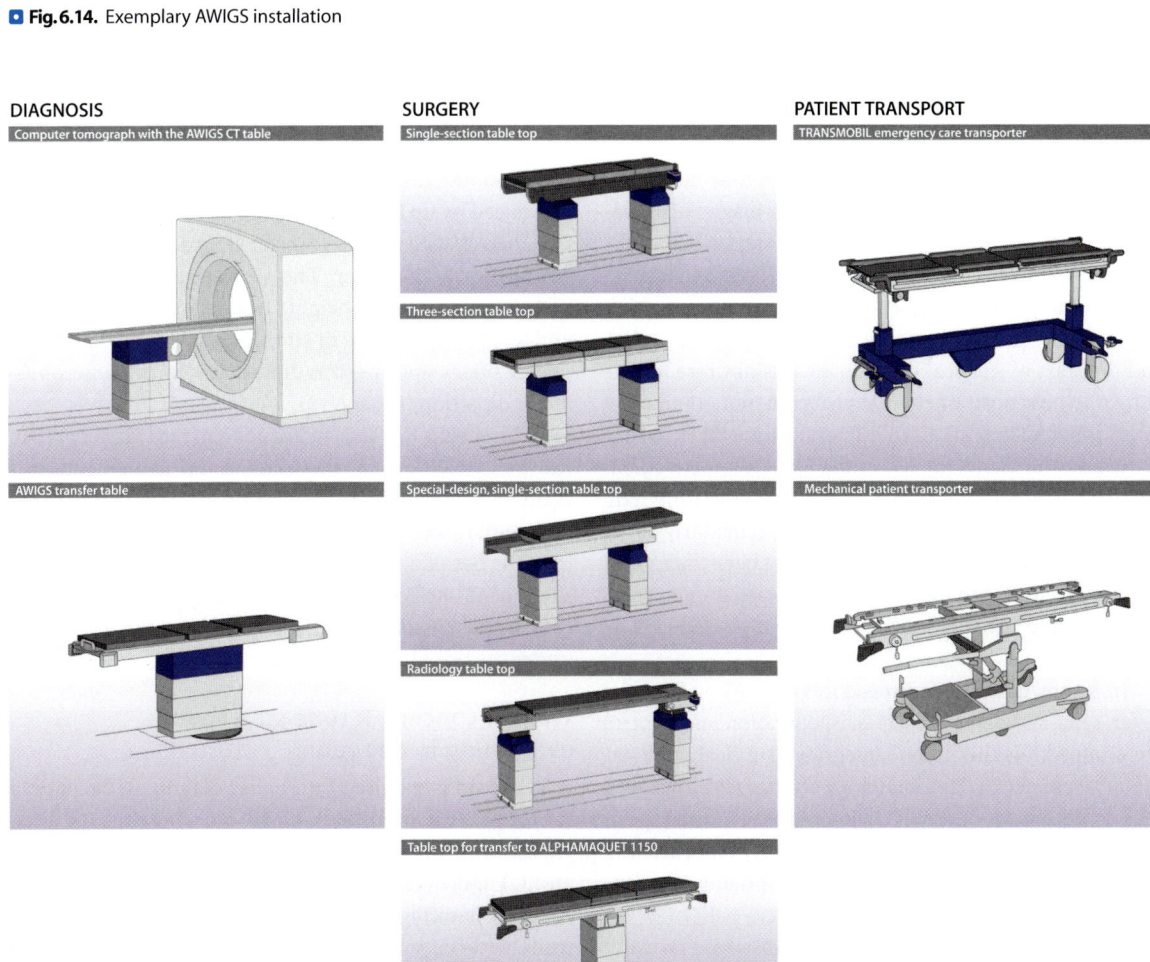

6.2 · AWIGS/VIWAS – new systems for image-assisted surgery

Fig. 6.14. Exemplary AWIGS installation

DIAGNOSIS
- Computer tomograph with the AWIGS CT table
- AWIGS transfer table

SURGERY
- Single-section table top
- Three-section table top
- Special-design, single-section table top
- Radiology table top
- Table top for transfer to ALPHAMAQUET 1150

PATIENT TRANSPORT
- TRANSMOBIL emergency care transporter
- Mechanical patient transporter

Fig. 6.15. Overview of the components

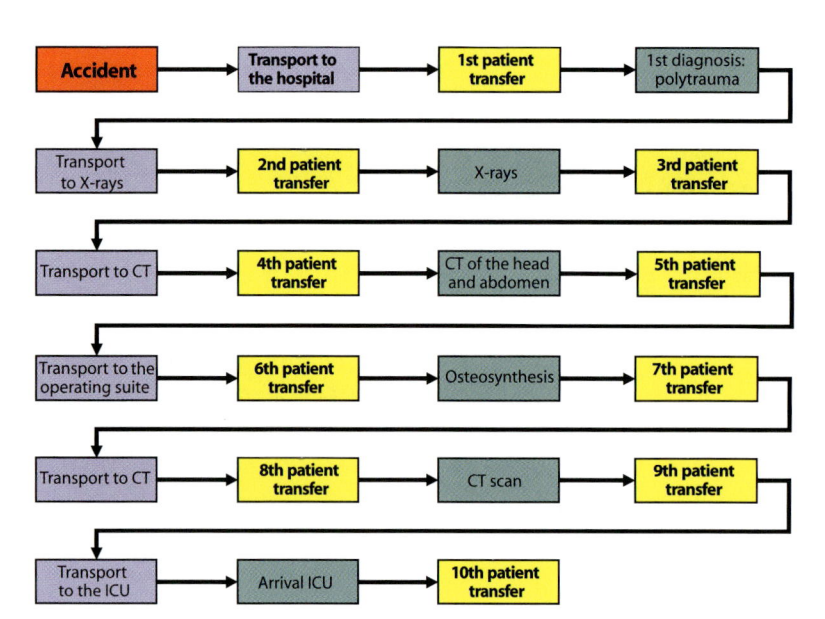

Fig. 6.16. Case study of a trauma patient (conservative). Manual transfer of the patient is necessary up to 10 times (Kantonsspital Basle, CARCAS Group)

first aid and transport, this period is still considerable in view of the subsequent time taken up by diagnostic measures in hospital until an operation can start. Manual patient transfers are still common practice today and take up a great deal of time, which could otherwise go to looking after the patient. Between arrival in the emergency room and the start of surgical procedures, it is not rare for the patient to be repositioned or transferred more than eight to ten times, taking about 10 min every time (Fig. 6.16).

On the one hand, the use of the AWIGS system considerably reduces the physical burden on the operating staff. On the other hand, the time savings are particularly beneficial for patients whose injuries have not been diagnosed yet. If there are only 2 instead of 4 h between accident and operation, the lethality[1] of the polytrauma is reduced by 70%.

In future, therapeutic procedures with AWIGS can be faster, safer and gentler. Diagnosis, operation and control are grouped together in one integrated surgical workstation. The use of CT in traumatology offers a 70% improved therapy decision for the polytrauma. Another advantage of this concept is the drastic reduction in risky repositioning for the patient which always ties up corresponding personnel resources.

The traumatised patient is only transferred twice in the hospital: from the ambulance or helicopter onto a special, radiolucent surface of carbon fibres (CRP), the so-called transfer board which is multifunctional for the system components patient transporter, operating table and computed tomography. The patient now stays on this transfer board from imaging diagnosis and initial care in the shock room through to the operation, until the emergency care is completed and it is time to transfer the patient to a bed in intensive care. The number of manual repositioning tasks or patient transfers for a polytrauma is reduced by up to 80% (Fig. 6.17).

The AWIGS/VIWAS transfer board is placed on the emergency transporter. The various positions include raised back, adjusted height, Trendelenburg adjustment and length adjustment; in addition, the emergency transporter offers optimised radiolucency in the anteroposterior direction (Fig. 6.18).

This means that initial diagnosis of the trauma patient can be carried out on the transporter. To this end, it is equipped with adapters for monitoring and therapy units on lateral rails. The design of the transporter not only allows for use of a C-arm but also for conventional X-rays. The board surface of the patient transporter is radiolucent. X-ray cassettes can be pushed into the guide rails under the board surface.

Trauma concept 1: »one stop shop« – everything in one room

If a CT scan is required for further diagnosis, the patient is brought to a multifunctional room where the CT is installed with the AWIGS duplex column operating table and CT table. The patient transporter is coupled to the AWIGS operating table. The transfer board on the patient transporter is pushed (with the patient on it) onto the operating table. Further transport from the operating table to the CT is automatic with push-button control. A whole-body scan is possible for body heights of up to

---

[1] The lethality rate is the relationship between the number of those who have died due to a specific disease and the number of new cases. (It only makes sense to determine this ratio in cases of acute disease.) Cf. mortality.

6.2 · AWIGS/VIWAS – new systems for image-assisted surgery

Fig. 6.17. Case study of a trauma patient with AWIGS. With AWIGS, manual transfer of the patient is only necessary on arrival and after treatment

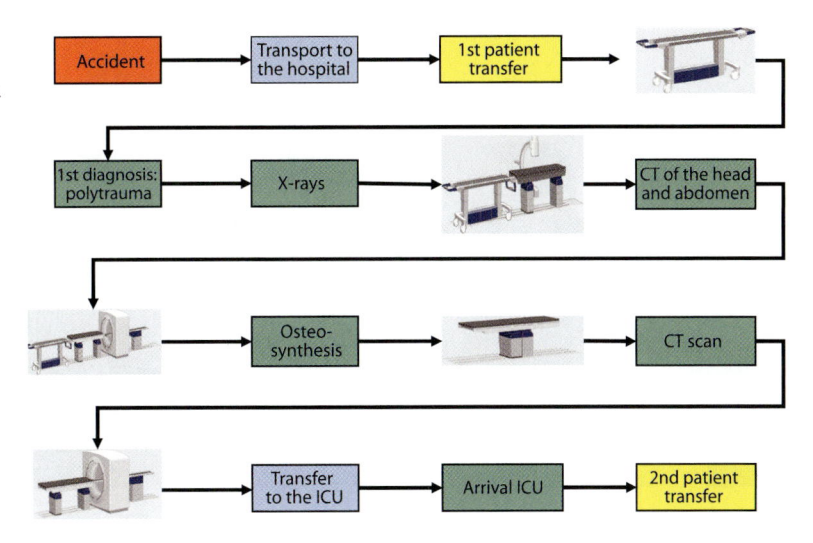

approx. 2.10 m. This concept describes an installation in the Kantonsspital hospital in Basle/Switzerland (Fig. 6.19).

Special attention was given to providing the user interface with an ergonomic design. All functions can be handled by infrared remote control or via a touch screen (Fig. 6.20).

Trauma concept 2: radiology requirements – utilisation of the CT

The version described above is very effective because everything is in one room. It is worth giving a special mention to two facts:
- In this version, the CT is used for traumatology and intraoperative X-ray control during surgery. The CT is therefore not used as much as a conventional CT for standard diagnostic purposes.
- Relatively long rooms are required for the whole system to be docked together in line.

The AWIGS transfer board not only allows for optimum use of the space available, but the AWIGS-CT can also be used for pure diagnosis.

The operating table and scanner unit can be accommodated in two separate rooms. The AWIGS transfer board is in front of the AWIGS CT table, so that it can be docked onto the operating table or a patient transporter can dock onto it in turn. This means that the AWIGS CT can be used for both standard diagnosis and for traumatology without having to transfer the patient.

The AWIGS transfer board swivels manually through +/− 130° and can be lowered to 50 cm. Patients capable of walking can position themselves comfortably for pure diagnosis (Fig. 6.21).

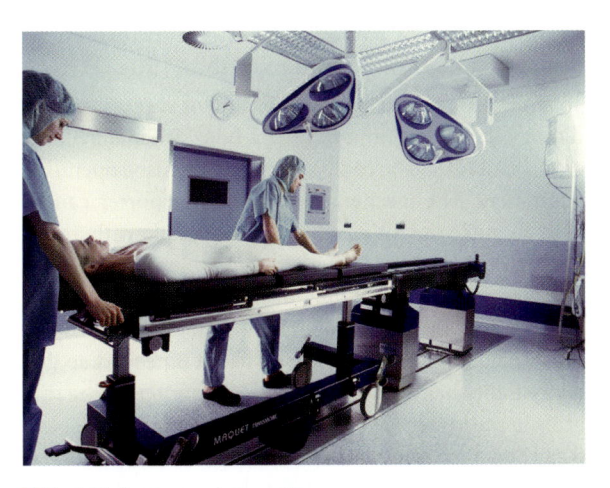

Fig. 6.18. Emergency transporter

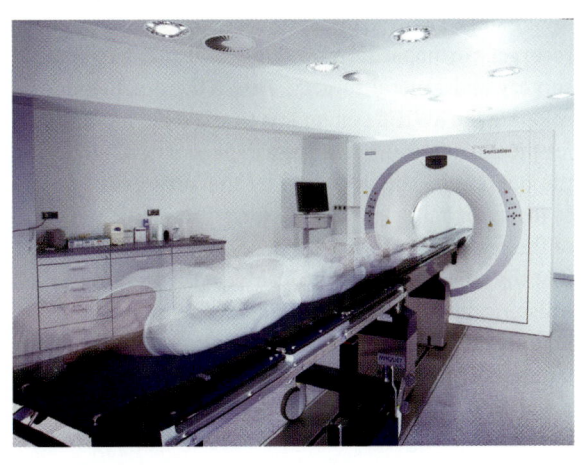

Fig. 6.19. The patient is transferred between the components without any need for manual repositioning

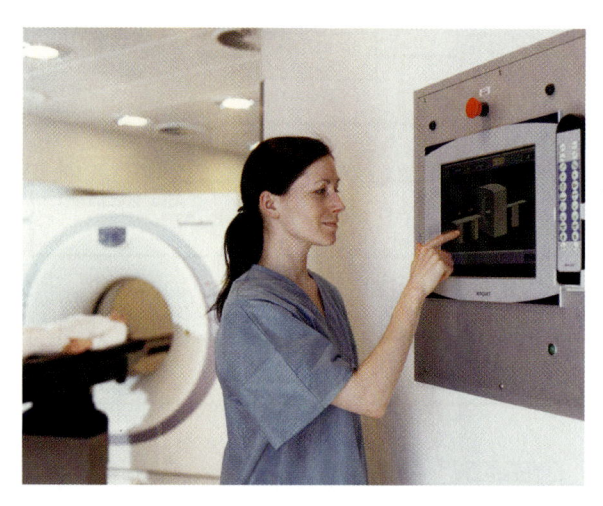

Fig. 6.20. Touch screen and IR remote control

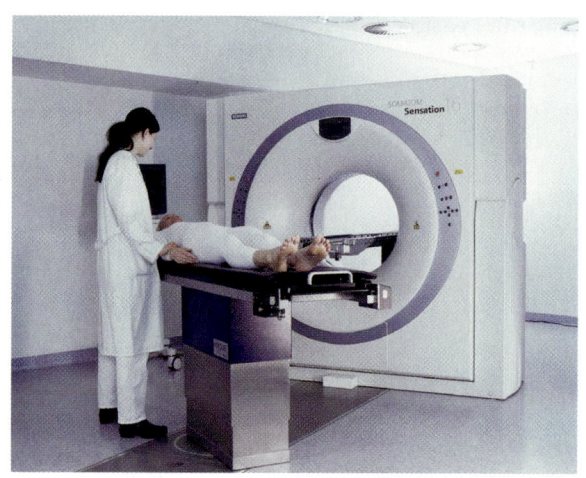

Fig. 6.21. AWIGS transfer table turned

Both cases offer the advantage of being able to do a whole-body scan.

Compatibility of AWIGS with the standard operation column »Alphamaquet 1150«

To allow for interdisciplinary working of surgery and radiology, it is also important for new systems such as AWIGS/VIWAS to be compatible with standard operating equipment. The mechanical patient transporter can be used to make the AWIGS system compatible with an Alphamaquet 1150 standard operating table column. Polytraumas cannot be planned to schedule, and it is always possible that the AWIGS operating suite with the duplex column operating table is in use when it is needed, so that a possibility has been created to use other operating theatres in the same way. The illustrations in Figs. 6.22 and 6.23 show the compatibility and flexibility of both systems without having to transfer the patients.

Elective surgery, illustrated by neurosurgery

When it comes to elective surgery, AWIGS can save life-saving time. The system can be used for example for neurosurgery, orthopaedic procedures, oral and maxillofacial surgery and general surgery. The basic idea behind developing the AWIGS system was to avoid having to transfer the patient to the radiology department at all during the operation. This is joined by the surgeons' demand to make digital data available for an immediate control of the results of the operation, so that they can be sure that the operation was a positive success already on finishing the procedure. Intraoperative use of a CT in neurosurgery is one possible example here: at the moment, a tumour is removed on the basis of CT data taken a few days before and after the operation. But not even the most experienced surgeon can see from these data whether the tumour has shifted during the operation as a result of the situation.

The patient is operated on the AWIGS operating table. If an intraoperative CT scan is required, the patient can be moved straight into the CT gantry on the same board without having to be transferred (Fig. 6.24). If necessary, the operation can be continued immediately, depending on the results.

The advantages offered by this new link between surgery and radiology include:
— high-precision operating procedures because the results are controlled directly,
— the possibility of avoiding secondary operations,
— effective use for neuronavigation.

Another advantage of using the AWIGS system in neurosurgery comes from the radiolucent head plate units. The patient's head can be adjusted to the ideal position for the operation. To take a CT scan during the operation, the pa-

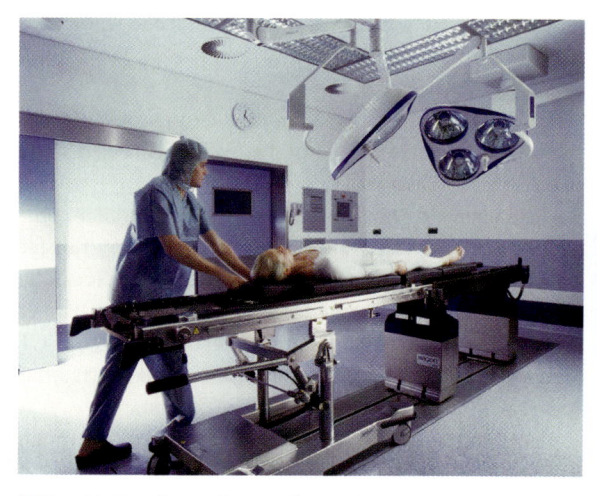

Fig. 6.22. Transferring the transfer board with patient onto the AWIGS operating table

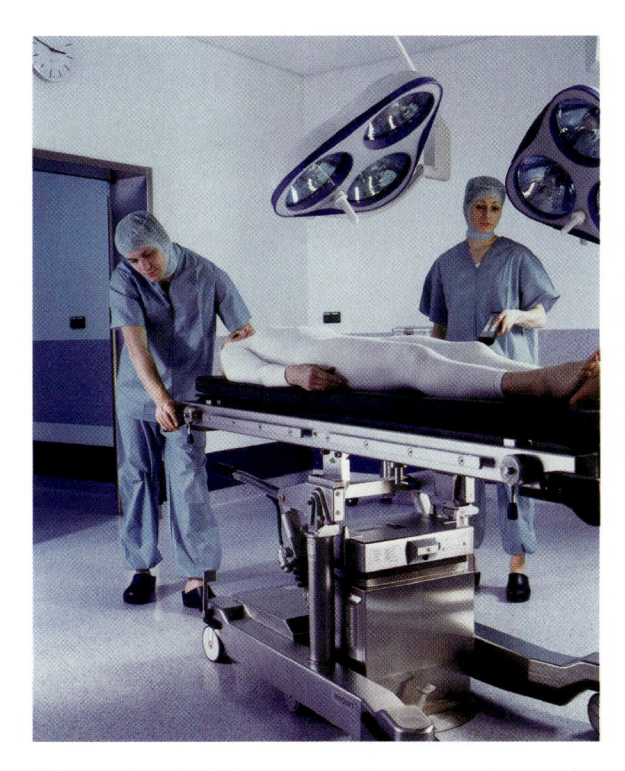

Fig. 6.23. Transferring the complete table top with patient onto the operating table column

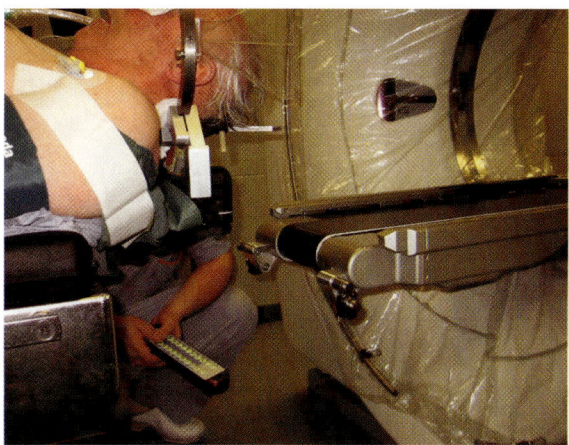

Fig. 6.24. Docking procedure with stereotactic frame of operating table and CT table

tient remains on the head plate without having to be re-bedded. All head plates developed for the AWIGS and VIWAS system are radiolucent. This means that CT scans, C-arm scans and angiograms can be carried out without any interfering artefacts. All head plates are adapted directly to the transfer board, so that the patient does not lose his position between the head plate and the table top.

Practical application in Innsbruck clinic – 18 months of clinical experience

»The system was used from January 2002 to the end of June 2003 for 1058 patients. The CT was used intraoperatively in 15% of the cases. Stereotactic procedures (biopsies, deep brain stimulation, abscess drainage, radiosurgery) were the main areas of application. Here the AWIGS system allows for intraoperative acquisition of top quality CT scans, with the following positive effects on neurosurgery:

- The operating time for stereotactic procedures can be reduced because it is no longer necessary to re-bed the patient.
- Intraoperative imaging with identification of residual tumours and at-risk structures. Here intraoperative use of the CT takes less than 20 min« [1].

6.2.4 VIWAS

VIWAS (Vascular Interventional Workplace for Advanced Surgery), brother to the AWIGS system, was specially developed for interventional radiology, vascular surgery and cardiosurgery. The system makes it possible to use imaging procedures such as C-arm or angiography system directly at the operating table without having to interrupt the procedure to change the positioning of the patient.

6.2.4.1 VIWAS in combination with an angiography system

Special functions for the VIWAS system such as longitudinal and transverse displacement offer optimum possibilities for positioning the scanning units.

As with the AWIGS system, the patient is placed on the radiolucent transfer board, which is compatible with the transporter and with the operating table. The transfer functions between transporter and operating table are the same as for the AWIGS.

The VIWAS system avoids the problems encountered with previous operating tables in the intraoperative use of scanning units. This is thanks to two columns which carry the table top. Both columns can be moved under the table top independent of each other, leaving generous scope for using the C-arm. The scanning unit can be placed once between the columns. Instead of the arduous procedure of manoeuvring the C-arm, the patient is »floated« on the table top to the scanning unit by a joystick with longitudinal and transverse movements, as on an angiography table. The completely radiolucent one-section table top offers artefact-free scanning through 360° specially for intraoperative scanning of aortic aneurysms.

The table top moves longitudinally on a linear guide system; transverse movements of up to 10 cm are possible

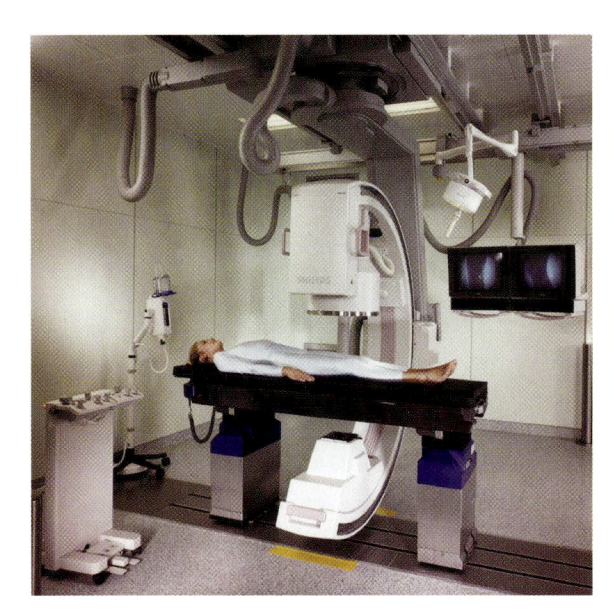

Fig. 6.25. Single-section table top VIWAS with angiography system

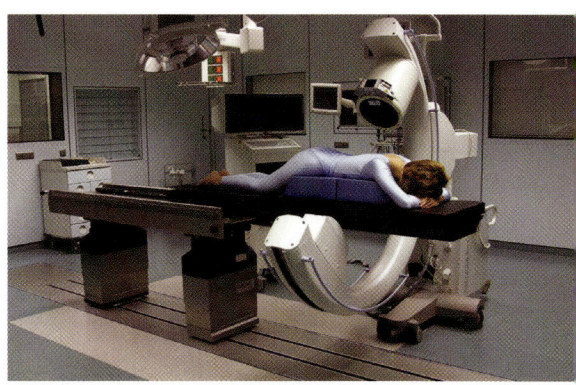

Fig. 6.26. Special table top for sliding gantry or C-arm

to both sides. Individual rails can be fitted to the frame of the table top to take accessories (Fig. 6.25).

6.2.4.2 VIWAS in combination with a sliding gantry

The VIWAS can be extended in combination with a mobile CT unit, a so-called sliding gantry. Here the transfer board is pulled out to a scan length of 1.50 m for intraoperative scanning, and the CT unit moves to the patient accordingly. Subsequently the operation can be continued on a specially developed one-section table top. This brand new product was presented for the first time at the Medica 2002.

Both systems work without mutual monitoring. The patient is held manually at the scanning position under the fresh air panel. After the interlocking device of the table top has been released, the operating table columns are moved away from under the patient by the sliding gantry. The patient board is now available in a length of 1.50 m for scanning under the laminar flow. To take the pictures, the sliding gantry moves across the patient on the extended transfer board.

In addition, the special board can also be used for procedures with a C-arm or angiography system (Fig. 6.26).

6.2.5 Prospects

The compatibility of the AWIGS and VIWAS systems with a standard Alphamaquet operating column makes them suitable for a wide range of surgical applications. Depending on the type of operation and the surgeon's requirements in terms of positioning the patient, the table top can be chosen before the operation: the one-section or three-section table top or the special table top for a sliding gantry and the one-section table top for a standard Alphamaquet column 1150.

Intraoperative updates of the image data and the possibility of producing a new set of primary data offer both the surgeon and the patient an enhanced quality of care, together with a reduction in patient transfers and the integration of improved workflows.

References

1. Fiegele T et al. (2003) Abstracts zum Vortrag der 39. Jahres-tagung der Österreichischen Gesellschaft für Neurochirurgie, 03.–04. 10. 2003, Klagenfurt
2. Ruchholtz S (2000) Das Traumaregister der DGU als Grundlage des interklinischen Qualitätsmanagements in der Schwerverletztenversorgung. Unfallchirurg 103: 30–37

7 Technical equipment

H. Colberg, D. Aschemann, B. Kulik, C. Rösinger

7.1 Operating table – 68
7.1.1 Introduction – 68
7.1.2 Historical development – 68
7.1.3 Classification criteria according to technical design – 73
7.1.3.1 Operating table systems – 73
7.1.3.2 Mobile operating tables – 75
7.1.4 Classification criteria according to purpose – 78
7.1.5 Classification criteria according to the school of surgery – 78
7.1.6 Production, production control and safety – 78

7.2 Positioning accessories and aids – 79
7.2.1 Pads – 79
7.2.1.1 Pads with viscoelastic foam core – 79
7.2.1.2 Gel pads – 81
7.2.2 Operating table accessories – 82
7.2.3 Extension table accessories – 86
7.2.4 Special devices – 88
7.2.5 Vacuum mats – 88
7.2.6 Patient warming system – 90

7.1 Operating table

H. Colberg, D. Aschemann

7.1.1 Introduction

The centrepiece of every operating theatre is the operating table. The operating table or the position in which it is erected is the basis for arranging all other high-tech devices, such as ceiling mounts for anaesthesia systems and surgery, operating lights, possibly ceiling-mounted X-ray image intensifiers or surgical microscopes, together with air-conditioning ceilings and panels.

What exactly is an operating table? An attempt to explain this with the help of a dictionary is sure to fail: operating table cannot be found in most dictionaries, although it is the central element of an operating theatre. The patient is positioned (in an anatomically correct fashion) for his operation on this »table«. In other words, an operating table has to satisfy the needs of the surgeon, the anaesthetist and the patient. These needs are essentially those shown in ◘ Table 7.1 (▶ see also Fig. 7.1):

In time, various special surgical disciplines have developed from so-called »general surgery«, so that special operating tables have been designed and produced to suit these requirements.

7.1.2 Historical development

The days in which surgeons operated on their patients while they lay in their hospital bed go back more than 160 years. Initially it was sure to be just the low bed height and instable positioning of the patient which surgeons objected to back then (◘ Fig. 7.2).

Remedies were found, resulting in the first »operating furniture«, which already took account of the salient anatomic points of the human body – the hips and the knees. There were far more operating tables throughout the years of development than just those shown here.

The development from »operating furniture« via operating table to operating table system consisted of the following stages:

◘ Figure 7.3 shows an early operating table made of wood, in part with artistically designed details, which only played a visual role, for example turned legs.

◘ Figure 7.4 features a mobile operating table on small castors with a metal structure. The device for Trendelenburg and reverse Trendelenburg adjustment would become standard in the next generation of operating tables.

The operating table according to Hahn with metal structure (narrow operating table foot), which included the device for Trendelenburg and reverse Trendelenburg adjustment, introduced the possibility of adjusting the height (◘ Fig. 7.5).

Further development of operating techniques made procedures more specific and extensive, with far greater requirements for adjusting the operating table and the patient's positioning. The operating table »Heidelberger 3000« with multi-section patient board, hydraulic height adjustment, Trendelenburg and reverse Trendelenburg adjustment already fulfilled many of these requirements (◘ Fig. 7.6).

The demand for better hygiene at the operating table resulted in all hand wheels for intraoperative adjustments being moved to the head end, so that the actual operating

◘ **Table 7.1.** Properties and requirements of an operating table

Height adjustment	to adapt to the surgeon's height to allow for ergonomic working
Slanting (Trendelenburg/reverse Trendelenburg)	to allow for immediate measures during crash/ileus intubation, risk of shock or embolism, and to control such measures during conduction anaesthesia
Tilting right/left	to give a better insight into the body cavity and for organ positioning during minimally invasive procedures
Adjusting the individual segments of the patient board	to allow for the body to be bent in the anatomically correct positions and to position the extremities as required for the operation, e.g. bending, spreading, etc.
Radiolucent patient board	to work with the X-ray image intensifier without any problems
SFC padding, soft and radiolucent (special foam core)	to avoid damage from pressure sores
Mobility	to bring the patient from the hospital bed or patient transfer board to the anaesthetic preparation room and operating theatre without having to transfer the patient

7.1 · Operating table

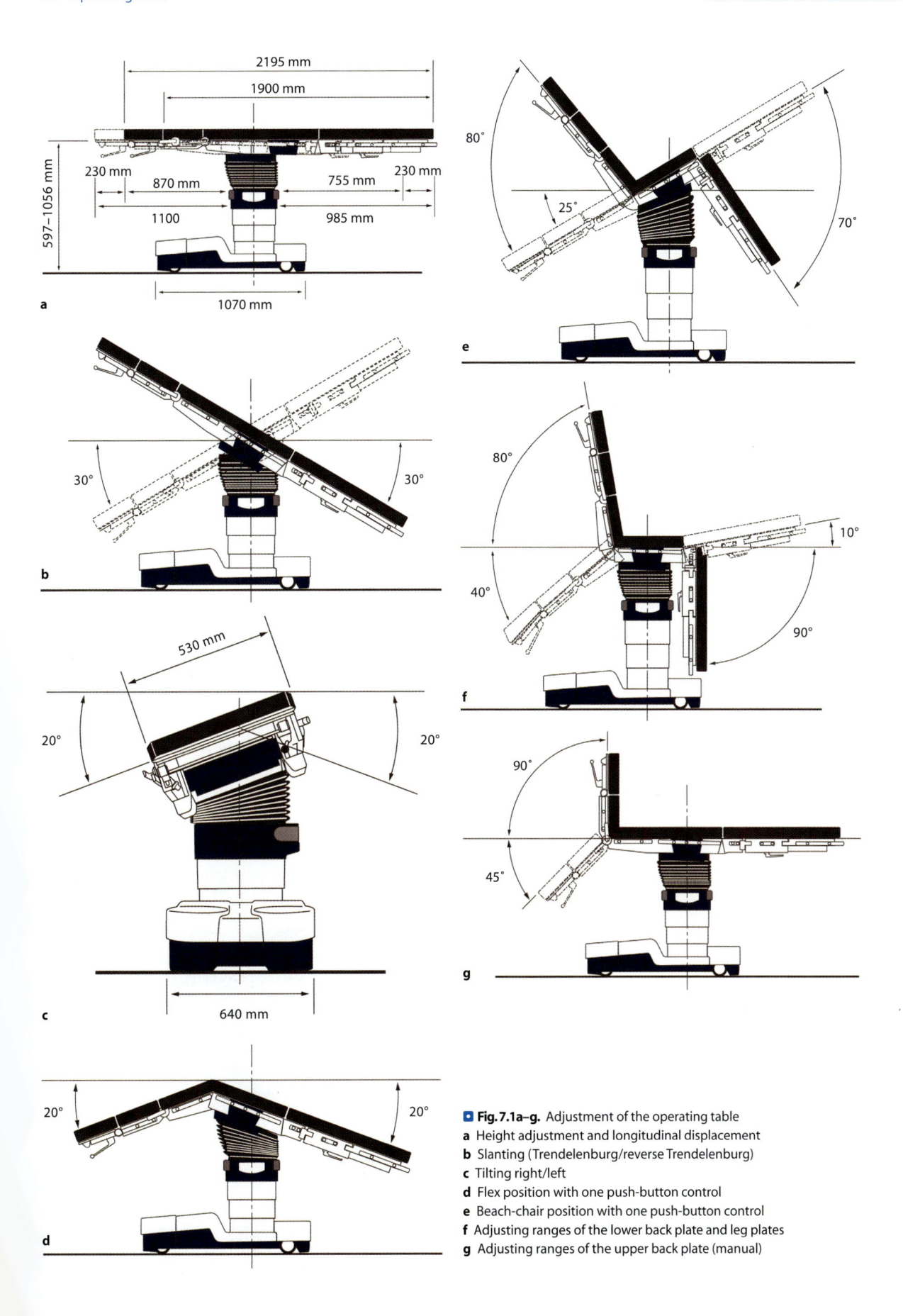

Fig. 7.1a–g. Adjustment of the operating table
a Height adjustment and longitudinal displacement
b Slanting (Trendelenburg/reverse Trendelenburg)
c Tilting right/left
d Flex position with one push-button control
e Beach-chair position with one push-button control
f Adjusting ranges of the lower back plate and leg plates
g Adjusting ranges of the upper back plate (manual)

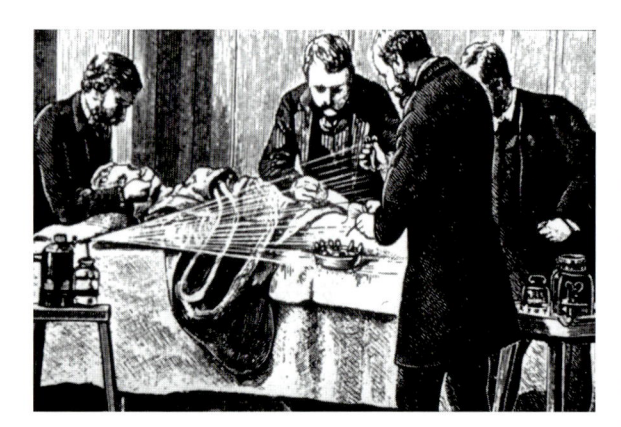

Fig. 7.2. Operation with Lister carbolic acid mist

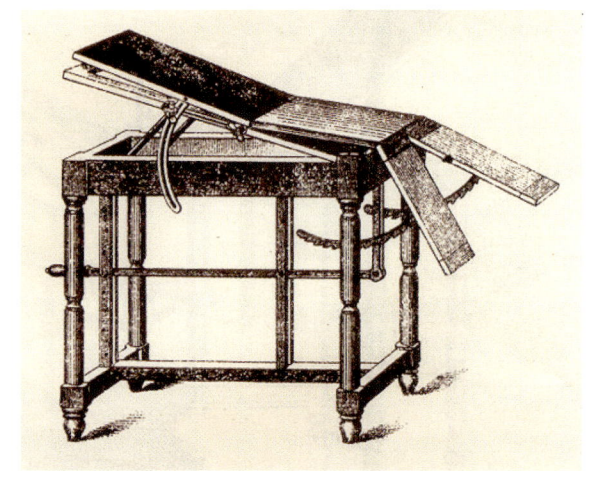

Fig. 7.3. Operating table made of wood, around 1840

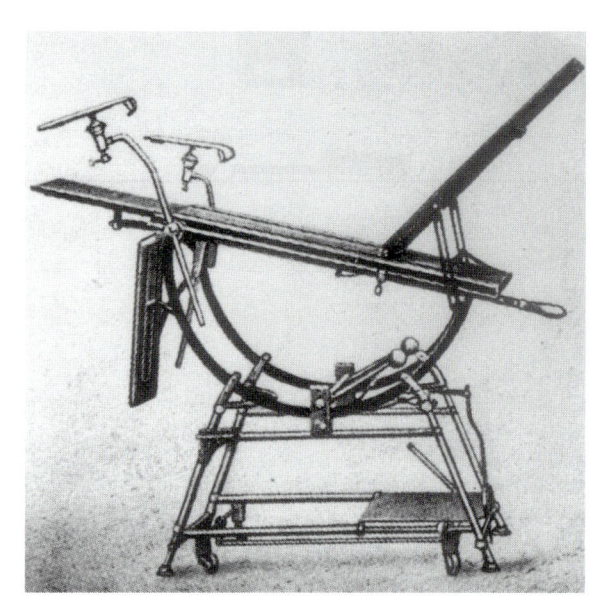

Fig. 7.4. Operating table according to Stelzner, around 1890

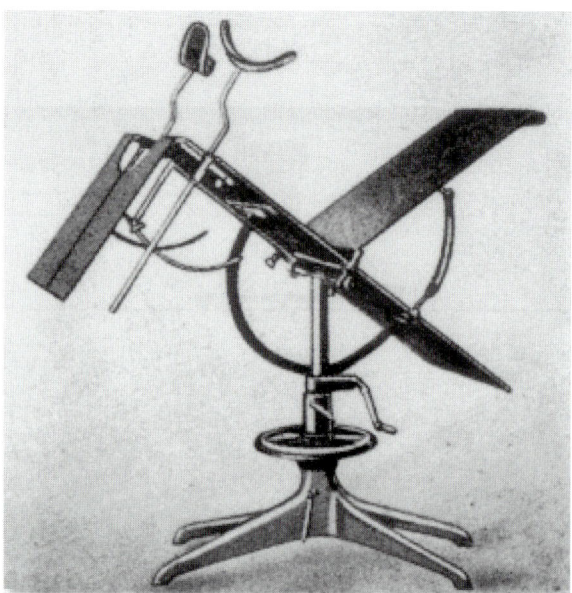

Fig. 7.5. Operating table according to Hahn, around 1910

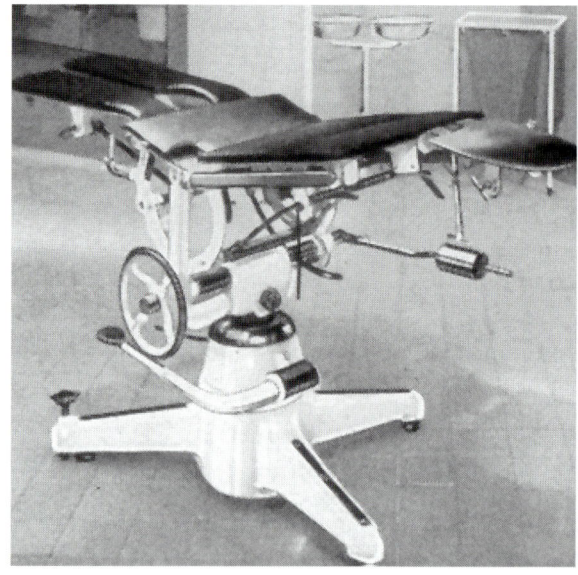

Fig. 7.6. Operating table »Heidelberger 3000«, around 1930

region remained sterile throughout. As a universal operating table, the »large Heidelberger« fulfilled all the demands made of an operating table for general surgery. It was divided into an upper and lower back plate, seat plate, body bridge, divided leg plates (4-section leg plates as an option) and hydraulic height adjustment so that it was possible to adjust the ideal position for the patient in the operation (Fig. 7.7).

Meanwhile, development of X-ray image intensifiers began. The prerequisite for intraoperative scanning is that in contrast to previous X-ray systems, the operating table

7.1 · Operating table

Fig. 7.7. Operating table »Large Heidelberger 1111« around 1960

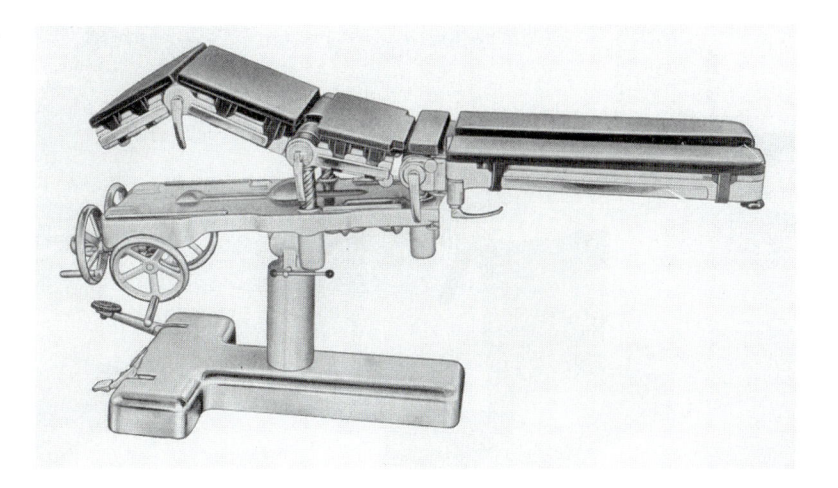

surface has to be radiolucent for X-rays. Up to then, X-ray film cassettes were simply pushed under the patient or the padding surface and exposed from above. Now the demand was to be able to scan through the patient and operating table surface, to see the results of this scan immediately.

The world's first operating table system, *the new Maquet 1120*, was presented at the surgeon's congress in Munich (Fig. 7.8). This operating table system, consisting of stationary operating table columns, removable patient board and transporter, revolutionised functional workflows in the operating suite, at least in Germany and Europe. This was the start of the circulation concept. It was easier to move the patient board with the transporter than the old, heavy mobile operating tables on small castors. The hygienic properties of this operating table system are still valid. In some cases, the »1120« is still fully functional and in use.

The »Heidelberger 1130« (Fig. 7.9) is an electrohydraulic operating table with battery operation. The patient board is divided into 8 sections and is radiolucent to X-rays. The upper back is moved by motors.

The electrohydraulic drive had proven effective for many years and was also successful with the Betastar 1131 (Fig. 7.10). The patient board is divided into 4/7 sections and is radiolucent to X-rays. The patient board can be displaced longitudinally by hand and is equipped with a hydraulic back plate as an option.

The operating table system Betamaquet 1140 is an electrohydraulic operating table system with stationary and, alternatively, mobile operating table columns together with nine different patient boards with manual adjustment (Fig. 7.11).

The Alphamaquet 1150 is an electromechanical operating table system with stationary and, alternatively, mobile operating table columns together with 12 different patient boards with microprocessor drives (Fig. 7.12).

An *extension table* had to be developed to treat fractures of long, tubular bones and for fractures to the neck of the femur. The operating table should make it possible to extend and reset the fractured extremity under X-ray control for it then to be stabilised for example with an intramedullary nail. It should also be possible to position patients for shoulder operations on a special back plate. These requirements are fulfilled by the special operating

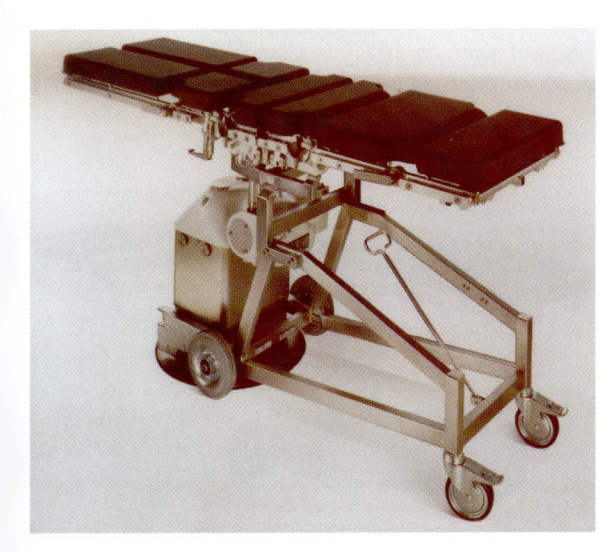

Fig. 7.8. Operating table system Maquet 1120 from 1964

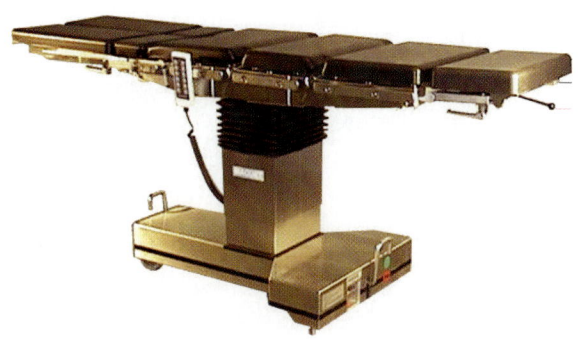

Fig. 7.9. Mobile universal operating table »Heidelberger 1130« from 1984–2003

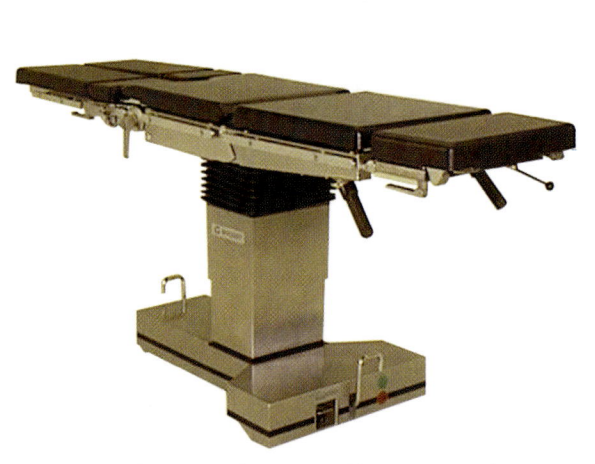

Fig. 7.10. Mobile universal operating table Betastar 1130 from 1990–2000

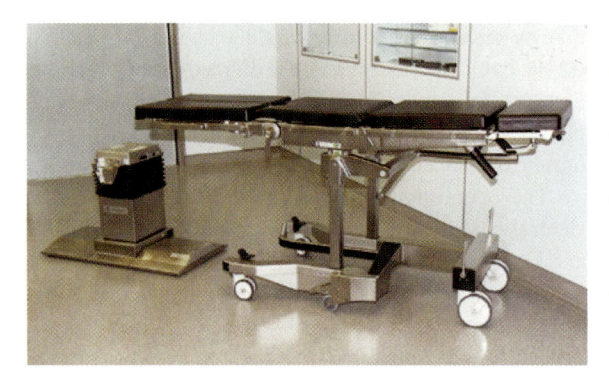

Fig. 7.11. Operating table system Betamaquet 1140 from 1994

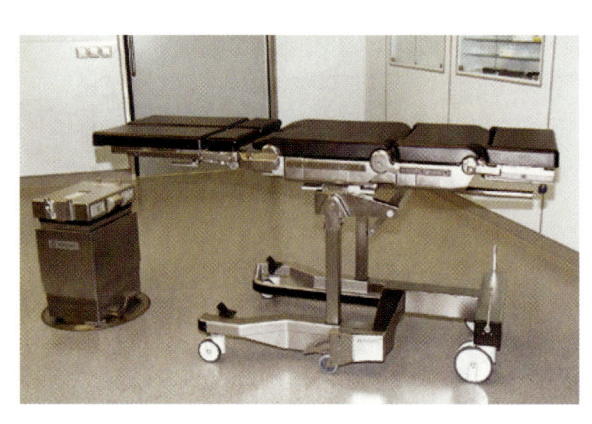

Fig. 7.12. Operating table system Alphamaquet 1150 from 1995

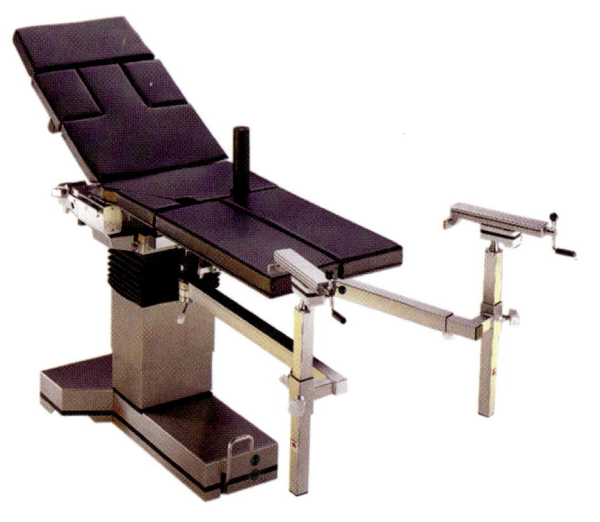

Fig. 7.13. Mobile special operating table Orthostar 1425 from 1997

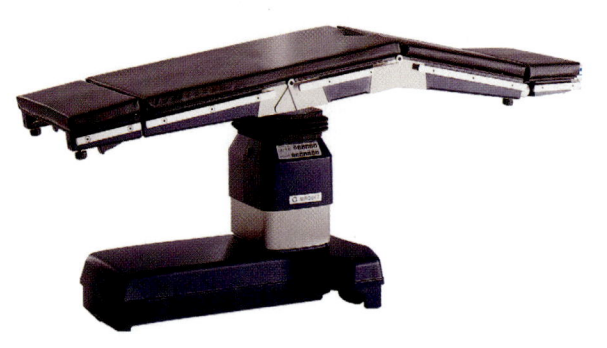

Fig. 7.14. Mobile universal operating table Alphastar 1132.01/02/03 from 1997–2003

table Orthostar 1425 (Fig. 7.13, not illustrated: Orthostar 1420 from 1985–1997).

The Alphastar series has an electrohydraulic drive for all movements (Figs. 7.14, 7.15). Since 2002, the patient board has a 3-section structure with short reverse back, seat and leg plate. The short reverse back plate can be used for fitting other modules, such as a shoulder plate. A headrest can be fitted on as an additional element, together with extension segments. Patients are placed on the patient board in *normal* or *reverse* position. The following versions are currently available: 1132.11, 1132.12 low version and 1132.13 plus. The plus version can take patients with a body weight of up to 450 kg. From 1997, for the first time these versions were offered with an optional electric travel drive.

The Classic series was launched in 1998 with the Betaclassic 1118.01, and the Alphaclassic 1118.02 was added in 1999. The Betaclassic is adjusted just manually and with pedals. In 2003, the handling concept for the Alphaclassic was revised, resulting in the 1118.03 (Fig. 7.16), with electrohydraulic adjustments in the column. The patient board is adjusted manually and the back and leg plates are supported by pneumatic springs. The series is extended by various versions with body bridge or longitudinal displacement.

The Alphamaxx combines the advantages of the modular patient board Alphamaquet 1150.30 and the load rating of Alphastar 1132 plus. All movements of the Alphamaxx are adjusted by electrohydraulic means (▶ see Fig.

7.1 · Operating table

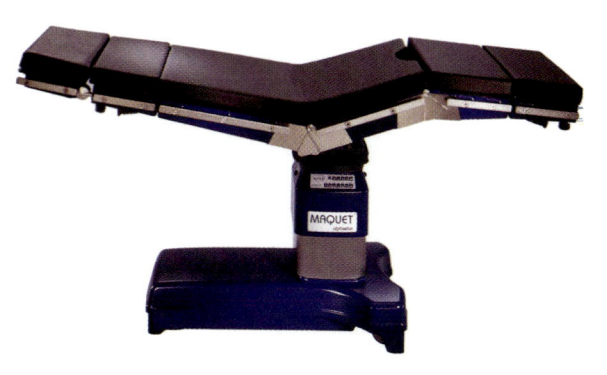

Fig. 7.15. Mobile universal operating table Alphastar 1132.11/12/13 from 2002

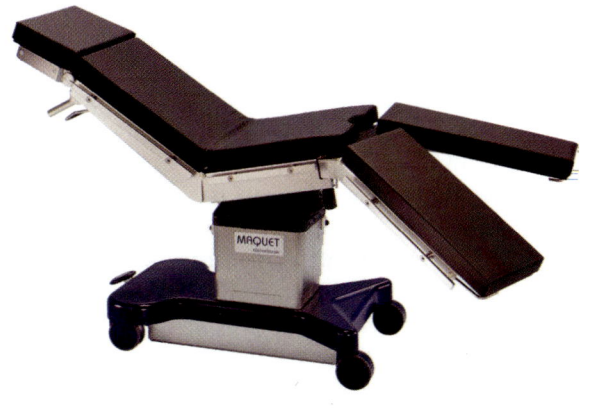

Fig. 7.16. Universal operating table Alphaclassic 1118.03 from 2003

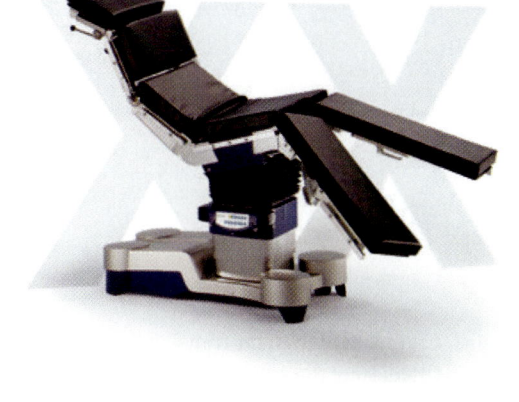

Fig. 7.17. Mobile universal operating table Alphamaxx 1133 from 2001

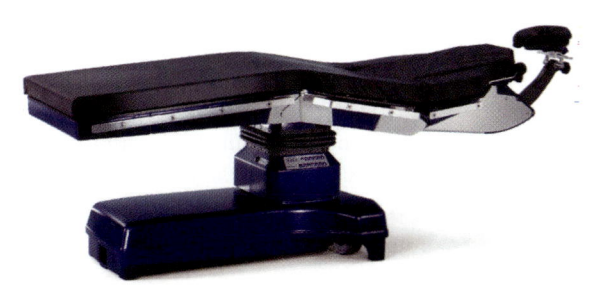

Fig. 7.18. Mobile special operating table Alphastar top 1132.17 from 2003

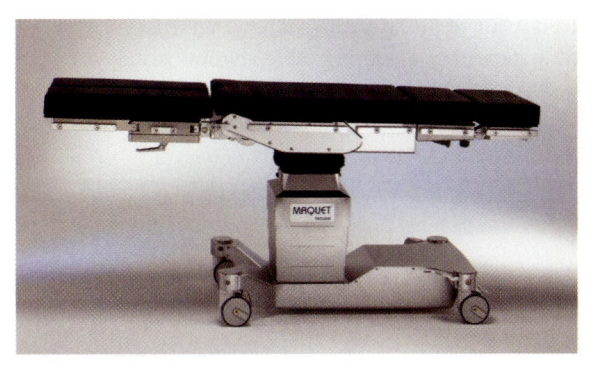

Fig. 7.19. Mobile universal operating table Betastar 1131.12 from 2004

7.1a–g). The patient board also has longitudinal displacement and divided, separately adjustable leg plates. The Alphamaxx can take patients with a body weight of up to 450 kg (Fig. 7.17).

The mobile special operating table Alphastar top 1132.17 with travel drive is moved electrohydraulically in all directions. The patient board is in 4 sections with headrest, longitudinally adjustable back plate, seat and leg plates. The head is adjusted by an »anatomy arm« which moves the cervical spine in anatomically correct positions without stretching and compression, in every phase of the treatment (Fig. 7.18).

The mobile universal operating table Betastar 1131.12 has an electrohydraulic drive for all movements. It is equipped with a new patient board geometry. The new interface is compatible with modules from the Alphamaxx and Alphastar series (Fig. 7.19).

New operating procedures and requirements for patient positioning will continue to make new demands of operating tables in future. Mobile operating tables and operating table systems will have to be developed further in order to satisfy the expectations and demands of operating teams and patients.

Operating tables are always classified as shown in Table 7.2.

7.1.3 Classification criteria according to technical design

7.1.3.1 Operating table systems

Back in the early 1960s, developments in surgery, anaesthesia and new hygiene know-how demanded new concepts for the operating suite. Hospital beds and nursing staff from the wards were not allowed into the aseptic area as germ carriers. The »bed transfer« room was created which was divided into *clean* and *unclean* to prevent the entrainment of germs (Fig. 7.20).

Table 7.2. Classification criteria for operating tables		
Technical design	Purpose	School of surgery
Operating table systems	Universal operating tables	»German«
Mobile operating tables	Special operating tables	»Anglo-American«
		»French«

Transfer rooms with patient transfer sluices were invented and fitted. Here the patient was handed over to the operating staff in the aseptic part of the operating suite, thus essentially preventing the entrainment of germs.

In addition, patient anaesthetising and post-anaesthesia recovery rooms were planned and furnished, together with scrub rooms for the operating staff, each allocated to a specific operating theatre.

New demands were also made of the operating table, covering the following points in particular:
- **Small castors:** they make it difficult for staff to move the table and often damage the floor covering, thanks to the weight of the table which can frequently reach 300 kg
- **The patient board surface:** it should be radiolucent across the whole surface to allow for unhindered intraoperative X-ray scans.

All these requirements were fulfilled in 1964 with the introduction of the operating table system 1120. It consisted of a stationary operating table column installed in the operating theatre which turned through nearly 360°C, had two removable radiolucent patient boards and two motorised joints (back and leg plates), together with two transporters for the patient boards.
- **Less weight:** the heaviest components of the operating table, the foot and column, no longer have to be moved when the patient is being transported. The foot is omitted completely, and the column is installed in a stationary position in the operating theatre.
- **No small castors:** the transporter has large, wide castors which run easily and protect the floor covering.
- **No interfering foot:** the stationary, slim-line operating column turns through nearly 360° and offers ideal free foot space.
- **Radiolucent patient board:** thanks to the use of radiolucent materials.

The invention of the operating table system not only remedied the prevailing disadvantages but also invented the *circulation concept*:

In the patient transfer room or sluice, the patient is transferred to the operation patient board with transporter and brought into the preparation room where the anaesthetic is induced.

Three different transporters are available:
- Rigid transporter
- Transporter with adjustable slant (Trendelenburg/reverse Trendelenburg adjustment),
- Transporter with adjustable slant and height.

> Remarks: experience recommends for example that for an expected emergency/ileus intubation, there should always be a transporter with integrated one-hand fast adjustment for Trendelenburg/reverse Trendelenburg adjustment under the patient board!

When using modern operating table systems, the procedure for positioning the patient can begin in the preparation room. The patient is then brought into the operating theatre with the easily rolling transporter and positioned over the stationary operating table column. The operating table column is raised to accept the operating patient board with the patient on it. The transporter is removed and the procedure for positioning the patient can be concluded with specific details.

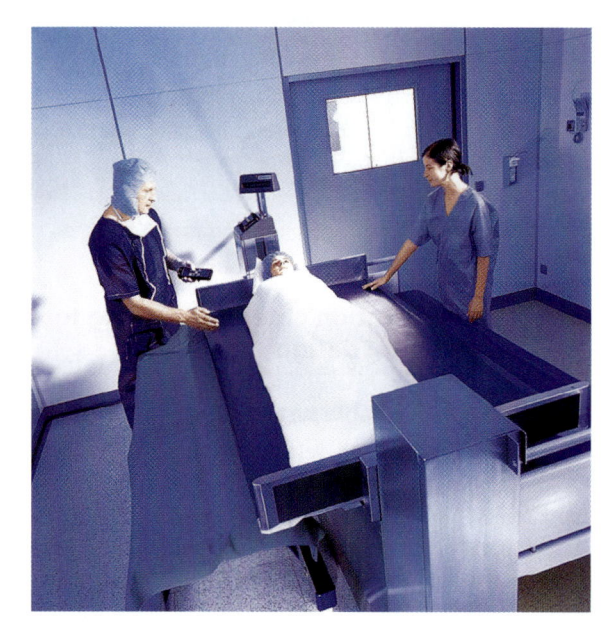

Fig. 7.20. Transfer room with patient transfer sluice Transmaquet

7.1 · Operating table

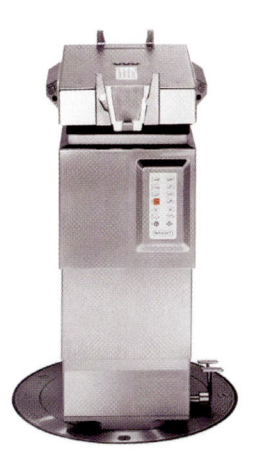

Fig. 7.21. Stationary operating table column

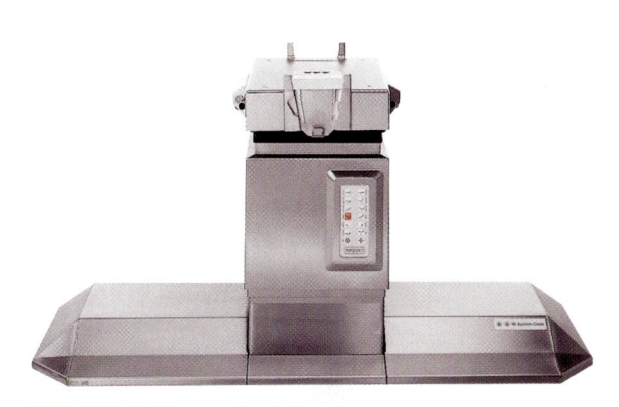

Fig. 7.22. Mobile operating table column

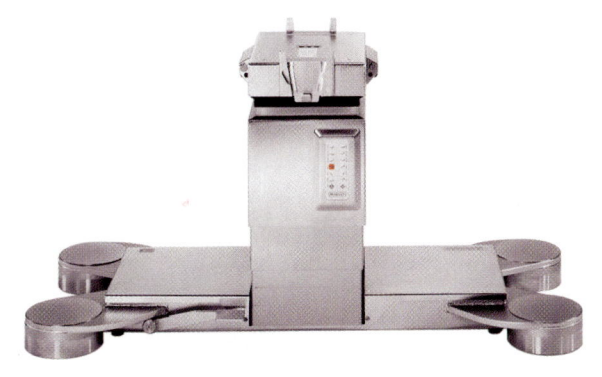

Fig. 7.23. Rolling operating table column

To provide more flexibility and varied use, 3 different operating table columns are in use worldwide with an integrated »override panel«:
- the **stationary** operating table column (Fig. 7.21),
- the **mobile** operating table column (Fig. 7.22) and
- the **rolling** operating table column (Fig. 7.23).

Every operating table system has two patient boards and two transporters, so that this kind of *circulation concept* (Fig. 7.24) reduces waiting times between operations. Some hospitals work safely, successfully and efficiently with 3 patient boards and 3 transporters per operating table column.

The patient boards have been specially developed for effective use in modern operating theatres. They can be brought to the operating table column by the transporter from both head ends.

This means for example that the Alphamaquet operating table system has 12 universal and special operation patient boards (Fig. 7.25).

The decontamination system Cleanmaquet reliably cleans and disinfects the patient boards, transporters and accessories which are washable as a standard feature (Fig. 7.26).

7.1.3.2 Mobile operating tables

Generally it can be said that mobile operating tables consist of 3 main elements:

Base	Consisting of a *robust foot with castors*
Operating table column	With additional tilting and slanting function
Patient board	Generally with various divisions and adjustments

Adjustments are made:
- manually and with pedals or
- by electrohydraulic means, battery driven or
- by electromechanical means, also battery driven

The movements of the electric operating tables and the operating table systems are transmitted by a cable or cordless infrared remote control. Other control elements include a wall control panel and foot switch; a voice-controlled system is also available to the surgeon. This means that generally the adjustments are performed outside the sterile operating area without affecting the operating team at all and preserving sterility.

Today, mobile operating tables also have a kind of »emergency control«, the so-called »override panel« integrated in the operating table column (Fig. 7.27).

The optional travel drive allows for the circulation concept at mobile operating tables (Fig. 7.28). The large wheel diameter no longer causes any damage to the floor covering and some models are even capable of taking patient weights of up to max. 450 kg. But machine washing is not permitted.

Chapter 7 · Technical equipment

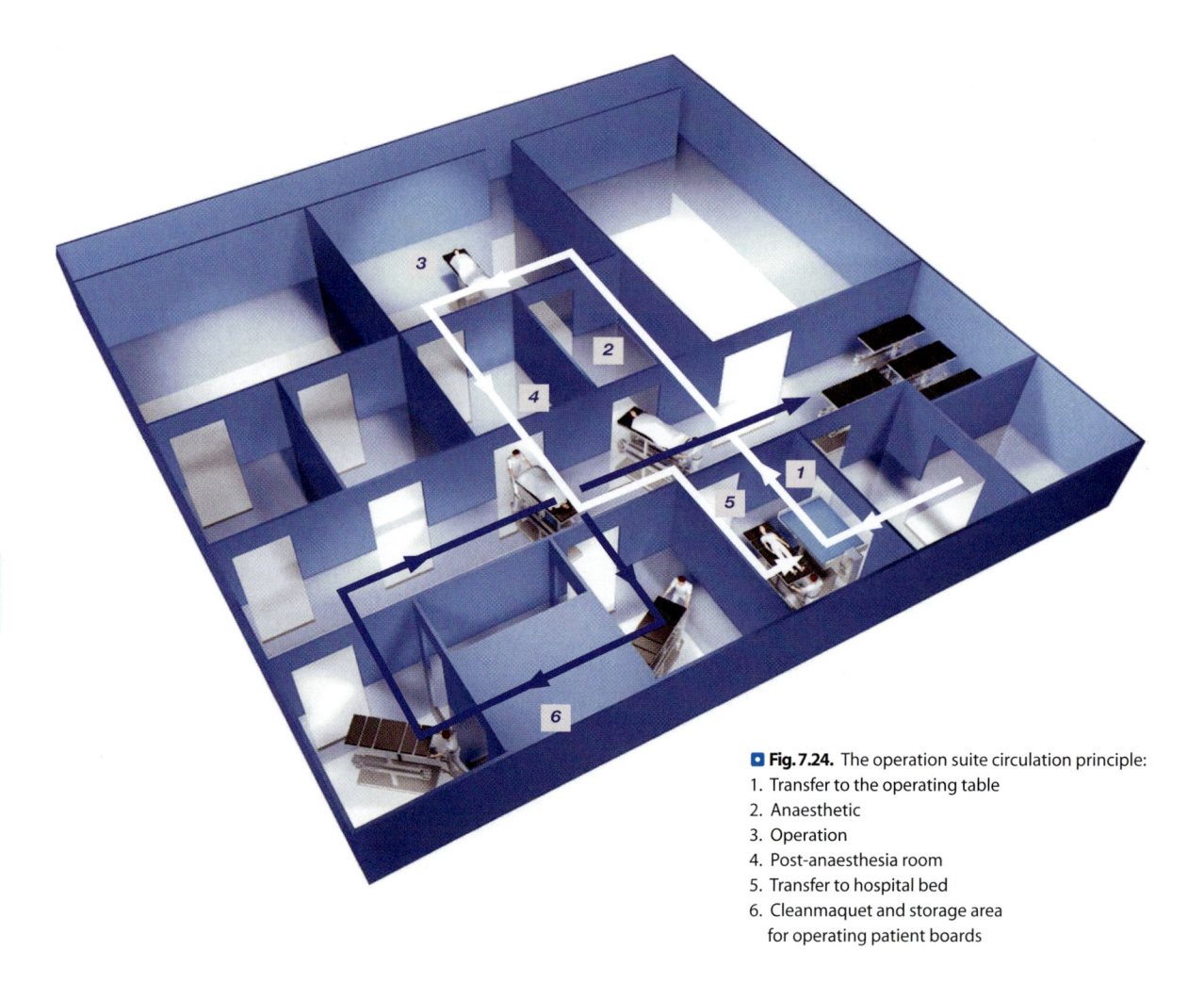

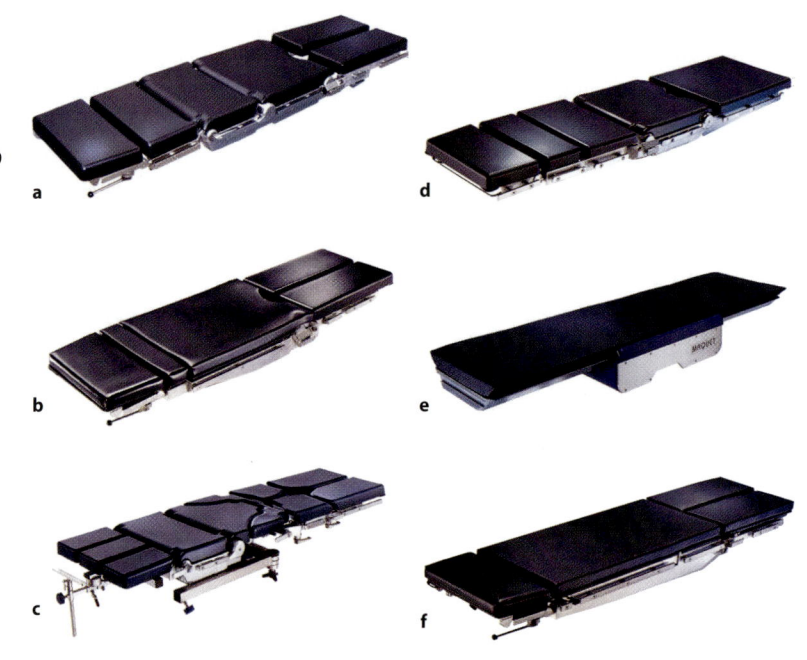

Fig. 7.24. The operation suite circulation principle:
1. Transfer to the operating table
2. Anaesthetic
3. Operation
4. Post-anaesthesia room
5. Transfer to hospital bed
6. Cleanmaquet and storage area for operating patient boards

Fig. 7.25a–f. A selection of universal and special operating patient boards Alphamaquet 1150/1140 from 1994/95
 a Modular universal operating patient board 1150.30
 b Universal operating patient board 1150.19
 c Modular universal operating patient board 1150.20 for orthopaedics and traumatology
 d Operating patient board 1150.25 for operations to the head
 e Operating patient board 1150.16 for vascular surgery, interventional radiology, orthopaedics and traumatology
 f Operating patient board 1150.23 for urology, orthopaedics and vascular surgery

7.1 · Operating table

Fig. 7.25g–j. A selection of universal and special operating patient boards Alphamaquet 1150/1140 from 1994/95
g   Operating patient board 1150.22 for general surgery and minimally invasive surgery
h   Operating patient board 1150.15 for orthopaedics, vascular surgery and traumatology
i   Operating patient board 1140.14 for paediatric surgery
j   Operating patient board 1140.17 for ophthalmology

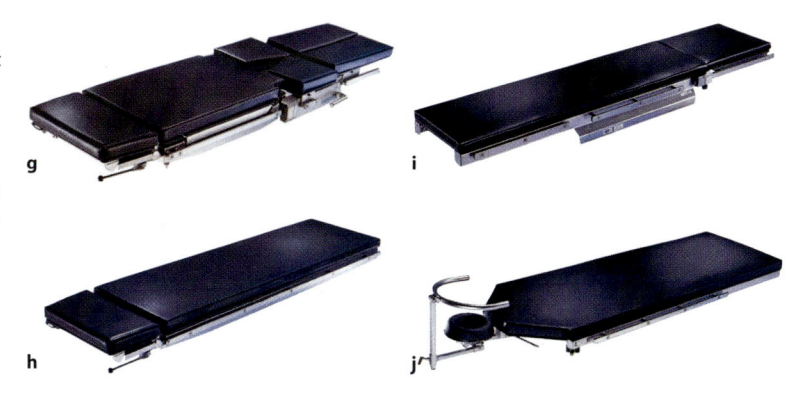

Fig. 7.26. Highest possible hygiene standard thanks to machine cleaning with Cleanmaquet

Standard program operating patient boards
End/start of cycle

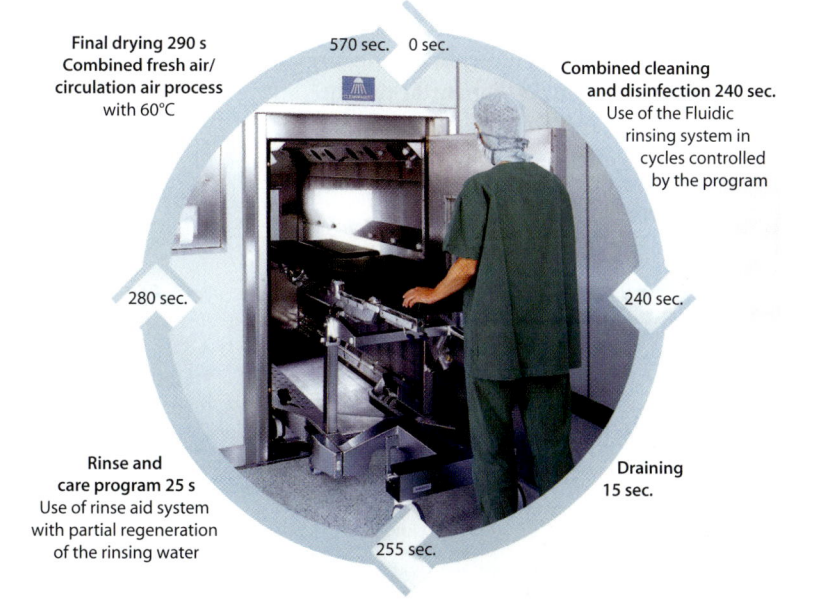

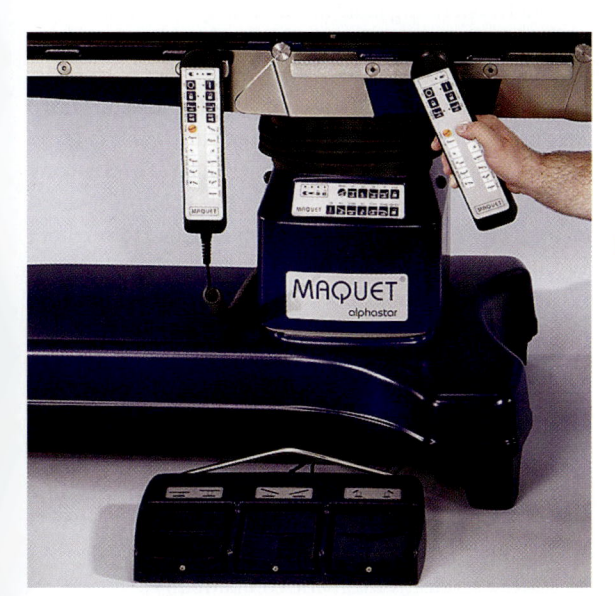

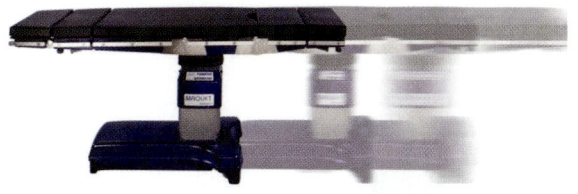

570 sec.   0 sec.

Final drying 290 s
Combined fresh air/
circulation air process
with 60°C

Combined cleaning
and disinfection 240 sec.
Use of the Fluidic
rinsing system in
cycles controlled
by the program

280 sec.

240 sec.

Rinse and
care program 25 s
Use of rinse aid system
with partial regeneration
of the rinsing water

Draining
15 sec.

255 sec.

Fig. 7.28. Travel drive for mobile operating tables

Fig. 7.27. Controls

7.1.4 Classification criteria according to the purpose

Universal operating tables. The patient boards for the »universal operating tables« are divided into up to 9 sections and can be adjusted in such a way that the patient can be positioned according to the surgeon's requirements specifically for the pending operation (Figs. 7.29, 7.30).

Special operating tables. Ongoing developments in general surgery as a result of new findings and new operating methods have produced new surgical disciplines. As a result of this specialisation in surgery, new, different demands have been made of the operating table (Figs. 7.31, 7.32).

Multifunctional universal operating tables have developed into special operating tables which comply with the specific requirements of the corresponding surgical discipline when it comes to positioning the patient.

7.1.5 Classification criteria according to the school of surgery

- German school of positioning (Fig. 7.33),
- Anglo-American school of positioning (Fig. 7.34),
- French school of positioning (Fig. 7.35).

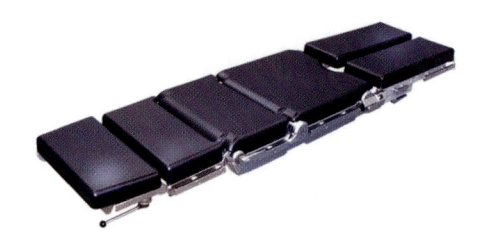

Fig. 7.29. Example of a universal operating patient board at the system

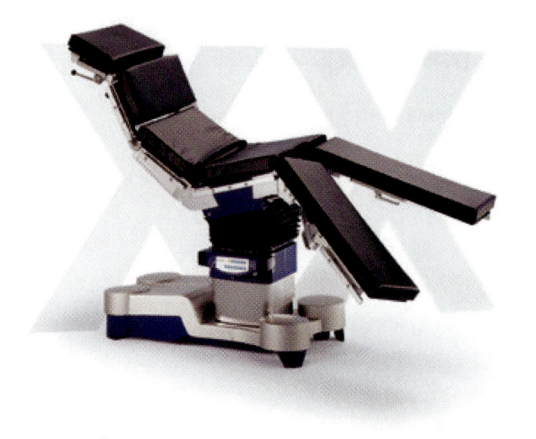

Fig. 7.30. Example of a universal operating patient board on the mobile operating table

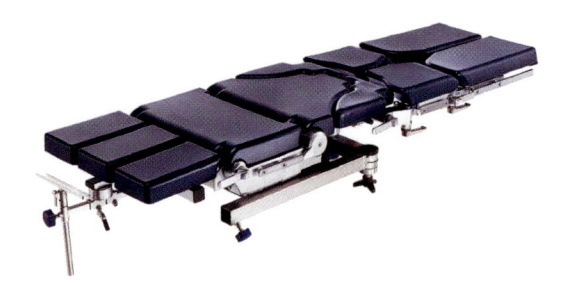

Fig. 7.31. Example of a special operating patient board at the system

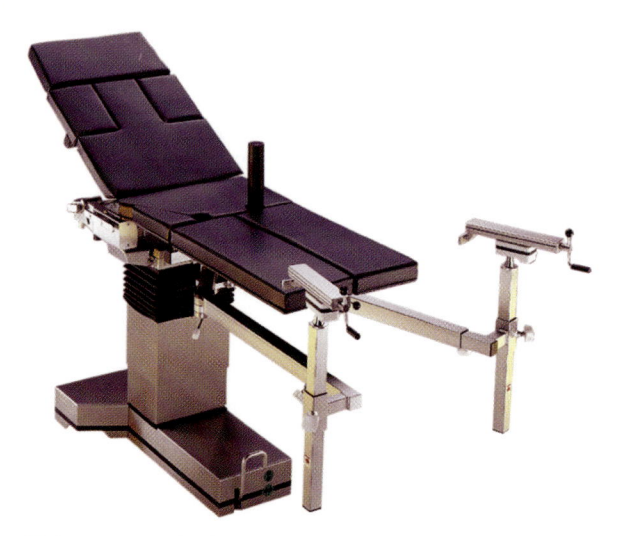

Fig. 7.32. Example of a special operating patient board on the mobile operating table

7.1.6 Production, production control and safety

A modern operating table or modern operating table system today is without doubt a high-tech product that complies with the strictest safety requirements.

In Germany, special laws and testing specifications have been passed for *medical devices*. Since 13.06.1998 the *Medical Product Law* (MPG) has been in force in Germany as a result of the EU *Council Directive 93/42/EEC* about medical devices which had to be implemented throughout Europe.

The operating table is a *class 1* medical device.

A Maquet operating table conforms to the CE regulations. The high safety and quality standard of an operating table is also a result of the company being certified to DIN EN ISO 9001 or EN 46001.

Various regulations, specifications and standards have to be fulfilled in the design and production of an operating table, for example:
- AN test (anaesthesia test),
- EMC test (electromagnetic compatibility),
- Test of tilting stability (to a 5° or 10° slant),

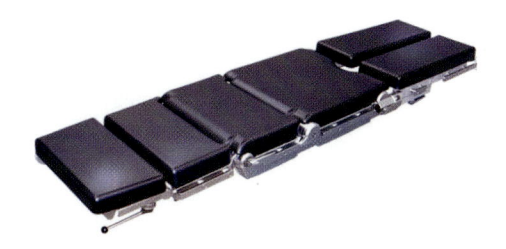

Fig. 7.33. 6/9 segments in the operating patient board

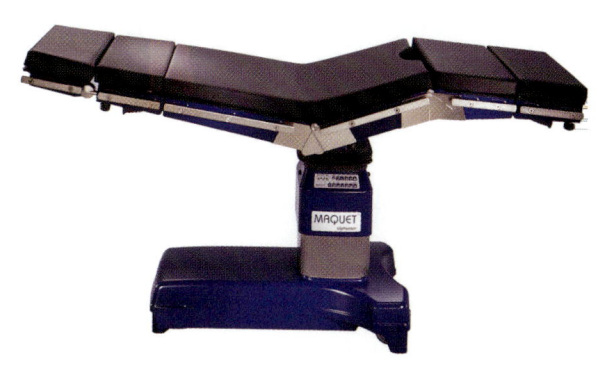

Fig. 7.34. Three basic segments in the operating patient board with reverse positioning (possibly with extension plates and head plate)

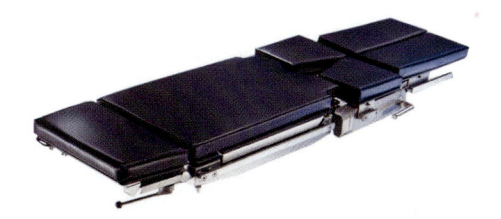

Fig. 7.35. Body patient board with large longitudinal displacement and 4-section special leg plates

- Test for deformation (2.2× safety = 135 kg × 2.2),
- Test for failure (4× safety = 135 kg × 4).

Detailed information can be found for example in the following standards:
- IEC 60 601-1: 1998 + A1: 1991 + A2: 1995
- IEC 60 601-2-46: 1998
- IEC 60 601-1-2: 1993 and IEC 60 601-2-46

The German version of the MPG also makes reference to the *Ordinance for erecting, operating and using medical products* (medical product owner ordinance – MPBetreibV). This ordinance contains detailed rules which the owner of the product has to observe, for example:
- Using the device according to the manufacturer's instructions
- Keeping the user manual available on site
- Keeping records of corresponding instructions issued to the staff
- Keeping a medical product logbook
- Reporting any incidents
- Only allowing authorised skilled staff to proceed with servicing and repairs, etc.

The MPBetreibV basically contains aspects which were already required in the previously valid MedGV.

7.2 Positioning accessories and aids

D. Aschemann, B. Kulik, C. Rösinger

7.2.1 Pads

The clever use of suitable positioning aids, such as pads with viscoelastic foam core or gel pads, together with the right positioning technique, can effectively reduce and even prevent the risk of positioning damage. Positioning the patient correctly for the operation makes assistance during the operation much easier or at all possible. The following sections list some frequently used positioning aids together with the corresponding operating positions.

7.2.1.1 Pads with viscoelastic foam core

Cushions. In various sizes (e.g. 40×15×10 cm) to support the heads of adult patients in the supine position in the pre-, peri- and postoperative phase.

Head rings. In various sizes to hold the head firmly in child and adult patients in the supine and lateral position. Particularly for goitre positioning and secure positioning for operations to the face or head.

Special cushions. In various sizes for firm positioning of the head in the lateral and prone position. The cushion has cut-outs for the patient's nose and eyes and lateral cut-outs for the respiratory tube (Fig. 7.36).

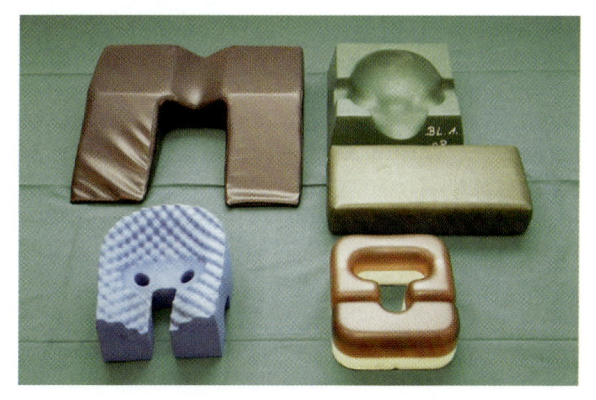

Fig. 7.36. Cushions for positioning the head in the supine, lateral and prone position

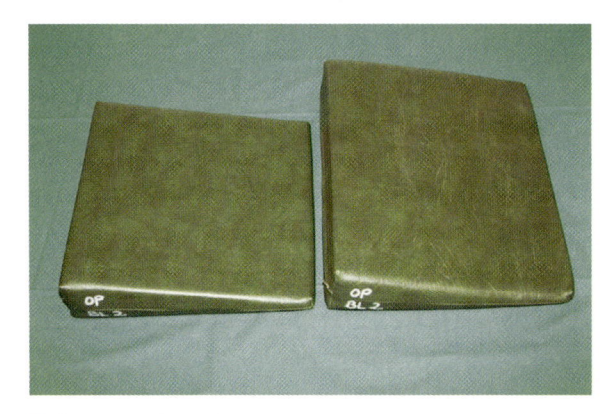

Fig. 7.37. Wedge cushions

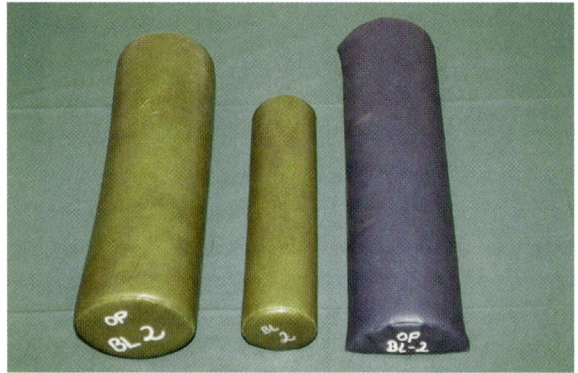

Fig. 7.38. Rolls and semi-rolls

Wedge cushions. In various sizes (e.g. 45×35×8 cm). Placing a wedge cushion under the pelvis with the patient in the supine position means that the leg lies in inner rotation on this side. This gives easier surgical access to the ankle joint. Another possible use is to pad the knee and foot region for patients in the prone position (Fig. 7.37).

Rolls and semi-rolls. In various sizes to relieve the brachial plexus; they are placed under the patient's knees to achieve a relaxed, almost physiological positioning in the patient's hips and knees (Fig. 7.38).

Double wedge cushions. In wedge shape, with cut-outs for the cervical spine and V-shaped cut-outs for the head. Firm positioning of the head and shoulders with the patient in the supine position. The shoulders are raised slightly to relieve the plexus (Fig. 7.39).

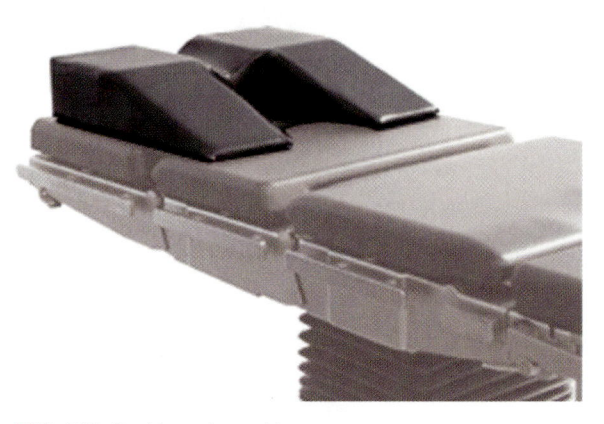

Fig. 7.39. Double wedge cushions

Padded cushions. For prone positioning of the patient. With abdominal cut-out and radiolucent, thermomodulating special foam. Removable padding elements for individualised adjustments to suit the patient's body (Fig. 7.40).

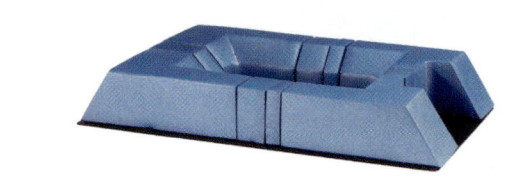

Fig. 7.40. Padded cushions for slipped disc operations

Bolsters (MHH). For prone positioning of the patient. Fitted with clamps to the lateral rails of the patient board (Fig. 7.41).

Tunnel cushion. Special U-shaped padding, positioned between the patient's legs in the lateral position to avoid pressure sores. The weight of the upper leg does not rest on the lower leg. The pressure on the fibular head of the lower leg is thus reduced to a minimum (Fig. 7.42).

Special knee positioning cushion. Positioning the healthy leg for arthroscopy of the knee, operations to the lower legs suspended on both sides. The cushion achieves a neutral position of the leg in the hip area (no hyperextension in the hip joint) and thus also relieves the lumbar spine.

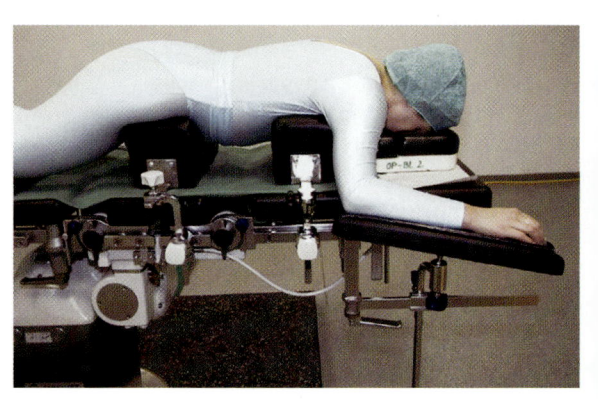

Fig. 7.41. Bolsters fitted with clamps

7.2 · Positioning accessories and aids

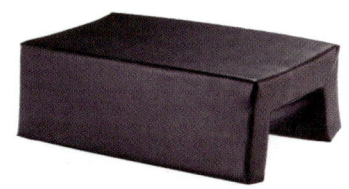

Fig. 7.42. Tunnel cushion

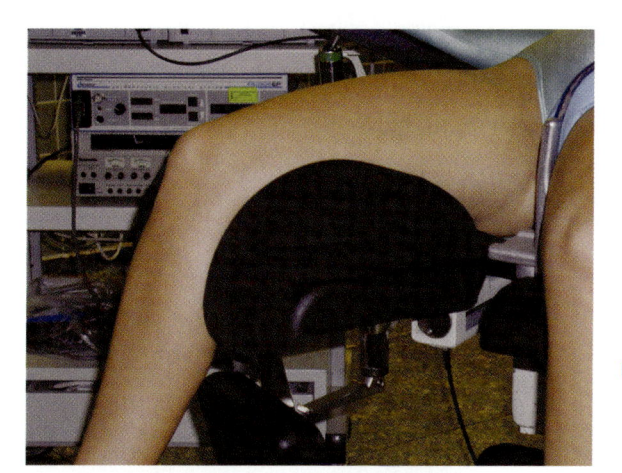

Fig. 7.43. Special knee positioning cushion (MHH)

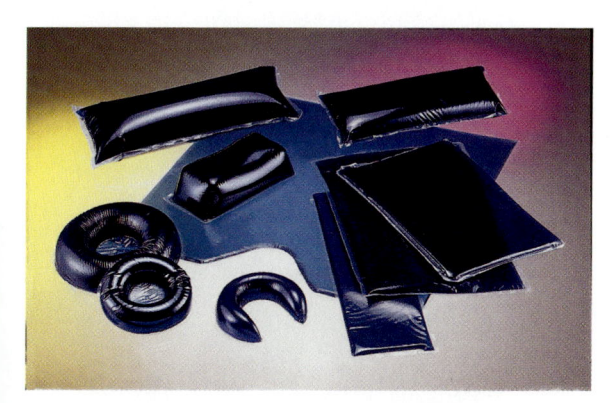

Fig. 7.44. View of the operating table mats, universal positioning aids and head rings

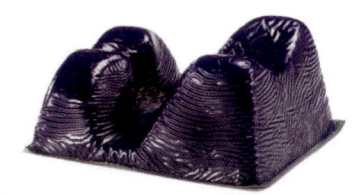

Fig. 7.45. Head cushion for prone position

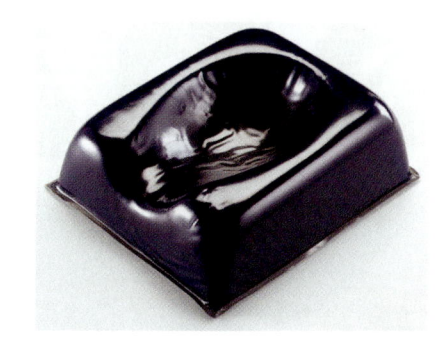

Fig. 7.46. Head cushion for supine position

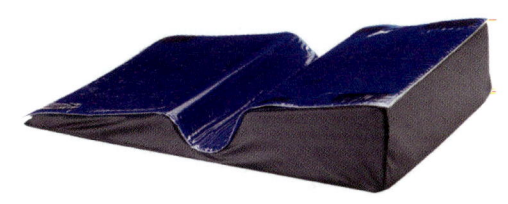

Fig. 7.47. Lateral positioning padding

The raised sides provide adequate lateral stability (Fig. 7.43).

7.2.1.2 Gel pads

Various positioning aids of special gel in a flat or specially shaped design offer good pressure distributing properties and thus help to prevent pressure sores. They can be heated to approx. 50°C.

Patient board mats. These mats cover the full length of the patient board and help to distribute weight evenly. They are ideal for universal use because they can be folded together or rolled up easily.

Universal positioning aids. Used as heel supports, shoulder supports and axilla rolls in various sizes.

Head rings. Available in closed and open design. Protect the head, face, neck and ears in all kinds of procedures (Fig. 7.44).

Cushion for prone position. Supports the head in an anatomically correct position and provides tube access on both sides (Fig. 7.45).

Cushion for supine position. For better fixing and positioning of the head with the patient in the supine position (Fig. 7.46).

Lateral position pads. Wedge-shaped positioning aids with a cut-out to relieve the lower arm specially for the lateral position, e.g. total hip replacement surgery or kidney operations (Fig. 7.47).

Heel protection. Provides support and maximum heel protection even during long operations with optimum pressure distribution.

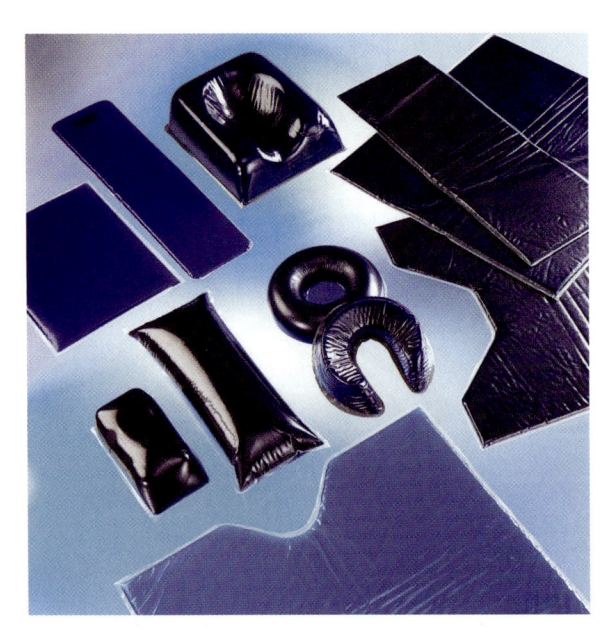

Fig. 7.48. Overview

The positioning aids described here should be available in an adequate quantity to ensure that every patient is positioned correctly, regardless of the patient's size (Fig. 7.48).

7.2.2 Operating table accessories

Fastening piece for head positioning elements. With star handles for adjustment in 3 joints with rail piece to take various head positioning elements, e.g. horseshoe headrest, headrest or skull clamp. Optimum adjustment thanks to the fine indentation of the joints (Fig. 7.49).

Horseshoe headrests. As adapters for fastening pieces (Figs. 7.50, 7.51).

Arm positioning device. Supports the arms in any position to give the best possible access for the anaesthetist. Maximum adjustments in all levels to prevent plexus damage when adjusted to the right height. The arm support is padded to avoid paralysis (ulnar nerve). A belt prevents the arm from being moved unintentionally (Fig. 7.52).

Arm protection. For positioning the arm firmly to the body with L-pad and 2 belts. The patient's arm is protected from the operating team standing at the side of the operating table and from unintentional movement when adjusting the position of the operating table during the operation (Fig. 7.53).

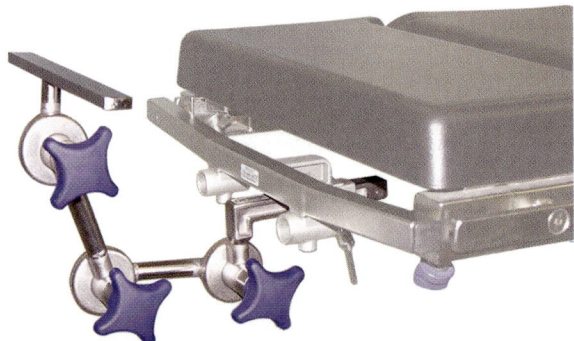

Fig. 7.49. Fastening piece

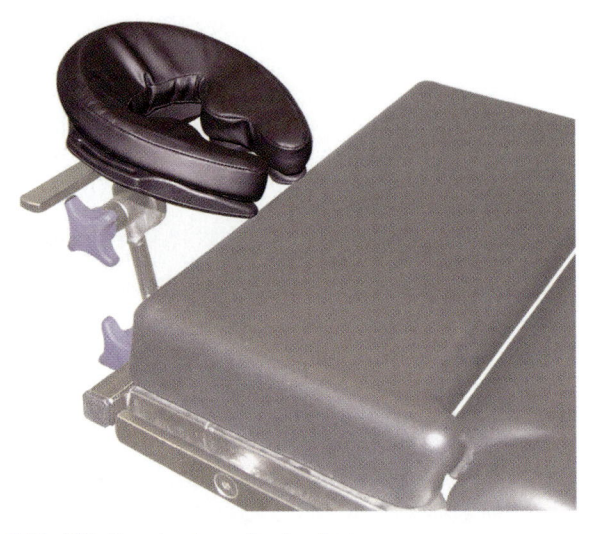

Fig. 7.50. One-piece horseshoe headrest

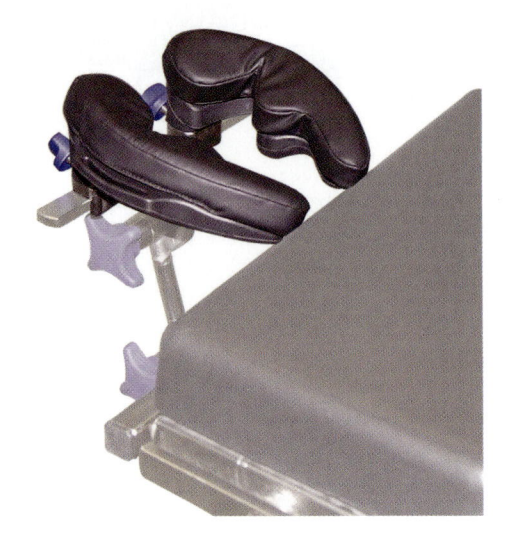

Fig. 7.51. Two-piece horseshoe headrest

7.2 · Positioning accessories and aids

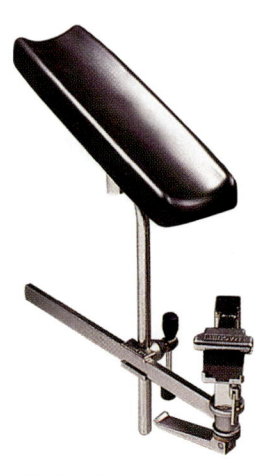

Fig. 7.52. Arm positioning device

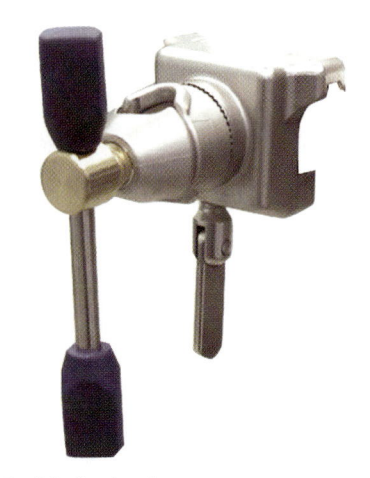

Fig. 7.54. Radial adjusting clamp

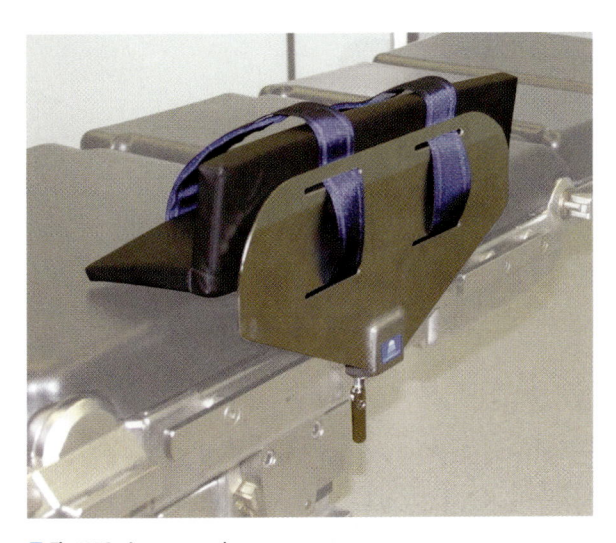

Fig. 7.53. Arm protection

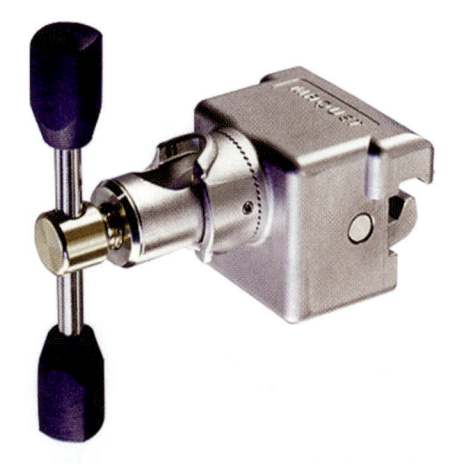

Fig. 7.55. Radial adjusting clamp with one-hand control

Anaesthesia screen. For screening the sterile area. Adjustable height fitted with a radial adjustment clamp on a rail.

Arm restraint straps for anaesthesia screen The arm restraint straps are fastened to the anaesthesia screen for suspending the patient's arm (supine position).

Radial adjustment clamp. Fastening element for accommodating and safely fastening accessories to the rails of the operating table. A radial adjustment mechanism facilitates optimum placement of the accessories (Figs. 7.54, 7.55).

Upper arm positioning plate. Fitted to the lateral rail of the operating table. For treating humerus fractures in the prone and supine position; radiolucent (Fig. 7.56).

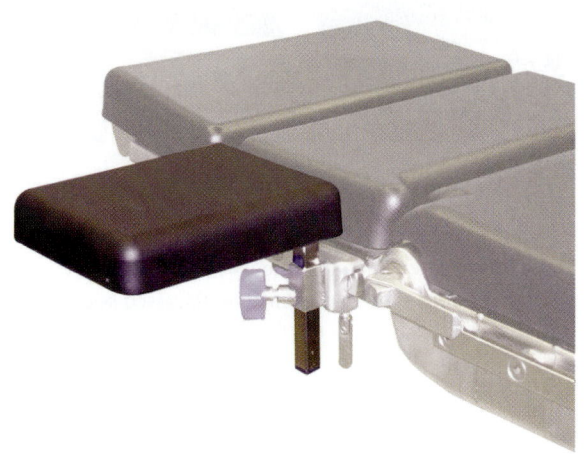

Fig. 7.56. Upper arm positioning plate

Hand operating table. Fitted to the lateral rail of the operating table. For surgery to the arm and hand. Radiolucent

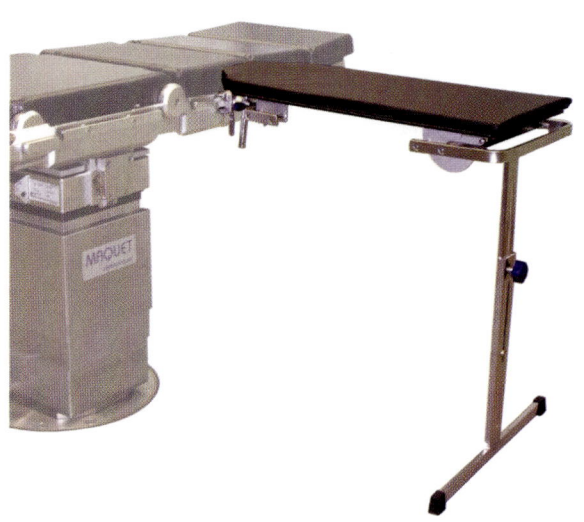

Fig. 7.57. Hand operating table

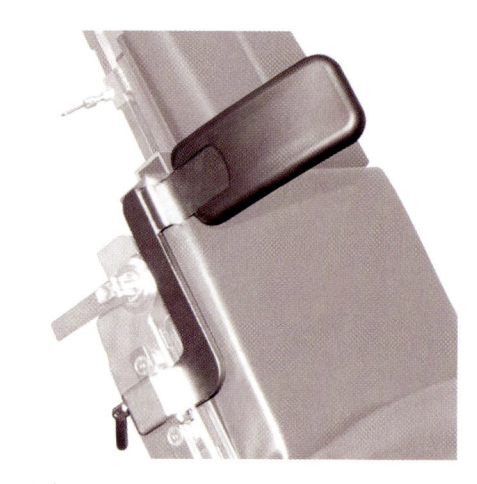

Fig. 7.59. Thorax support

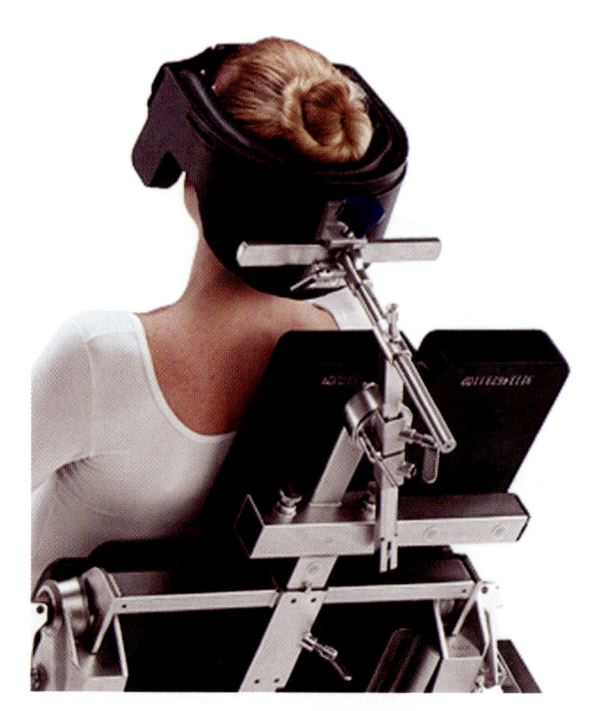

Fig. 7.58. Back plate for shoulder operations

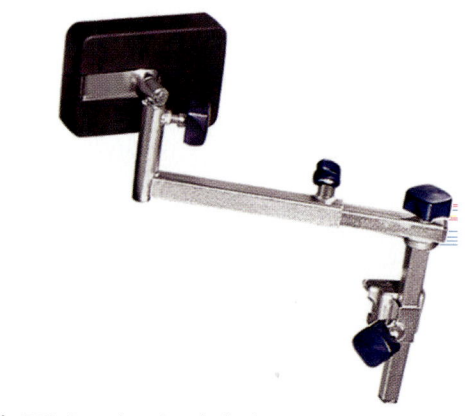

Fig. 7.60. Fastening piece for body supports

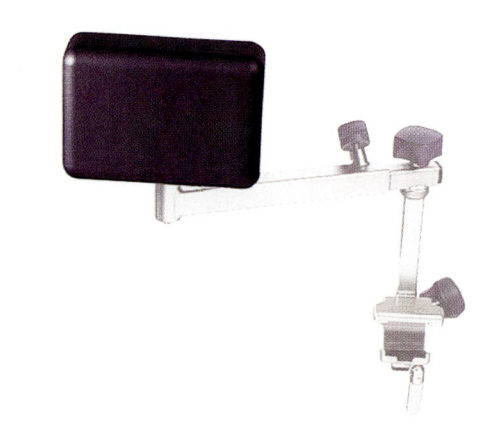

Fig. 7.61. Back/buttocks support

and with many varied adjustments for anatomically correct positioning of the patient also with raised back plate (Fig. 7.57).

Back plate for shoulder operations. Back plate with two laterally removable pads for exposing the shoulder being operated and free anteroposterior scanning with the image intensifier, with adapter at the head end for head positioning accessories (Fig. 7.58).

Thorax support. For supporting the body when positioning the patient in the sitting position (beach-chair positioning), fitted to the lateral rail of the lower motor-driven back plates (Fig. 7.59).

Fastening piece and body supports. Fitted to the lateral rails of the operating table to fix the patient's body in any position. Various pads are available for anatomically correct positioning, e.g. back/buttock support, pubis/sacrum/sternum support and lateral support (Figs. 7.60–7.63).

7.2 · Positioning accessories and aids

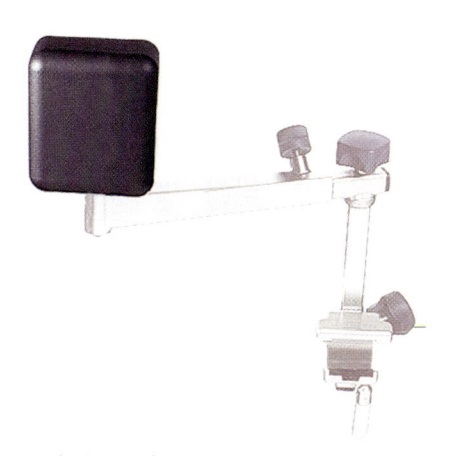

Fig. 7.62. Pubis/sacrum/sternum support

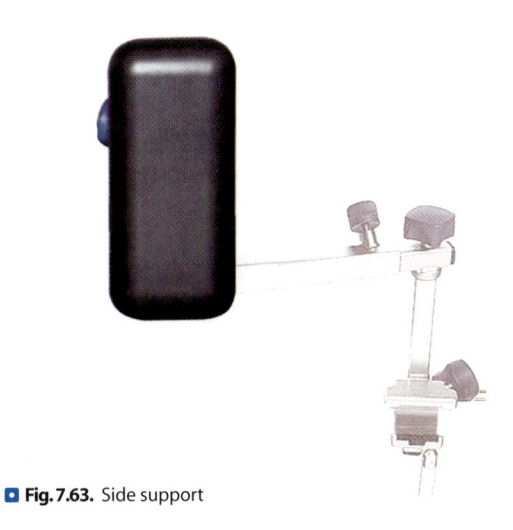

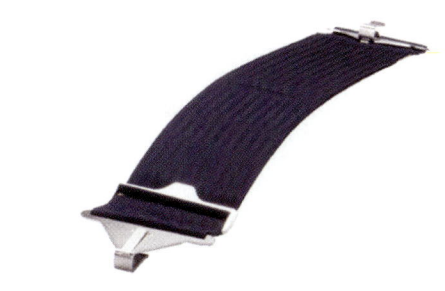

Fig. 7.63. Side support

Fig. 7.64. Body belt

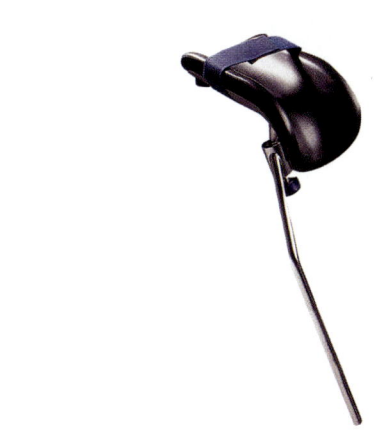

Fig. 7.65. Goepel leg holder

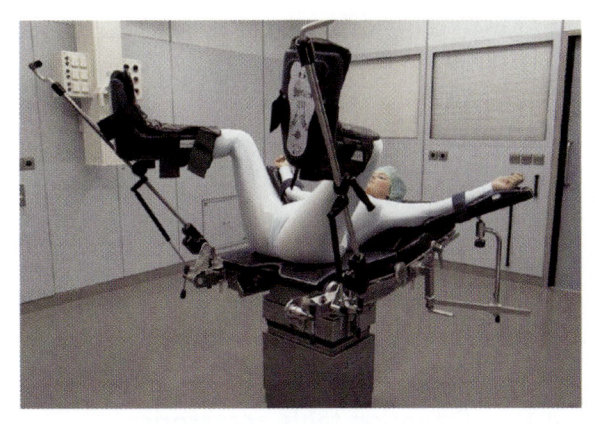

Fig. 7.66. Leg holder with one-hand control

Shoulder holder. To support the body when the patient is positioned with lowered head (e.g. Trendelenburg positioning). Fitted and adjusted in the lateral rail.

Side holder. To support the body when the operating table is tilted. Fitted and adjusted in the lateral rail.

Body belt. For fixing the body and holding it firmly in any position and also during patient transport (Fig. 7.64).

Goepel leg holder. For the lithotomy position. The *Goepel leg holder* is fitted to a rail with a clamp. The foam core pad with fastening belt holds the lower leg. The patient's upper arm can be supported as well when in the lateral position (Fig. 7.65).

Leg holder with one-hand control. Pressure assisted leg holder with padded boot to take or support the lower leg and foot. Pressure is moved to the sole of the foot away from the lower leg and fibular head (Fig. 7.66).

Knee supports. For knee/elbow positioning. Fitted to the lateral rails of the lowered leg plates.

Meniscus bar. Angled shape with foam padding roll, fitted with radial adjusting clamps to the lateral rail of the operating table and adjustable in height.

Manual knee support unit. For positioning the thigh for arthroscopy, arthrotomy and total knee replacement surgery. Fitted to a lateral rail of the operating table (Fig. 7.67).

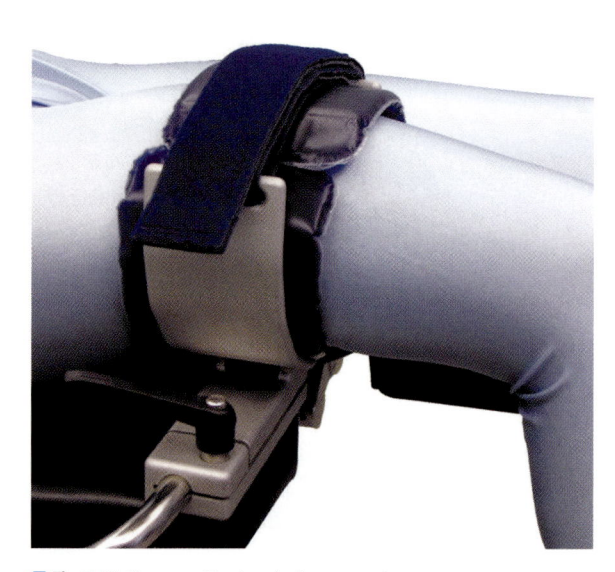

Fig. 7.67. Knee positioning device, manual

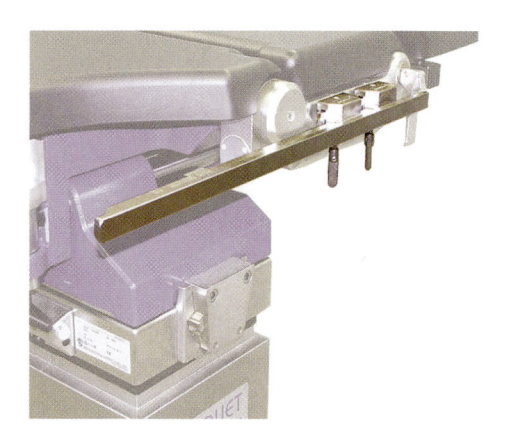

Fig. 7.68. Rail extension

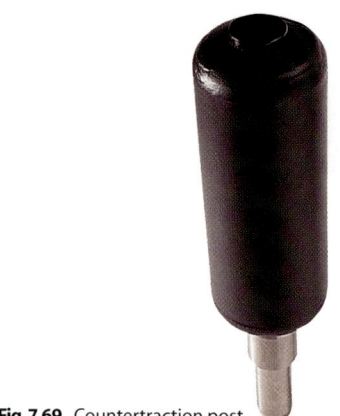

Fig. 7.69. Countertraction post

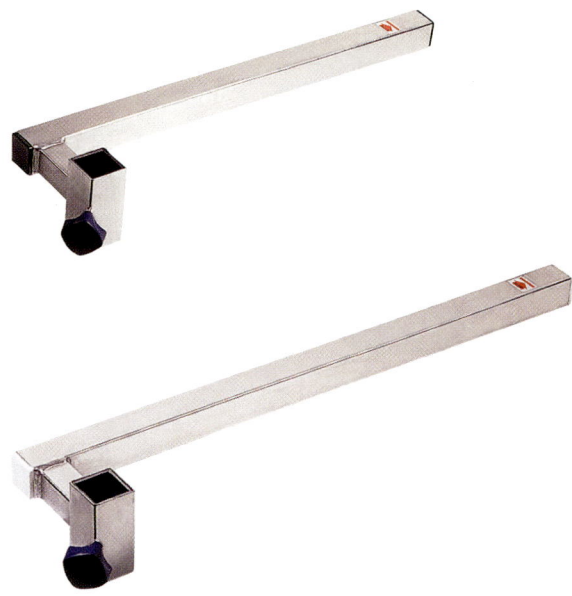

Fig. 7.70. Extension bars, short and long

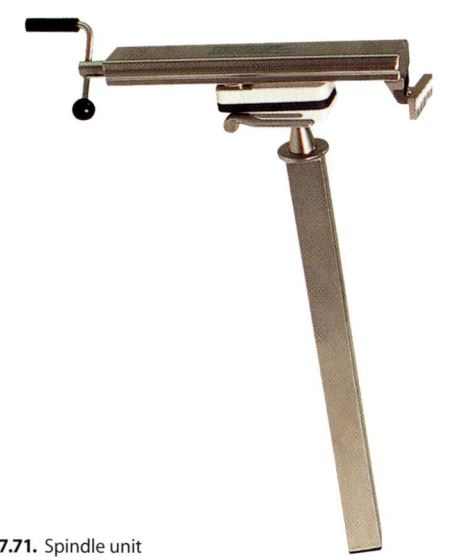

Fig. 7.71. Spindle unit

Operation accessory stand, mobile. With standard rails and wire baskets for positioning aids and small parts.

7.2.3 Extension table accessories

Sliding rail extension. Extends the lateral rail, e.g. at the extension operating table (Fig. 7.68).

Countertraction post. For supine positioning of the patient when performing surgery to the lower extremities. Fitted to the right or left bore of the cross bar at the end of the seat plate or extension table patient board. The countertraction post is fitted to the fractured side (Fig. 7.69).

Extension bars. For variable adjustment of the length when performing surgery to the lower extremities and to accommodate the spindle unit or foot plates. Standard accessories for extension tables always include a long and short exten-

7.2 · Positioning accessories and aids

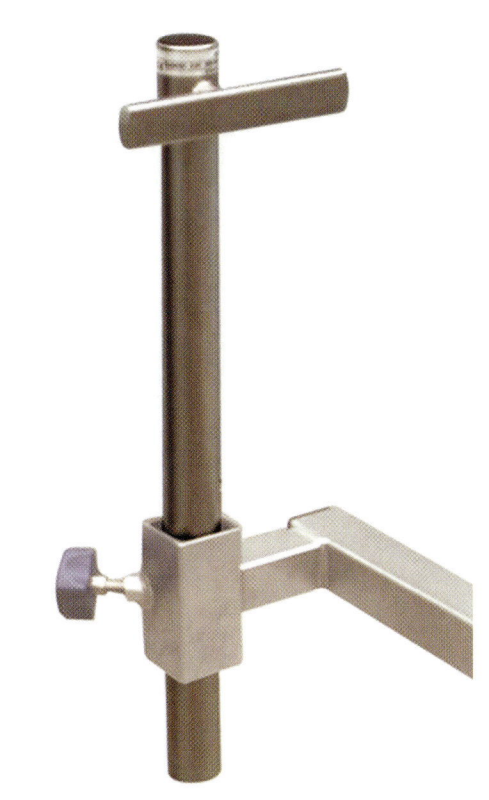

Fig. 7.72. Foot plate support

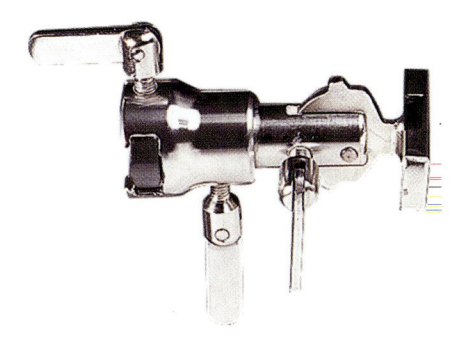

Fig. 7.73. Rotation tilt clamp

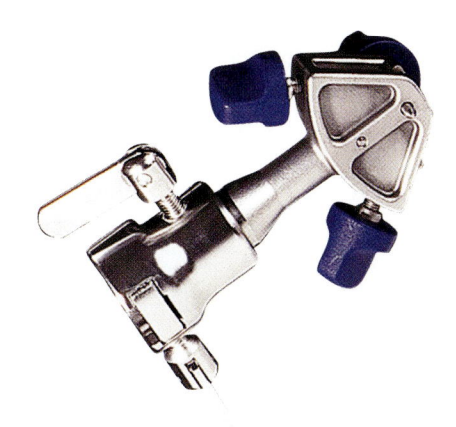

Fig. 7.74. Rotation bar clamp

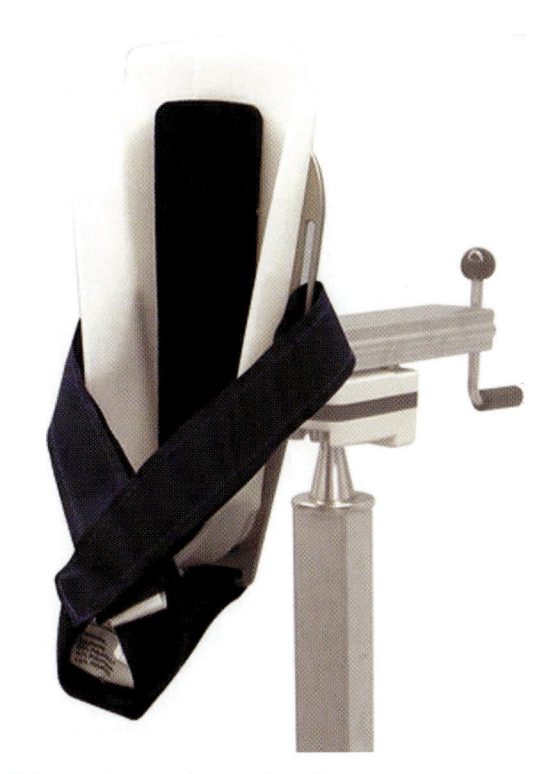

Fig. 7.75. Foot plate for extension table

sion bar. The short extension bar (black cap) can always be fitted to the fractured side (Fig. 7.70).

Spindle unit. Adjusts the extension length with a hand crank, with ball joint for anatomically correct alignment of the fractured extremity (Fig. 7.71).

Foot plate support. To support the non-fractured extremity with positioned foot plate (Fig. 7.72).

Rotation tilt clamp. Accommodates foot plates (extension shoes) for extensions to the lower extremities or Weinberger wristlets for hand/arm extensions (Fig. 7.73).

Rotation bar clamp. Accommodates the extension bar (Fig. 7.74)

Foot plate for extension table. Fixes the patient's foot to the spindle unit or foot plate support, possibly with rotation tilt clamp; can be adjusted in width to various foot sizes (Fig. 7.75).

Lower leg countertraction post. For positioning the fractured lower leg with CRP countertraction post and horizontal guide pipe for an extension bar (Fig. 7.76).

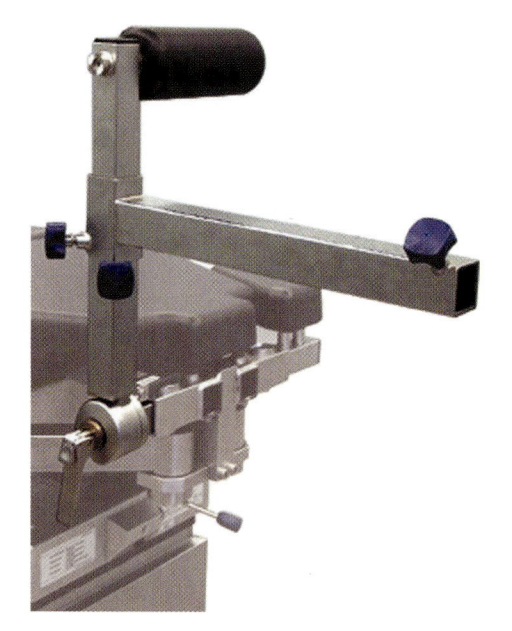

Fig. 7.76. Lower leg countertraction post

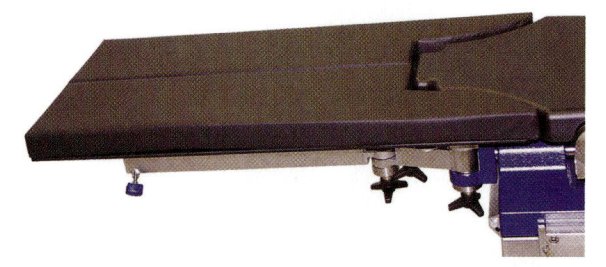

Fig. 7.77. Special leg plates

Fig. 7.78. Accessories stand

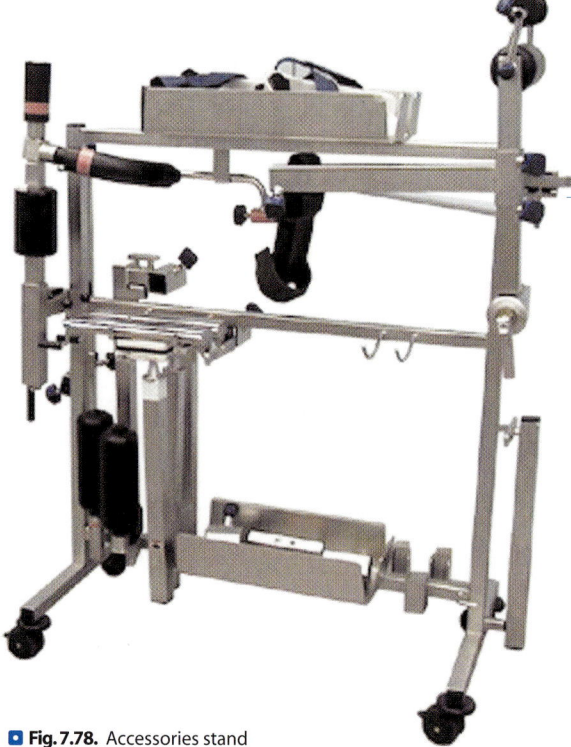

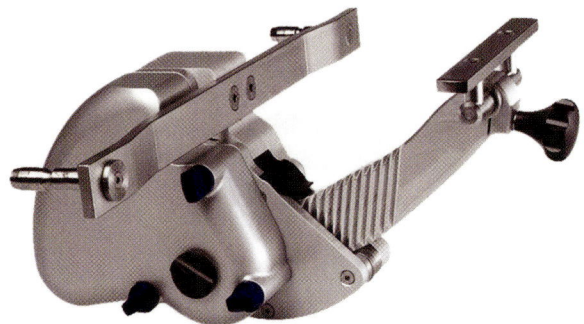

Fig. 7.79. Motor-driven headrest adjustment

Special leg plates for hip replacement. For positioning a patient in the supine position on the extension table, providing good access for the image intensifier to both hips (Fig. 7.77).

Accessories stand. Accommodates extension table accessories (Fig. 7.78).

7.2.4 Special units

Motor-driven headrest adjustment. Guarantees anatomically correct upwards and downwards movement of the horseshoe headrest/headrest to prevent compression and extension of the cervical spine. Motor adjustment in a range from +25 to -35°. Controlled by a separate foot switch so that the surgeon can sit to perform the procedure (Fig. 7.79).

Spinal support unit/head extension. For intraoperative repositioning and fixing for operations to the dorsal and ventral cervical spine in patients with halo fixator (Fig. 7.80).

Motor-driven knee positioning unit. The surgeon controls the electric knee positioning unit with a foot switch to facilitate the necessary bending and stretching movements particularly during knee replacement surgery (Fig. 7.81).

7.2.5 Vacuum mats

In various sizes for firm positioning of the patient through good distribution of pressure (Fig. 7.82).

7.2 · Positioning accessories and aids

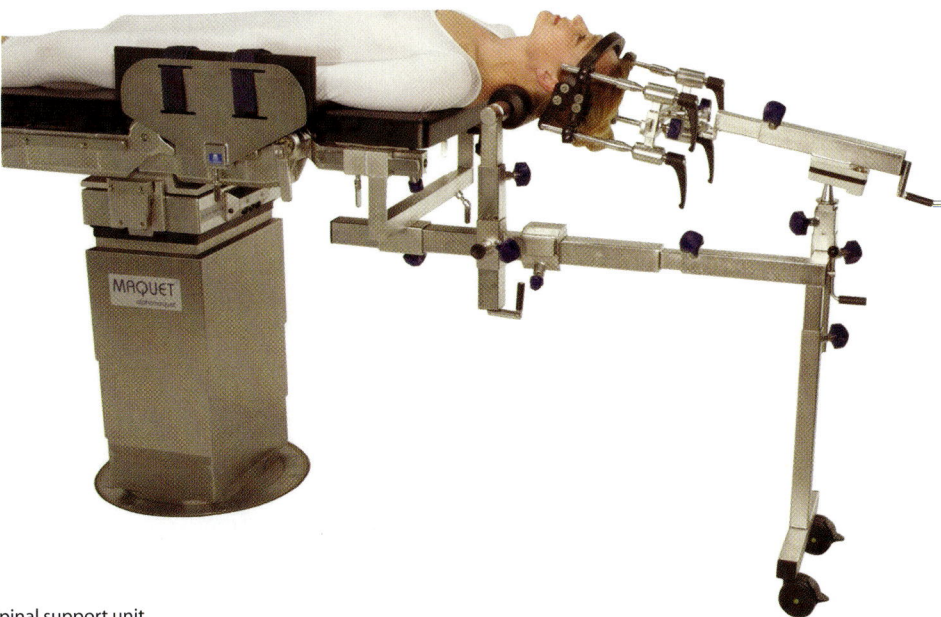

Fig. 7.80. Spinal support unit

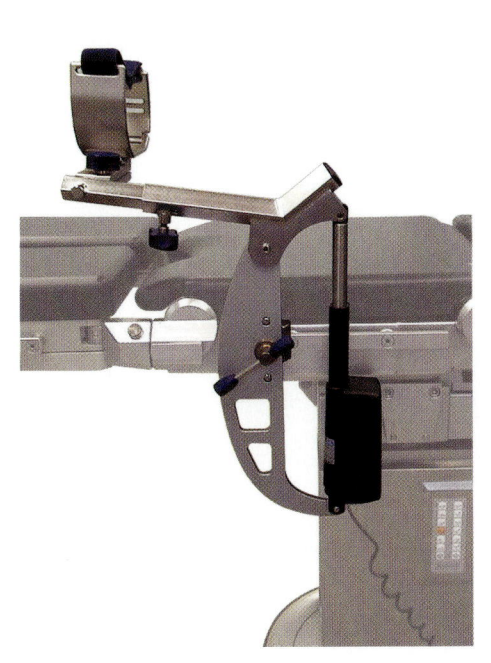

Fig. 7.81. Motor-driven knee positioning unit

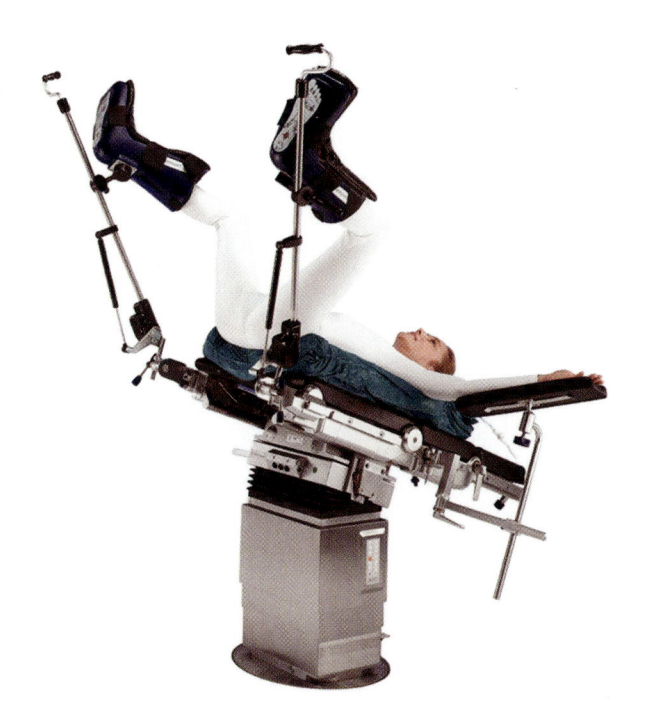

Fig. 7.82. Example of use

7.2.6 Patient warming system

The basic idea. Before surgery, it is decided which parts of the body can be covered without impairing the surgical activities. Heat is supplied from above (conductive method). The patient is covered outside the surgical/sterile area. Highly versatile, segmented and specially shaped blankets are ideal for individual use in every surgical discipline (Fig. 7.83).

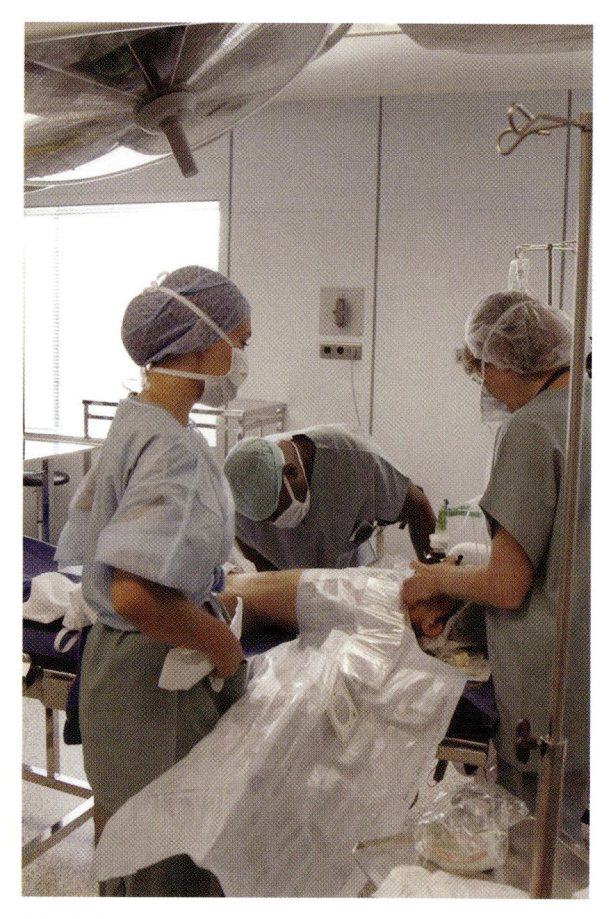

Fig. 7.83. Example of use

8 Standard positioning

D. Aschemann, A. Gänsslen

8.1 Introduction – 92

8.2 Preparation of the operating table – 92
8.2.1 Universal operating table Alphamaquet 1150.30 with water and gel mat for trauma surgery – 92

8.3 Supine position – 93
8.3.1 Head – 93
8.3.2 Shoulders and arms – 93
8.3.3 Back and pelvis – 94
8.3.4 Legs – 95

8.4 Lithotomy position – 96
8.4.1 Head, shoulders and arms – 96
8.4.2 Back and pelvis – 97
8.4.3 Legs – 97

8.5 Beach-chair position – 98
8.5.1 Head – 98
8.5.2 Shoulders and arms – 99
8.5.3 Back and pelvis – 99
8.5.4 Legs – 99

8.6 Prone position – 99
8.6.1 Head – 100
8.6.2 Arms – 100
8.6.3 Thorax and pelvis – 102
8.6.4 Legs – 102

8.7 The lateral position – 102
8.7.1 Head – 103
8.7.2 Shoulder and arms – 103
8.7.3 Thorax and pelvis – 104
8.7.4 Legs – 104

8.8 Final remarks – 105

8.1 Introduction

Avoiding pressure sores at the back of the head, at the shoulder blades, the coccyx and the heels are just as much a priority in preparing the operating table as positioning the patient so as to protect the nerves in the following steps. In the case of longer procedures or for intensive care patients with long stays in hospital, these are the parts of the body where bedsores can occur. The sequence in which protective and positioning materials are used to cover the operating table is directly related to care, safety and the operative procedure. Negligence in preparing the operating table and incorrectly performed positioning procedures will have a negative effect on the patient already during the operation.

8.2 Preparation of the operating table

8.2.1 Universal operating table Alphamaquet 1150.30 with water and gel mat for trauma surgery

An X-ray mat is placed on the operating table from the buttock plate to the headrest when permitted or required by the surgical procedure (X-ray protection against radiation from imaging equipment from below, here image intensifiers, ◘ Fig. 8.1).

The leg plates are not used for trauma surgery, as some procedures require the removal or lifting/lowering of a leg plate. Depending on the duration and type of procedure, the operating table can be prepared with a short water mat (e.g. 55×100 cm) with the mat always connected at the head end so that the C-arm can be moved without any problems in the scanning area and to provide better access to the patient in general (◘ Fig. 8.2). But generally the patient should always be warmed from above with a patient warming system (conductive method).

A short gel mat (e.g. 60×100 cm) is positioned to cover the water mat and, in turn, not cover the leg plates (◘ Fig. 8.3).

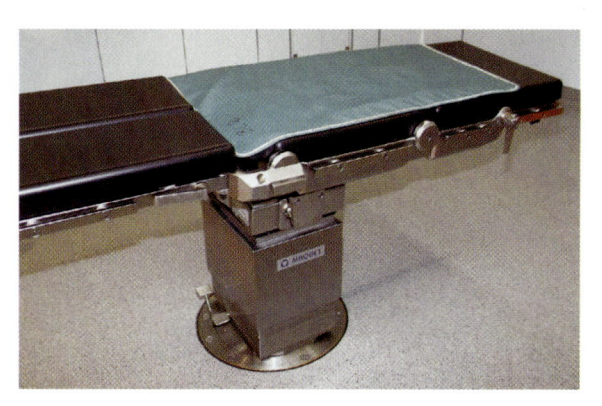

◘ **Fig. 8.1.** Universal operating table with X-ray protection

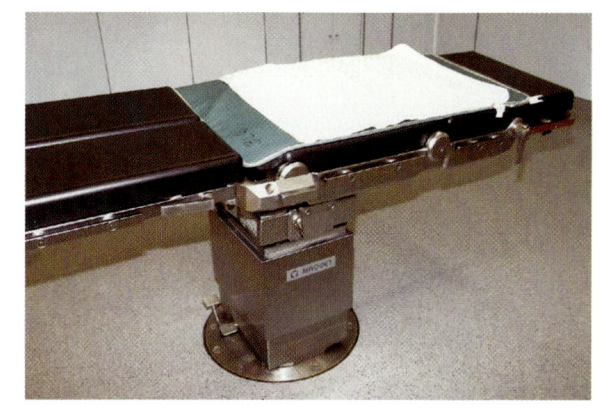

◘ **Fig. 8.2.** Water mat with connection at head end

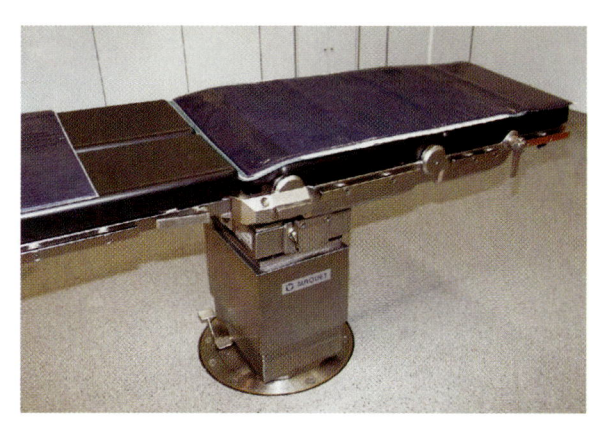

◘ **Fig. 8.3.** Gel mat for safe positioning of the patient

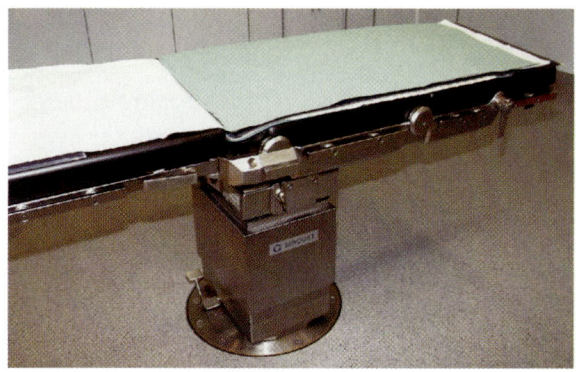

◘ **Fig. 8.4.** Paper sheet with water barrier and fabric sheet

A paper sheet with water barrier is spread as insulation over the complete operating table. A folded 120-cm fabric sheet is placed on the absorbent layer of the paper sheet and a neutral electrode is placed on the fabric sheet. All layers end flush with the edge of the table and the folds are smoothed down (◘ Figs. 8.4, 8.5).

It is also possible to use the gel mat as final cover on the operating table, so that the patient's body is in direct contact with the gel mat.

8.3 · Supine position

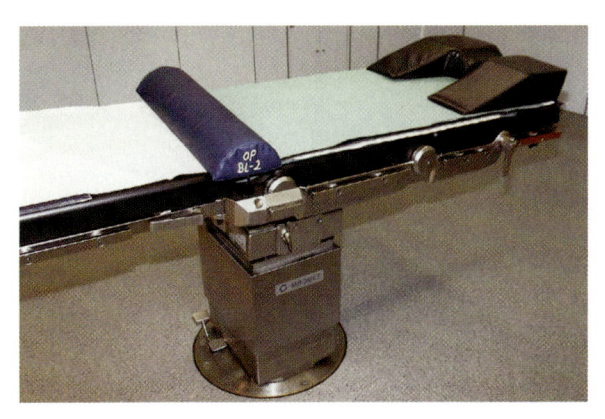

Fig. 8.5. Positioning aid (double wedge cushion and half-roll)

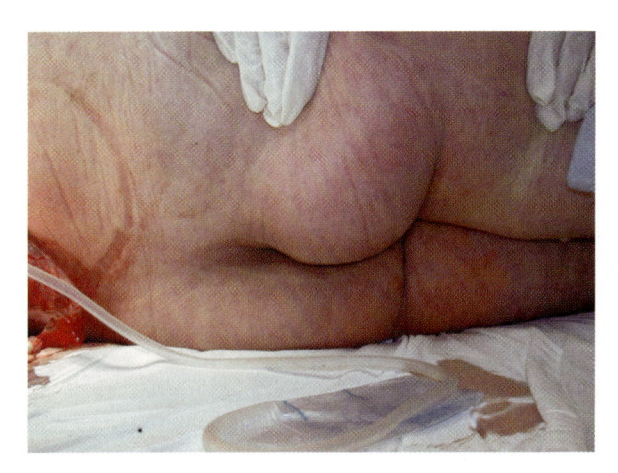

Fig. 8.6. Pressure marks from sheets and tubes

The number of additional layers between the patient and the operating table or padding should be reduced as far as possible as this otherwise limits usefulness and it is no longer possible to prevent bedsores (Fig. 8.6).

8.3 Supine position

8.3.1 Head

In the supine position, the head must be padded with various positioning aids so that the cervical spine is in the middle/neutral position (awake) and there is no local pressure on the back of the head (Figs. 8.7–8.9).

8.3.2 Shoulders and arms

Normally in general surgery, both of the patient's arms are spread out to the side. For pronation positioning, the spread arms should be put into abduction to approx. 60° bent at the elbows, and positioned and fixed with the lower arm on the arm positioning device. Support, for example with a short armrest, should always be provided for

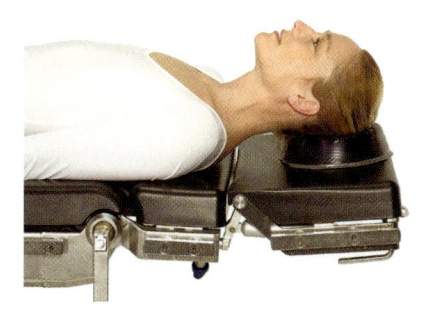

Fig. 8.7. Closed head ring

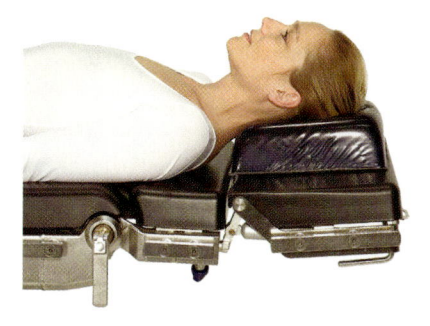

Fig. 8.8. Gel head cushion

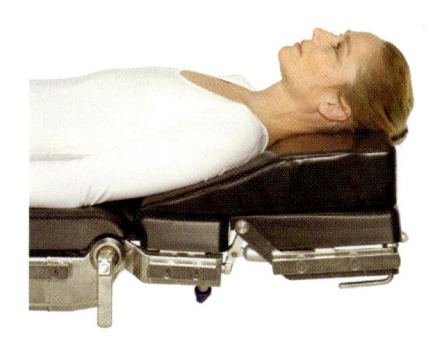

Fig. 8.9. Double wedge cushion with padding under the shoulders

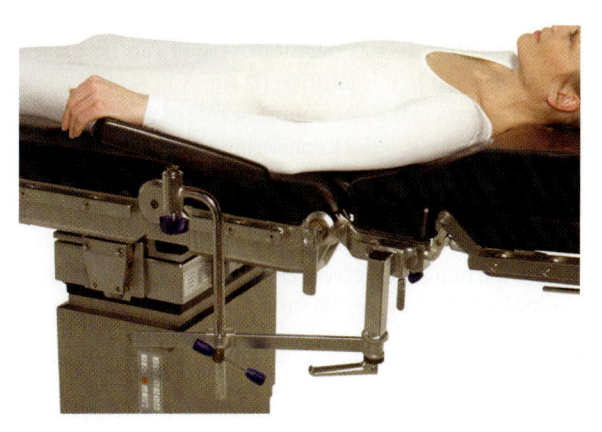

Fig. 8.10. Correct arm positioning with short armrest

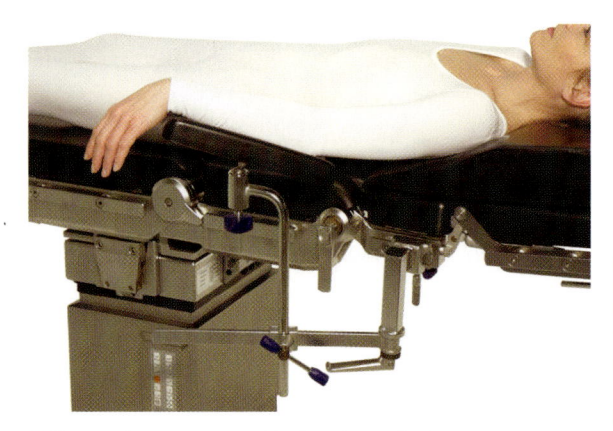

Fig. 8.11. Incorrect arm positioning, dropped wrist

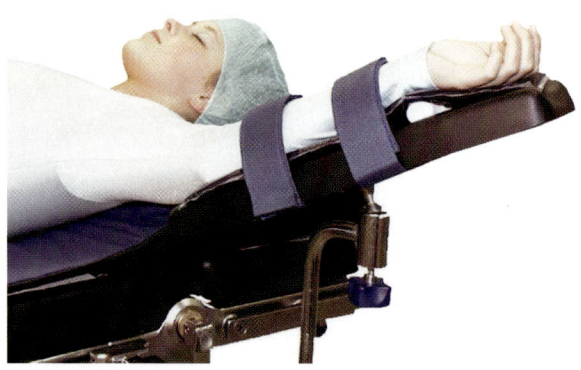

Fig. 8.13. Abducted arm with padding, fixed on a long arm positioning device

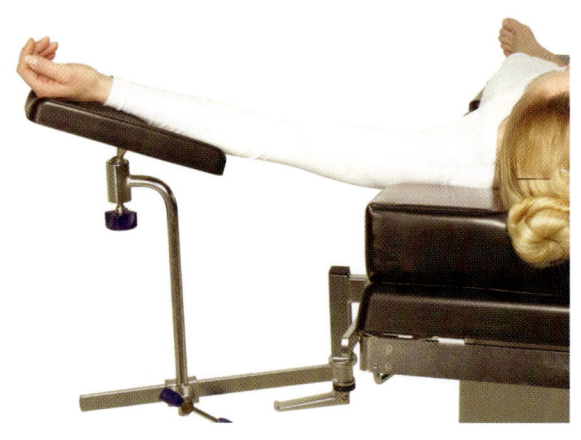

Fig. 8.12. Positioning the arm on short arm positioning device in abduction

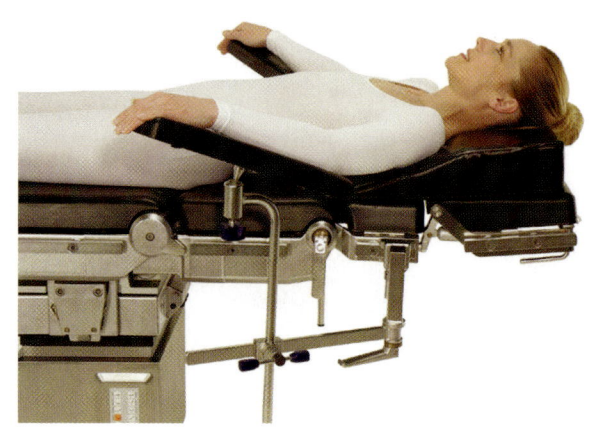

Fig. 8.14. Head and arm positioning with double wedge cushion

the lower arm and hand. This positioning of the arm prevents the so-called wristdrop (Figs. 8.10, 8.11).

For abduction of the arm between 60° and 90°, the patient should always be adjusted from pronation to supination position (Texas position). A pad can be placed under the wrist in this position (Figs. 8.12, 8.13).

The nerves in the elbow must lie free of pressure. Padding under the shoulder consisting of a special double wedge pad, gel pad or a 250/500 ml infusion bag raises the shoulder from the level of the table and enlarges the gap between clavicle and first rib, with a clear reduction in the risk of harming the nerves. The arm must be lifted over the level of the shoulder (Fig. 8.14).

The rule of thumb for positioning the arm in supine patients is as follows: place pads under the shoulder to lift it from the level of the table, with the distal joint higher than the proximal joint.

So the elbow is higher than the shoulder and the wrist higher than the elbow. The arm can be positioned at the body (e.g. heart surgery) using an arm holder (Figs. 8.15, 8.16).

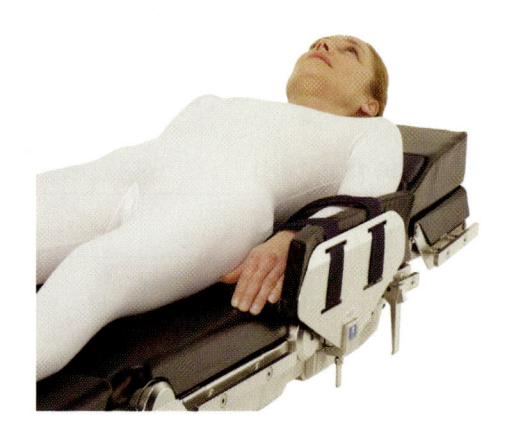

Fig. 8.15. Arm positioning with arm protection

8.3.3 Back and pelvis

Hips and knees should be preferably slightly bent; pads should be placed under the frequently exposed lumbar spine. The pads can consist of a small pile of cellulose, a small rolled/folded towel or an additional small gel pad. The thickness and position of the padding depends on

8.3 · Supine position

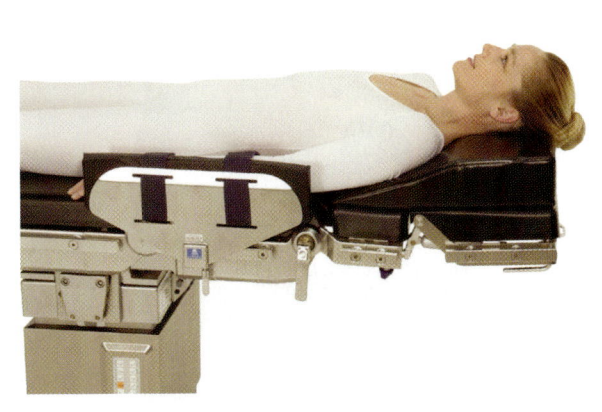

Fig. 8.16. Hand and elbow are protected

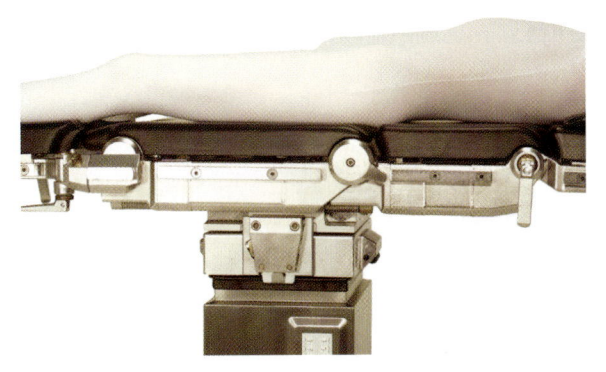

Fig. 8.17. Positioning without positioning aids and straight operating table

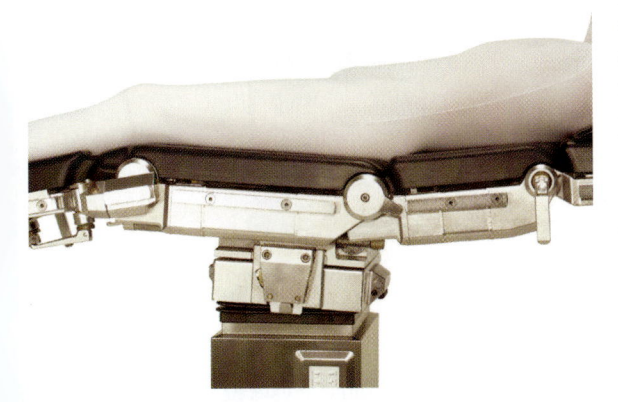

Fig. 8.18. Positioning without positioning aids with adapted adjustment of the operating table

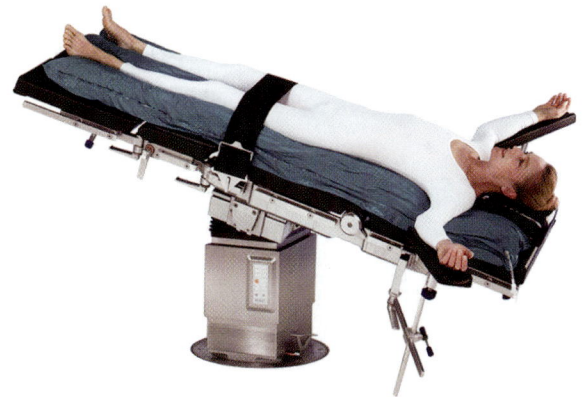

Fig. 8.19. Positioning with vacuum mat and operating table in Trendelenburg position and tilted to the left

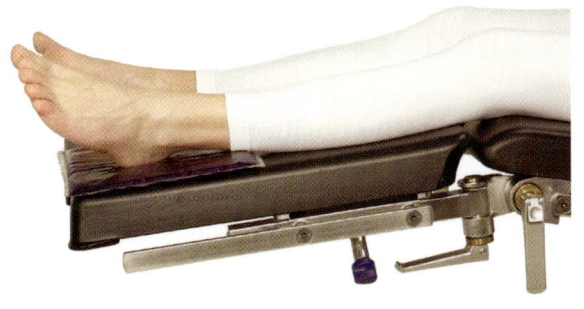

Fig. 8.20. Increased pressure on the heels

8.3.4 Legs

If necessary, a half roll is placed under the knees at the distal thigh. Another possibility is to adjust the leg plates at the knee joint. Pressure on the heels should always be reduced to a minimum. Figure 8.20 shows increased pressure on the heels with the use of a gel mat. One possibility is to use small gel mats placed under the lower leg (Fig. 8.21). But the leg should always have the greatest possible contact with the patient board with every kind of padding. These requirements can also be fulfilled by using a vacuum mat, as in Figs. 8.19 and 8.22.

the patient. The padding is placed *under* the top surface of the operating table (e.g. gel mat) so as not to interrupt the homogeneous top surface and impair its effect. If no positioning aids are available, the operating table should be adjusted to support parts of the body which are not flat on the table (Figs. 8.17–8.19).

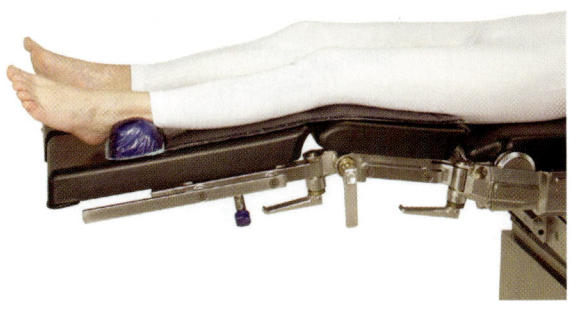

Fig. 8.21. Reduced pressure with clearance of the heels

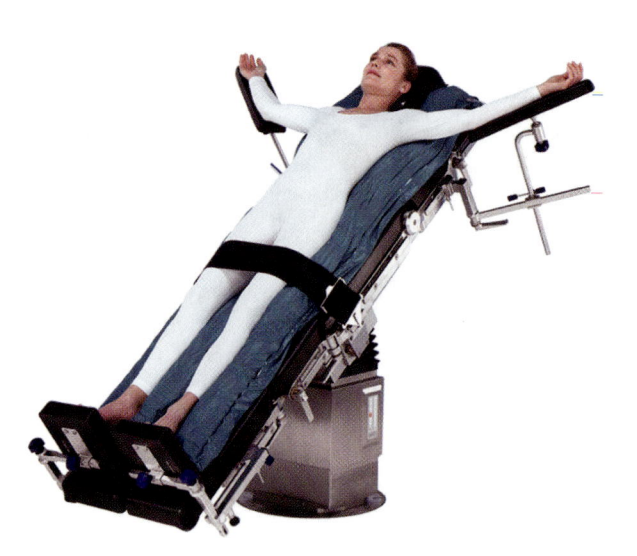

Fig. 8.22. Reduced pressure with clearance of the heels using a vacuum mat

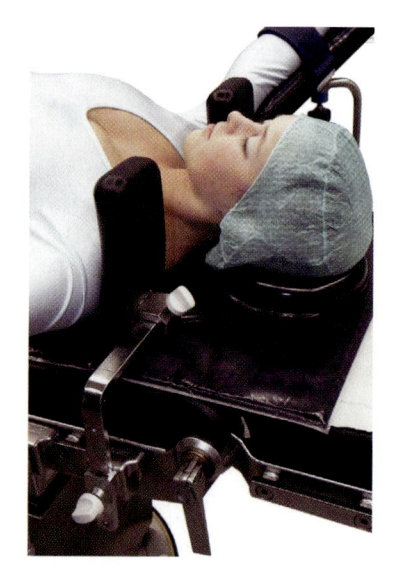

Fig. 8.24. Positioning with gel head ring and shoulder supports

8.4 Lithotomy position

8.4.1 Head, shoulders and arms

In the lithotomy position, shoulder supports are used in addition to position the head. Once again, the head should be held in the middle/neutral position (Figs. 8.23, 8.24).

The patient should be prevented from slipping if Trendelenburg positioning is required. It is also important to avoid a low position of the clavicle and to minimise pressure at the contact points, because not even well padded shoulder supports can always avoid damage to the plexus (Fig. 8.25).

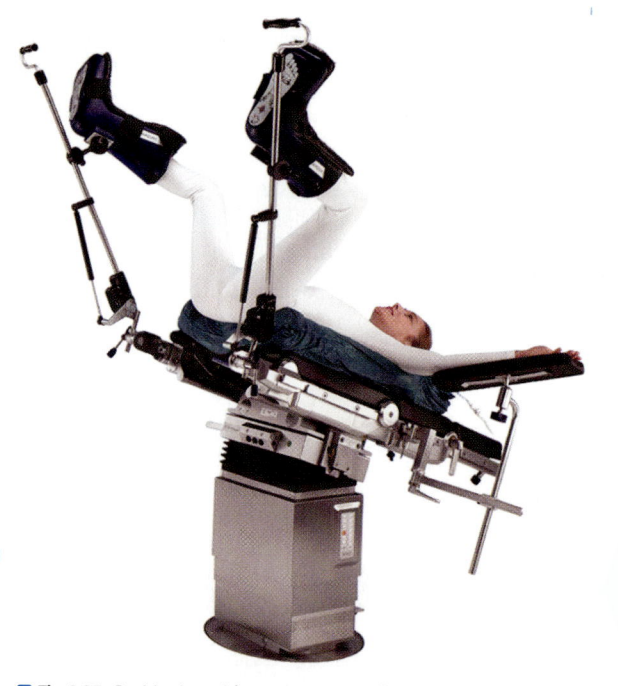

Fig. 8.25. Positioning with vacuum mat and operating table in Trendelenburg position

A short vacuum mat should always be used in this position as a standard procedure for longer operations or if required by the patient's size. This distributes the pressure across the back and relieves the pressure on the shoulders.

But if the patient is positioned as shown in Fig. 8.26, it is possible for the patient to slip in the Trendelenburg position. Without any positioning aids, the head has landed on an ECG lead. These »trifles« can lead to the onset of skin injuries.

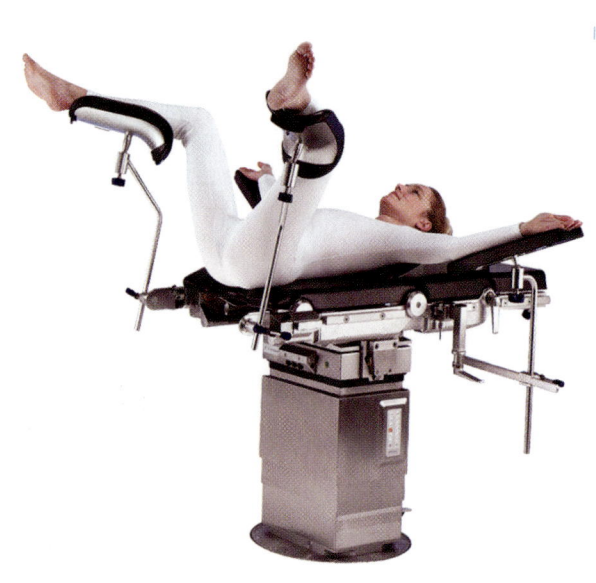

Fig. 8.23. Lithotomy position with Goepel leg holders

8.4 · Lithotomy position

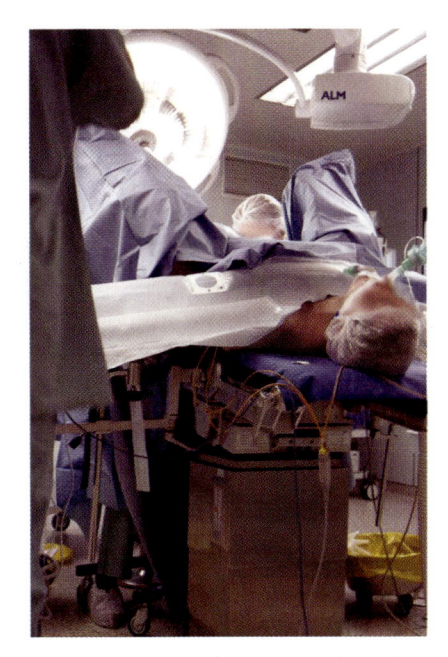

Fig. 8.26. Patient slides down the operating table with head lying on the ECG cable

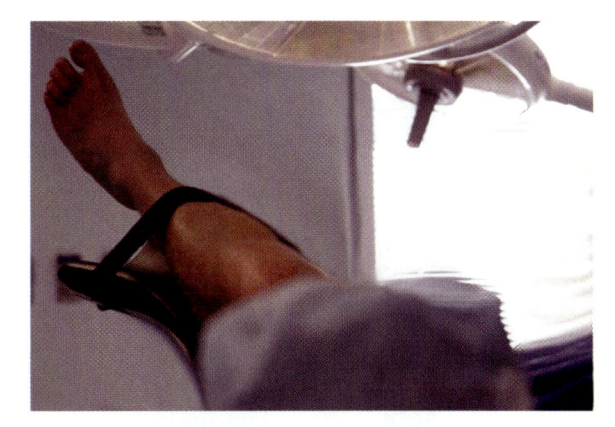

Fig. 8.28. Incorrect positioning of the leg in the Goepel holder, without padding and with pressure on the head of the fibula

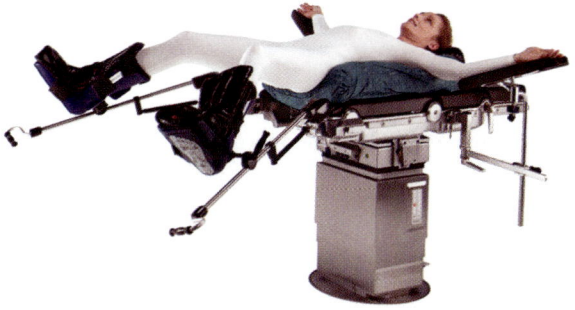

Fig. 8.29. Positioning the legs in special leg holders

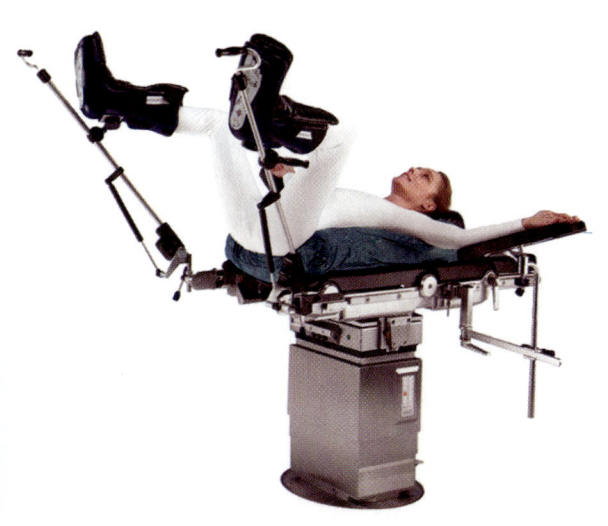

Fig. 8.27. Comfortable leg and back positioning

8.4.2 Back and pelvis

Special attention and care is required when positioning the pelvis/sacrum. Excessive warmth from water mats and local loads on the sacrum will encourage the development of pressure sores. Here again, the vacuum mat can be used as a suitable precaution, because the mat moulds itself to the whole back region, distributing the contact pressure which is thus also reduced at the exposed regions of the back. A dimpled gel mat with direct body contact can be beneficial for this kind of positioning because it distributes the contact pressure better. Furthermore, a drainage effect is achieved in case the drapes are inadequately adhered, so that the buttocks do not have to lie in disinfectants and body fluids.

8.4.3 Legs

The legs are normally positioned in Goepel leg holders (Figs. 8.23, 8.28). Another possibility is to use modern pneumatic leg holders with well padded calf boots (Figs. 8.25, 8.27, 8.29 and 8.30). These leg holders are recommended for longer operations, because the pressure is on the soles of the feet and less on the calves. Another version is to position with feet in leg holders with removable heel loops.

It is ideal if the leg holders are fitted at the level of the hip joint to prevent the patient from slipping on the operating table if the legs are moved. The end of the foot and knee of a leg should form an axis with the opposite shoulder. Unfortunately, compartment syndrome of the lower leg is not rare after an operation lasting several hours in the lithotomy position. Repeated, regular movement of the legs (not massage) during the operation by an assistant would help to prevent positioning complications and also reduce the risk of an embolism. Here it is sufficient to

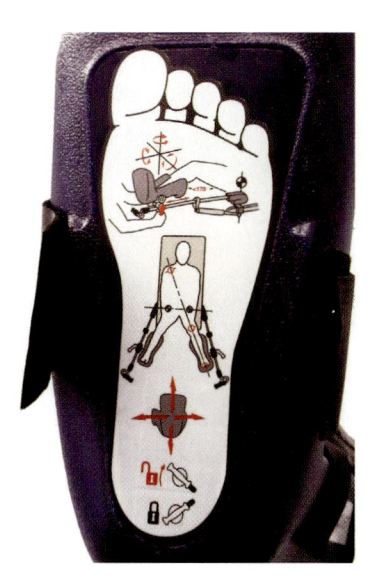

Fig. 8.30. Diagram to show positioning of the legs in the lithotomy position

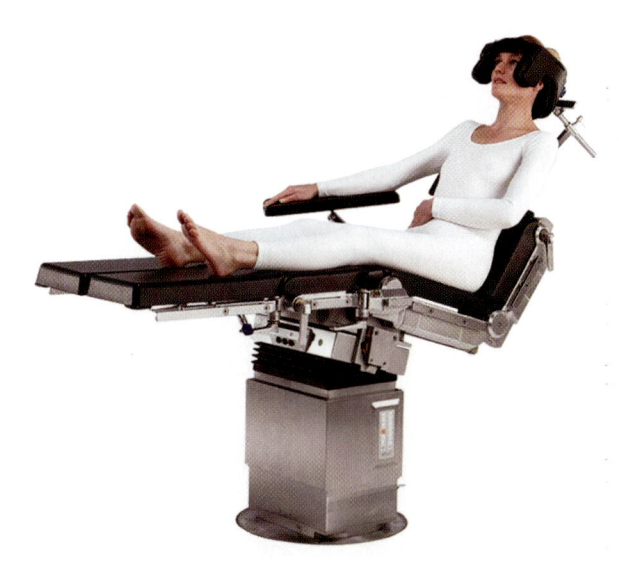

Fig. 8.31. Beach-chair position

apply slight pressure to the sole of the foot to relieve the calf briefly.

8.5 Beach-chair position

Three versions of the beach-chair position are common practice.

To prepare the operating table for the *first* version, it is sufficient to provide an operating table (here Maquet 1120 position II), but definitive positioning of the patient is time consuming, and requires physical effort and commitment on the part of the staff. After consulting the anaesthetist, the patient is positioned head-down on the fitted horseshoe headrest. After placing suitable positioning pads under the patient's buttocks (here: wedge and block pads depending on the patient's size), the operating table is brought gradually into the half-sitting position. The back plate is raised alternately with a low head movement of the whole operating table until the final position is reached. At the same time, the patient is pushed right over onto the operating side until the patient's side is on the edge of the table. Finally the leg plates are adjusted manually and the head is fixed.

Replacing the leg plates for a special shoulder plate in Maquet 1120 position I results in the *second* possibility for a sitting/half-sitting position. The operating table is adjusted by electromechanical means using the remote control. In this version, the positioning aids are already completely fitted to the table. The patient has been arranged in position and the table can be adjusted as usual until the final position is reached. It is rarely necessary to use positioning aids (wedge and block pads). In this case, the shoulder is exposed by removing a shoulder segment. This version involves minimum personnel and physical effort and takes up a minimum of time.

The *third version is described here for the universal operating table* 1150.30. The operating table is equipped with the *shoulder plate* component before the patient is brought into the operating suite. Once again, it is not necessary to fit additional positioning aids to the operating table, and the patient is already arranged with head and shoulders in position. After starting the anaesthetic and moving the patient board onto the operating table column, the patient board is aligned so that the operating side points towards the instrument nurse. To support sturdy, firm positioning, the buttocks are moved to the outer edge of the seat plate. The operating table can also be moved to the opposite side with the *tilting* function. There should therefore not be any protruding pins in the area of the seat plate bars to fasten operating table pads (Fig. 8.31).

8.5.1 Head

The distance between horseshoe headrest and the head end of the operating table depends on the patient's size. The head and cervical spine are positioned in the middle/neutral setting. The head should no longer be fixed and held to the horseshoe headrest with wide transparent plasters over the forehead. Today the head can be positioned comfortably in a helmet with special padding for the cervical spine and secured with a padded belt across the forehead (Fig. 8.32).

8.6 · Prone position

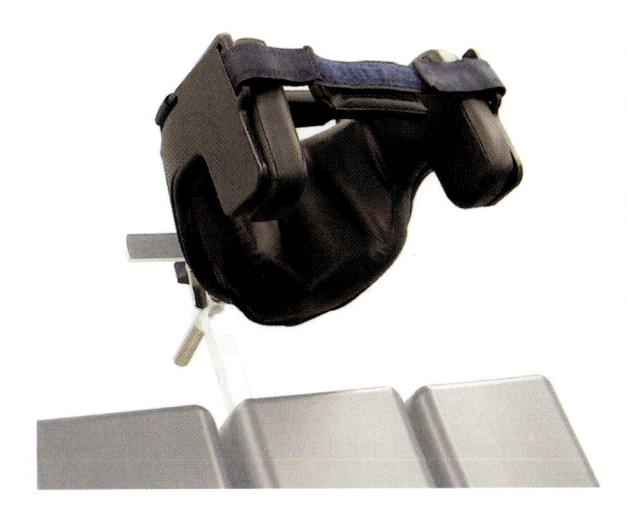

Fig. 8.32. Helmet for sitting position

8.5.2 Shoulders and arms

In the end, the patient should be positioned to give the surgeon suitable, free access to the operating site by removing the shoulder plate segment. If necessary, the arm can be positioned with abduction if required for the anaesthetic. On the operating side, the arm is usually positioned directly at the body (Fig. 8.33).

8.5.3 Back and pelvis

In this position, the upper body does not lie with its full weight on the back plate of the operating table but also puts pressure on the pelvis and thighs. Special attention must be given to distributing the contact pressure in this area. A thorax support can provide the patient with additional support on the side (Figs. 8.34, 8.35).

8.5.4 Legs

If necessary, a half roll is placed under the knees at the distal thigh. In other cases, a wedge pad can also be placed under the thighs. Pressure on the heels should always be reduced to a minimum, depending on the planned operation. One possibility is to use small gel mats placed under the calf. But the leg should always have the greatest possible contact with the patient board with every kind of padding (▶ see also Sect. 8.3.4).

8.6 Prone position

The patient is placed under anaesthetic while still supine and rolled into the operating theatre still supine. In the operating theatre, the arm positioning devices are brought into position and the patient is turned over onto the abdo-

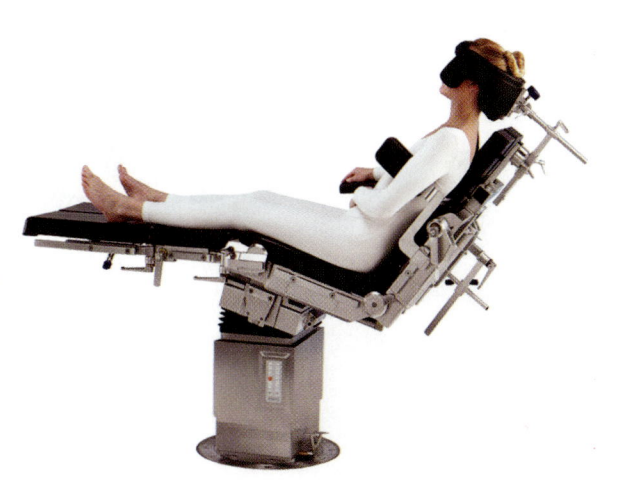

Fig. 8.34. Beach-chair position with thorax support

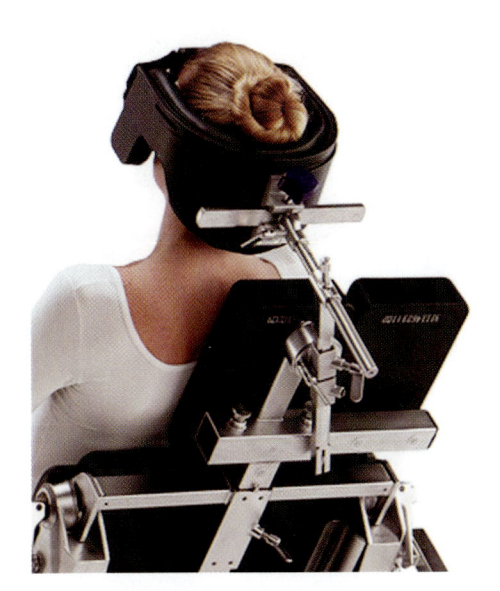

Fig. 8.33. Shoulder positioning with segment removed

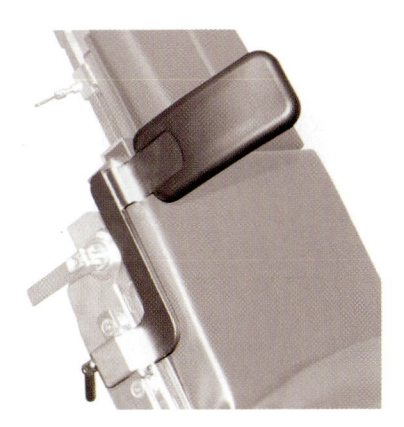

Fig. 8.35. Thorax support

men by at least four persons. The positioning aids are fitted in position.

Before placing the head on the positioning aid, padding must be placed under the thorax!

But the procedure for changing the patient's position can be much simpler for everyone involved by preparing a second operating table with the corresponding positioning aids, adjusting it in height to be lower than the first operating table, and the patient is then rolled over into the prone position (Figs. 8.36, 8.37).

In any case it is important to consult the anaesthetist to ensure that IV drips and monitoring leads (ECG) are secured or, preferably, disconnected while repositioning the patient.

8.6.1 Head

In the prone position, the head must be arranged using various positioning aids so that the cervical spine is in the middle/neutral position (awake, ▶ see. Figs. 8.38–8.41).

8.6.2 Arms

Both arms are lowered about 30° in the shoulder and brought forward by max. 90° with a bend of about 90° at the elbow. The lower arms are placed on the arm positioning devices, ensuring that the elbows are free (for short arm supports) or well padded (Fig. 8.47). The patient's upper arms must not be positioned at the lateral edges of the operating table (incorrect arm positioning Figs. 8.42–8.45).

The rule of thumb for positioning the arms in the prone position:
Position the distal joint of the arm lower than the proximal joint.

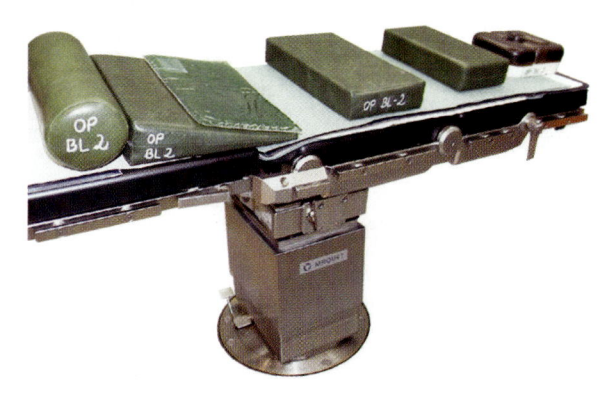

Fig. 8.36. Operating table with positioning aids ready in position

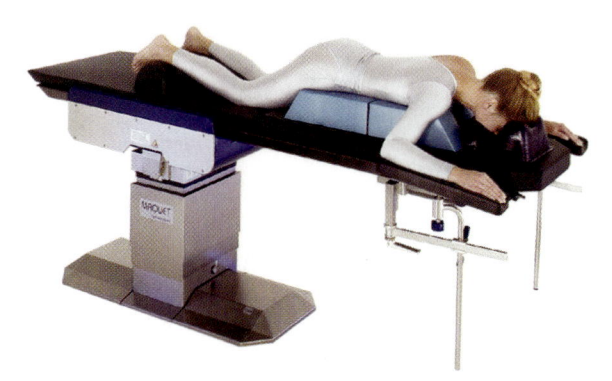

Fig. 8.37. Prone position on the CRP operating table

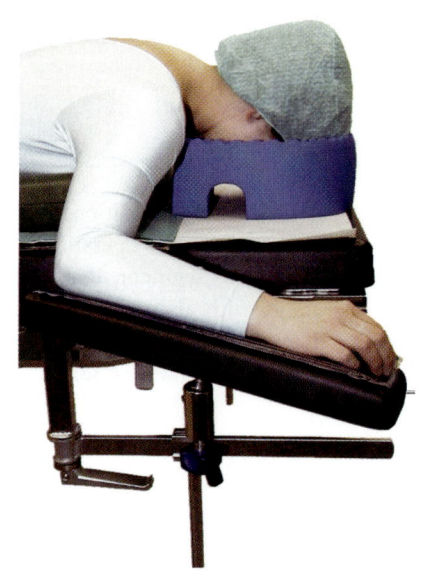

Fig. 8.38. Head position on dimpled foam cushion

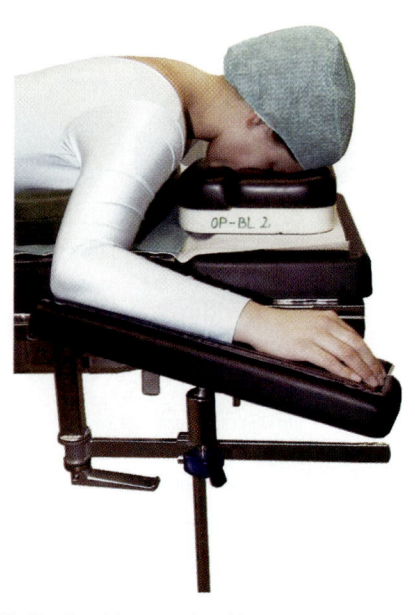

Fig. 8.39. Head position on gel cushion

8.6 · Prone position

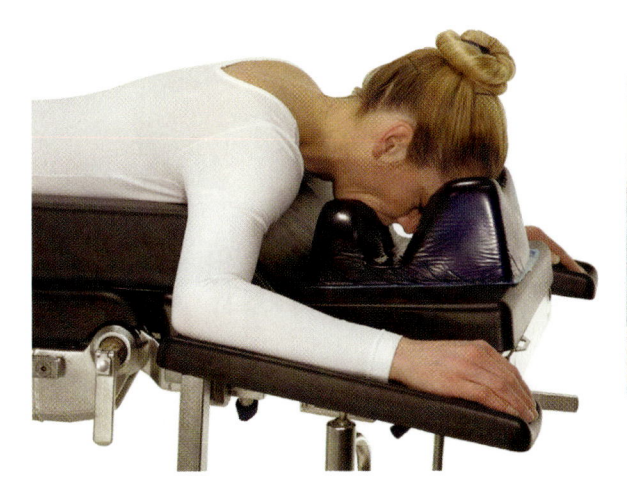

Fig. 8.40. Head position on gel cushion

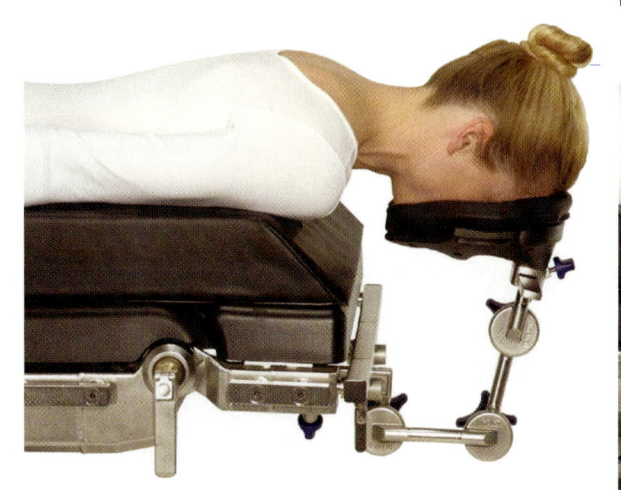

Fig. 8.41. Head position on one-piece horseshoe headrest

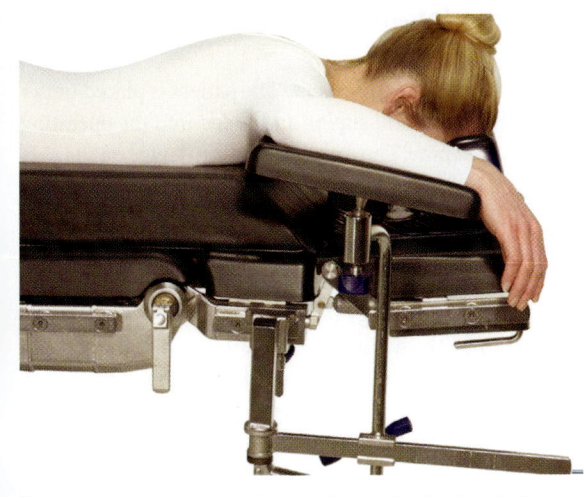

Fig. 8.42. Incorrect arm positioning. The arm is raised too high on the short armrest with *dropped wrist*

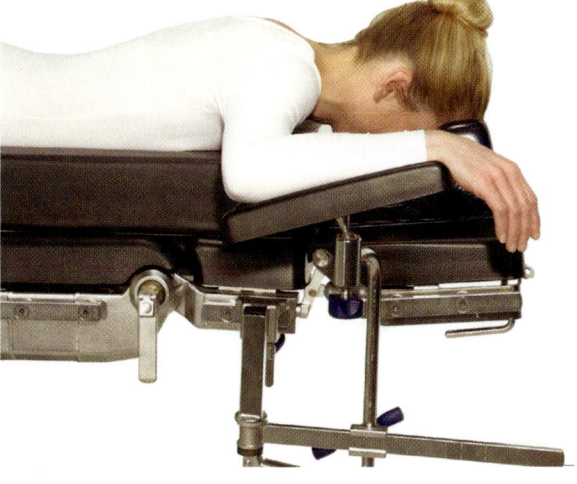

Fig. 8.43. Incorrect arm positioning. The arm is raised too high on the short armrest with *dropped wrist*

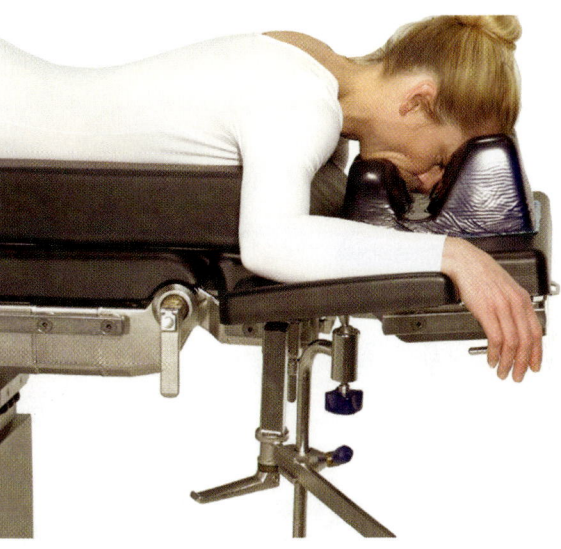

Fig. 8.44. Incorrect arm positioning, *dropped wrist* and unfavourable position of the shoulder

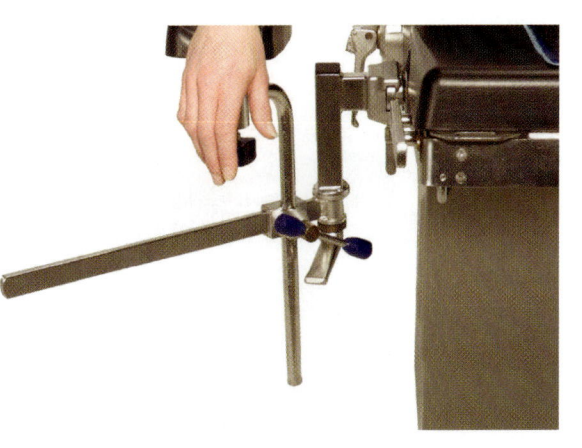

Fig. 8.45. Incorrect arm positioning, *dropped wrist* and unfavourable position of the clamps

This means the elbow is lower than the shoulder and the wrist lower than the elbow (Figs. 8.40, 8.46, 8.47).

8.6.3 Thorax and pelvis

The thorax and pelvis are raised using suitable positioning pads so that the abdomen is free and the patient's breathing is not affected. It is important that the pelvic pad does not to squash the blood vessels in the groin (*vena cava syndrome*). The dimensions for the positioning pads depend on the patient's size (Fig. 8.48).

8.6.4 Legs

The patient's knees and feet are positioned with protection from pressure sores by placing a wide wedge pad, roll and, if necessary, small gel mat under the knees (Fig. 8.49).

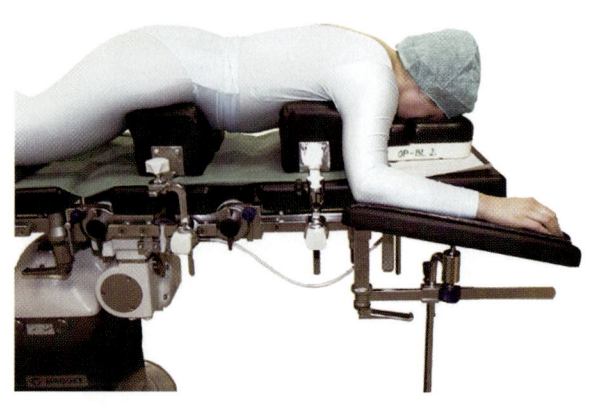

Fig. 8.48. Abdominal position on 4 special bolsters

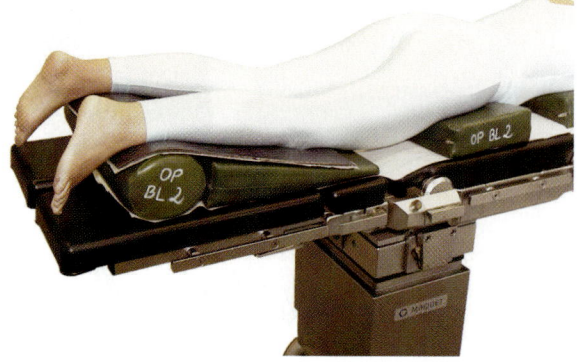

Fig. 8.49. Leg positioning with wedge cushion and roll

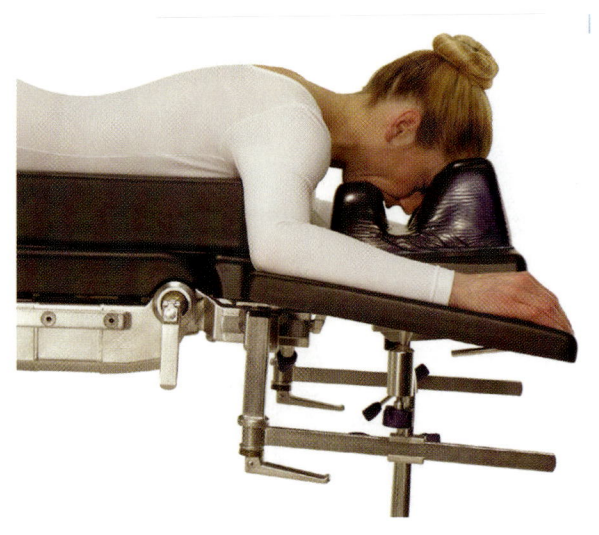

Fig. 8.46. Safe arm position and ideal shoulder position

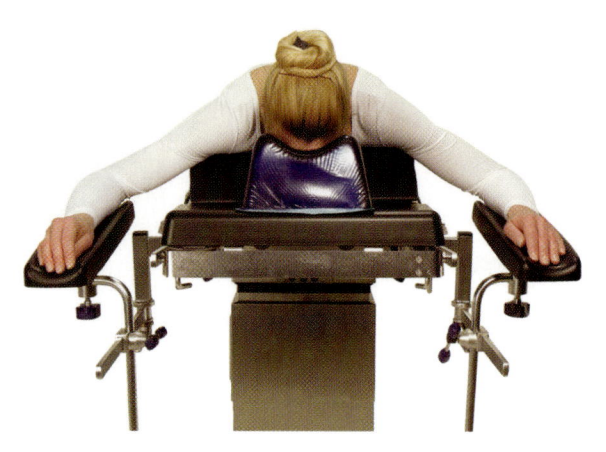

Fig. 8.47. Arm positioning to protect the nerves and optimum shoulder position on the arm positioning device

8.7 The lateral position

Version without vacuum mat. The patient is placed under anaesthetic while still supine and rolled into the operating theatre still supine. The arm positioning device on the side not being operated is positioned at an angle of 90° to the operating table. A Goepel leg holder is fitted to the rail of the headrest using a radial adjustment clamp, this is for the upper arm. The patient is brought into the lateral position using kinesiology (Fig. 8.50).

Version with vacuum mat. The vacuum mat is moulded to the body of the patient in the lateral position, then the air is withdrawn from the mat with a surgical suction unit or special pump. This means the patient is now lying in a bed fitted to his body shape. If before extracting the air a side support is fitted for safety reasons to either side on the level of the sacrum and symphysis if the operating table is expected to tilt to the side, as far as possible the support should not be in contact with the patient but support the vacuum mat (Fig. 8.51).

8.7 · The lateral position

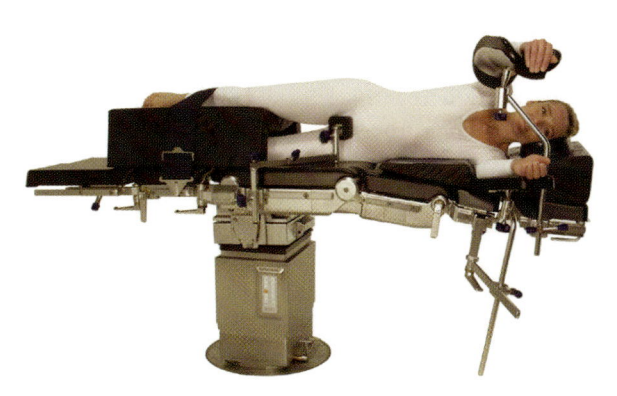

Fig. 8.50. Lateral position

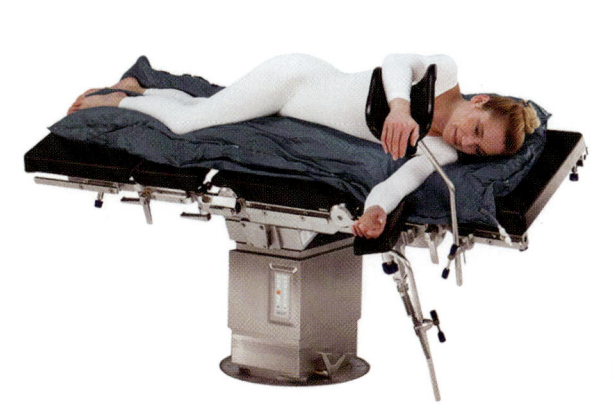

Fig. 8.51. Lateral position with vacuum mat

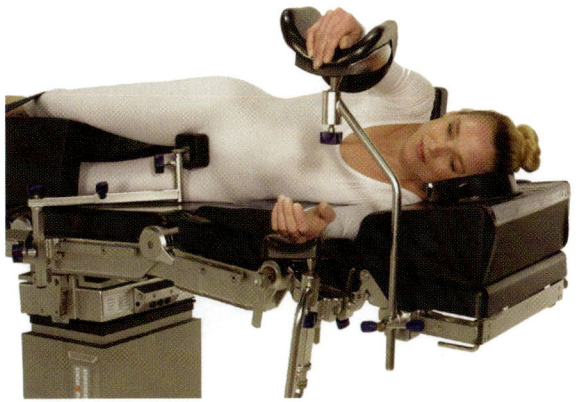

Fig. 8.52. Positioning the patient on a special cushion for lateral position

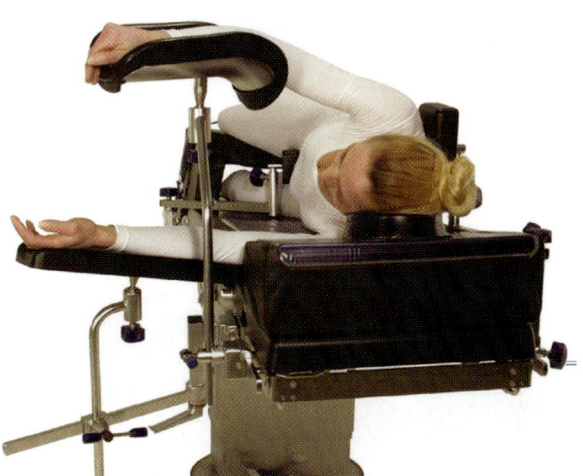

Fig. 8.53. The left ear is kept free with a gel ring

8.7.1 Head

The operating table headrest is adjusted in such a way that the patient's head is positioned with the spinal column in a straight neutral position in the area of the lower cervical spine. Another version is to use a gel ring as additional padding for the head (Figs. 8.52, 8.53).

8.7.2 Shoulders and arms

The lower arm is pulled forwards slightly and placed on the arm support device which stands at an angle of 90° to the operating table and reaches up to the table. The upper arm is abducted maximum 90° in the shoulder and positioned with the lower arm and slightly bent elbow on the Goepel leg holder. Both arms are padded with small gel mats (Fig. 8.54).

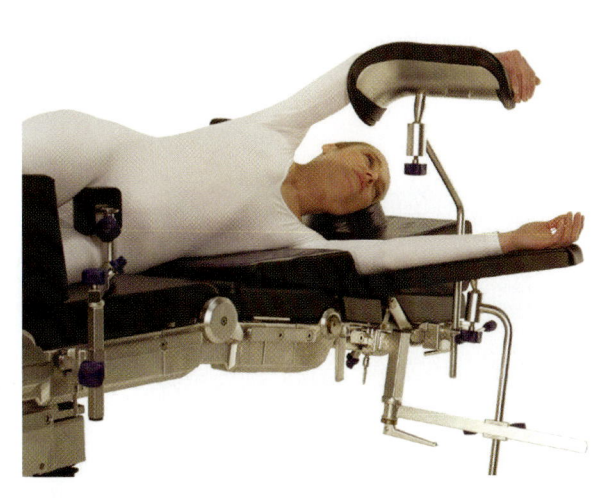

Fig. 8.54. Maximum 90° abduction of the arms with shoulders moved forwards

8.7.3 Thorax and pelvis

A foam or gel roll is pushed under the lower thorax side to relieve the shoulder. The special pad for the lateral position cushions the thorax to a large extent and supports the lower arm and shoulder with a padding effect (◘ Fig. 8.55).

The pelvis is supported with two side supports at the symphysis and sacrum. For operations to the lower extremities, the side supports are fitted to the rails of the lower back plate or seat plate from the head end, and for lateral thoracotomy, retroperitoneal access or procedures to the vertebral column, from the foot end, (◘ Fig. 8.56).

8.7.4 Legs

A tunnel cushion is positioned between the legs to prevent pressure sores. By using the tunnel cushion, the weight of the upper leg does not impair the position of the lower leg. One or two body belts fix the positioning of the legs and pads (◘ Fig. 8.57).

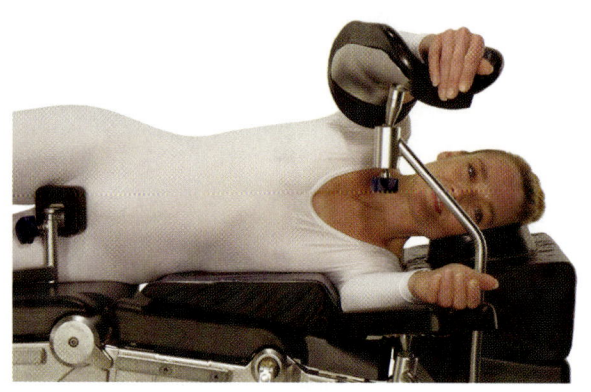

◘ **Fig. 8.55.** Padding under the thorax and positioning of the lower arm and shoulder so as to provide relief

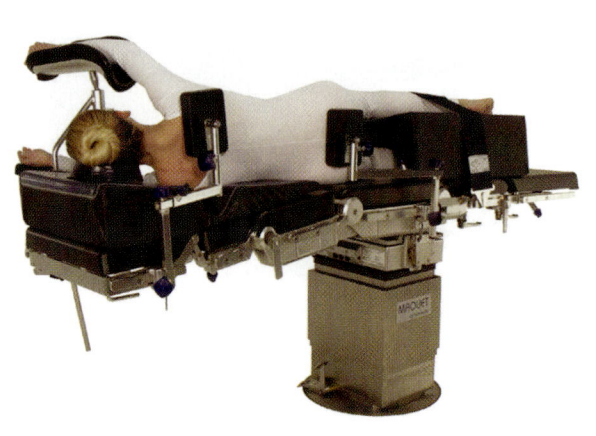

◘ **Fig. 8.56.** Support for shoulder and sacrum

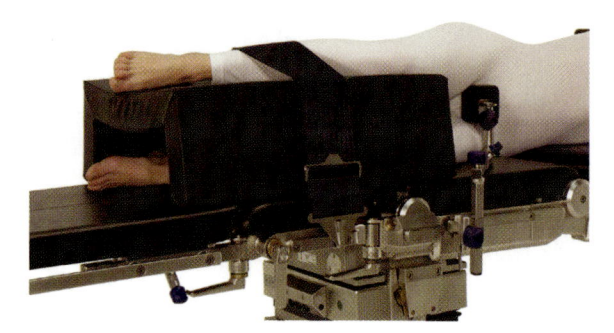

◘ **Fig. 8.57.** Tunnel cushion, patient safeguarded with body belt

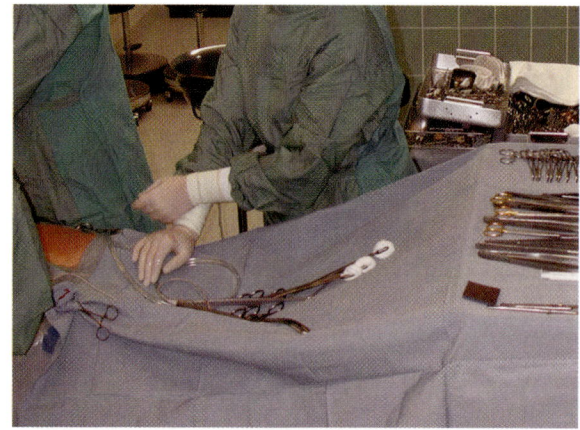

◘ **Fig. 8.58.** The surgical nurse is leaning on the patient's left knee

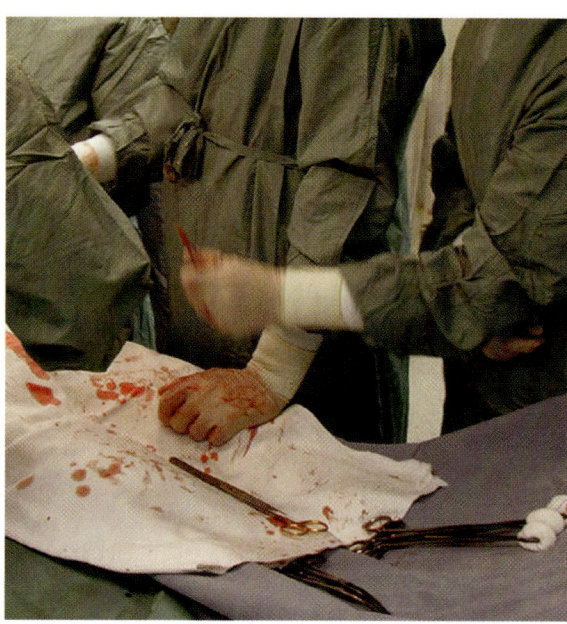

◘ **Fig. 8.59.** The surgeon is leaning on the patient's left knee

8.8 Final remarks

It is not only the standard positioning procedures, our positioning know-how and the positioning aids which protect the patient from positioning injuries. The operating team must be disciplined in continuing to support the prophylaxis measures during the operation. Frequently one of the team members will lean on the patient's knee without realising it. The patient in ◘ Figs. 8.58 and 8.59 has not been supported by a half roll under the knee. Here the left knee is straightened with increased pressure on the heels. Neither is it necessary for the instruments to lie on the legs.

Our aim is for the patient to be satisfied after the operation, having been well padded by the team during the operation, and kept in a dry, warm position (◘ Fig. 8.60).

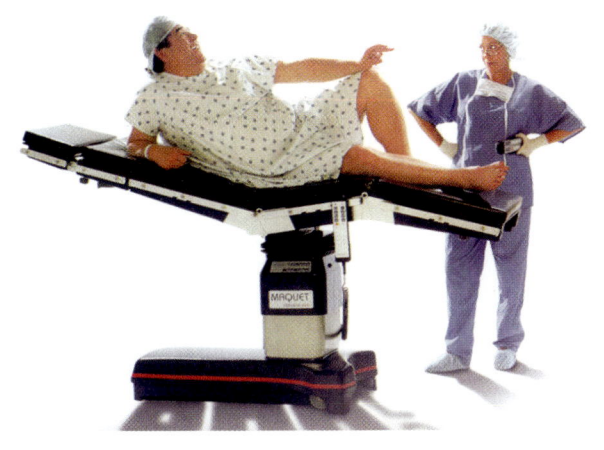

◘ **Fig. 8.60.** A satisfied patient after the operation

9 Function workflow in the operating suite

D. Aschemann, A. Gänsslen, L. Mahlke

9.1 Standard steps in the elective programme – 108
9.1.1 Patient reception – 108
9.1.2 Selection of the operating table and placing the patient on it – 108
9.1.3 Preparation of the patient in the anaesthesia induction room – 108
9.1.4 Definitive positioning – 109
9.1.5 Preparing the bed and measures at the end of the operation – 109

9.2 Preparations in an emergency (under time pressure) – 110

9.3 Preparations for open fractures – 110

9.1 Standard steps in the elective programme

Preparation of the patient for the planned operation begins on making the indication and planning the date. Special implants or special positioning aids, for example a cervical spine holder, must be ordered in plenty of time and be available in time for the operation, and be sterilised if necessary.

In our own procedures, it has become established practice for the medical director/senior doctor to check the indication on the day before the operation (preferably before informing the patient), with corresponding instructions for the operating nurse/orderly who is on duty with regard to the expected positioning (including position aids) or additional materials required (e.g., special implants, imaging intensifier, Iso-C3D). If necessary, the side being operated will also be indicated (for operations to the extremities or when there are two organs).

About 10–20 min before being called to the operating suite, the ward staff administer the patient's premedication and the transport staff bring the patient to the operating suite, bringing all the files with the findings and necessary X-ray pictures. It is normally not necessary to wash the patient at this point because as a rule, this will already have been done by the patient or nursing staff on the ward. The patient is wearing disposable pants and a surgical gown.

9.1.1 Patient reception

On arriving in the patient sluice, the patient is welcomed by the operating staff. Firstly unambiguous identification of the patient is checked verbally or according to the files. If this is not possible, a person must be called to identify the patient. The records of the surgeon and anaesthetist informing the patient about the procedure are checked for the patient's written documented consent before moving the patient. While the patient is still awake, the side being operated should be checked according to the operating schedule. If the patient is not conscious, this is checked together with the operating surgeon.

9.1.2 Selection of the operating table and placing the patient on it

The operating table and required positioning aids are chosen according to the kind of procedure and the special aspects clarified before the operation (▶ see Sect. 9.1).

The patient's bed and the operating table are adjusted to the same height. The patient can now either slide over onto the operating table from his bed; he should not have to stand up to do so, because the premedication can cause

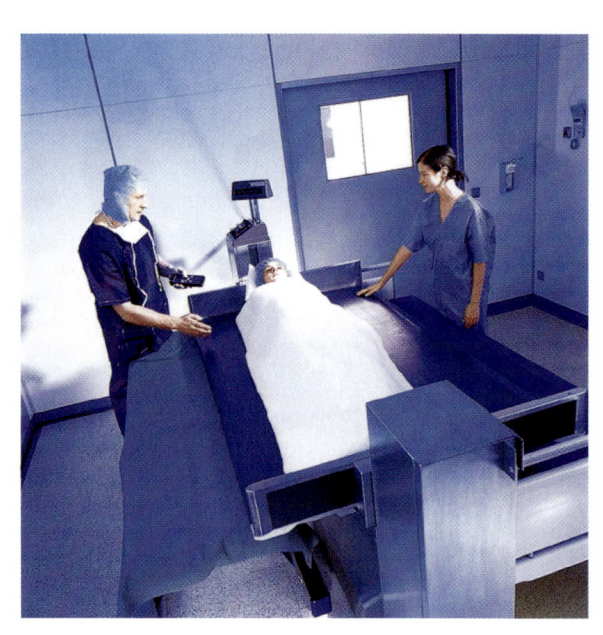

Fig. 9.1. Patient transfer system

orthostatic problems (e.g. circulatory collapse). Neither should the patient suffer from unnecessary pain during the transfer, to ensure that the anaesthetic can be started gently.

On the other hand, the patient can be moved with a roll board or patient transfer system. This method should be given preference in the case of instable, painful conditions. Well instructed staff are vital in both cases (◘ Fig. 9.1).

9.1.3 Preparing the patient in the anaesthesia induction room

In the anaesthesia induction room, the patient is placed under anaesthetic. While the patient is being prepared by the team of anaesthetists, the positioning aids are put at the ready. After intubation or completion of the local anaesthetic, work starts to prepare the patient for the operation. If necessary the disposable underwear is removed (e.g. hip operation). General body hygiene has already been completed on the ward. If necessary, the operating site can be cleaned again in the anaesthesia induction room. This is always the case after removing any bandages or plaster casts and in the case of dirty operating sites, for example in the case of open injuries. If the patient has to be shaved in the incision area and area for applying the neutral electrode, this is carried out with a dry, sparse procedure after placing an absorbent disposable cloth underneath. After replacing the cloth, the operating site is washed with a washing lotion and then dried with pads. The operating site is then rubbed with alcoholic disinfectant and covered with a sterile drape. Any necessary tourniquet can be applied now, taking great care to ensure that no residual moisture collects under the tourniquet. The neutral electrode is only applied after completing the definitive positioning procedure!

9.1.4 Definitive positioning

After moving into the operating theatre, the operating table is positioned on the column, the transporter removed from the theatre and the table brought to its final position (e.g. for surgery to the arm: operating table positioned crosswise in the room). Having made all positioning aids and accessories for special positioning available in advance, work can now begin promptly on positioning of the patient (◘ Fig. 9.2).

The definitive positioning is brought to its conclusion with application of the neutral electrode and connecting up to the HF surgery device, connecting the tourniquet to the pressure gauge, applying adhesive drapes for preparation of the operating site and, if necessary, replacing the absorbent sheet under the extremity to be washed. The patient is always covered with warm drapes or, at the latest in this preparatory phase, with a patient warming system (◘ Fig. 9.3).

The operating lights are positioned so that the sterile light handles can be plugged in quickly.

Skin disinfection by the surgeon must take place with the extremity held up high (◘ Fig. 9.4).

After disinfecting the skin, the operating site is covered correctly by several persons in sterile clothing, or a washed extremity is handed over to sterile staff (◘ Fig. 9.5).

The operation can begin (◘ Fig. 9.6).

9.1.5 Preparing the bed and measures at the end of the operation

Meanwhile the equipment for postoperative positioning of the patient is placed at the ready. The bed is chosen according to the patient's size. There is a choice between standard beds, children's beds, cots or intensive care beds,

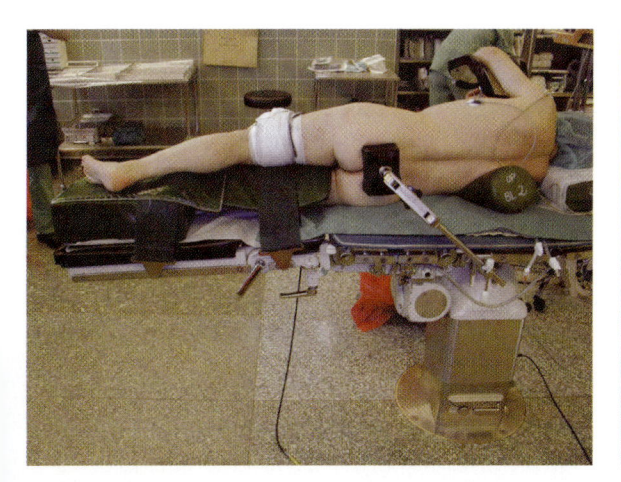

◘ **Fig. 9.2.** Definitive positioning of the patient

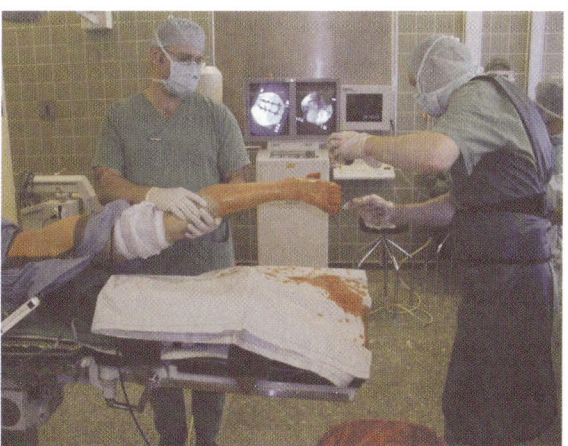

◘ **Fig. 9.4.** Skin disinfection

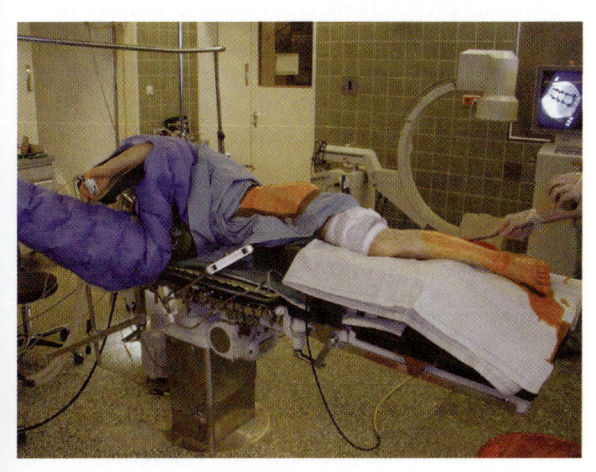

◘ **Fig. 9.3.** Patient warming system

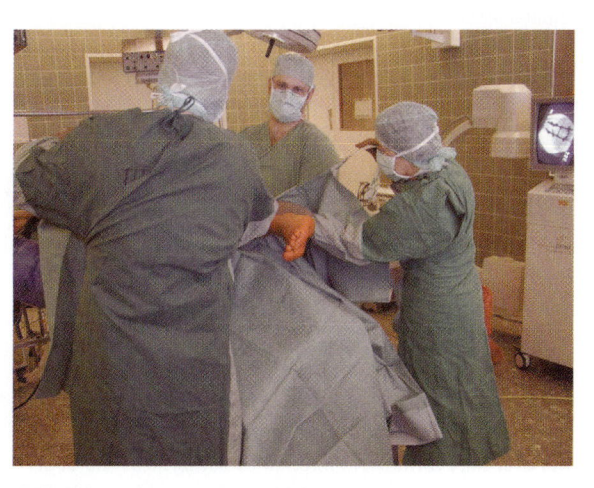

◘ **Fig. 9.5.** Handing over the washed extremity

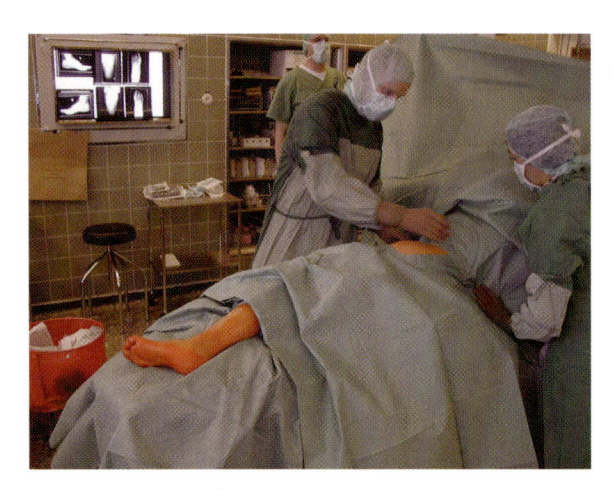

Fig. 9.6. At the end of the sterile covering phase

with bed extensions, extension devices or special rails which can be fitted if necessary. It has become indispensable practice to heat the bed for the patient after the operation using an electric blanket.

At the end of the operation, a sterile bandage is applied by the operating team, the patient is disconnected from the HF surgery device and any other connections are removed (e.g. tourniquet). Disposable or multiple use covers are disposed of in the normal containers. If necessary, postoperative X-rays are taken to allow for possibly necessary surgical corrections before bringing the patient round after the anaesthetic. For extubation, the patient is moved from the definitive positioning back into the supine position, and the extremities are held with body belts. It has proven effective to place the arms parallel to the body on the arm positioning supports in this phase. The patient can be extubated in the operating theatre or in the post-anaesthesia room to keep the circulation concept working in the surgical department.

If necessary, a postoperative plaster cast can be applied before the patient leaves the operating suite; for hygiene reasons, this should not be done in the operating theatre itself.

The patient is transferred to a preheated bed in the patient sluice by the surgeon and anaesthetist together. To do so, the bed is raised to the level of the operating table. Depending on the positioning and kind of anaesthetic, the patient should be transferred by sliding onto the roll board or using a patient transfer system, by rolling from the prone directly into the supine position on the bed or by the patient sliding over on his own. It is up to the surgeon to ensure that any peripheral drips, drainage tubes and thorax drains are securely positioned, even if the patient transfer phase consists of team work. The patient is placed in the middle of the bed without any contact with the edges. Any positioning cushions or rails are fitted and the drainage containers fixed to the outside of the bed. In the case of freshly extubated patients, padded side bars should be fitted to the bed initially and the patient should be monitored constantly.

The patient is then brought to the recovery room or intensive care station. In exceptional cases with regional or local anaesthetic, the patient can also be brought straight to the normal ward.

9.2 Preparations in an emergency (under time pressure)

Time and again situations occur where the patient's life can only be saved by acting immediately and starting to operate without delay, for example massive haemorrhaging, circulatory instability or resuscitation. These situations frequently demand improvisation because the normal planned procedure would take too long. Here it is important to weigh up the various risks to obtain the best outcome in each specific situation.

Fundamentally, an operating table prepared with a water mat or electric heating mat should always be at the ready in every operating department. The vital problem of cooling down can be reduced at least by the use of a heating mat or moving mat for operating tables. Recently, disposable covers with circulating hot air have proven effective on the non-operated regions. Similarly, a neutral electrode should also always be ready on the operating table for immediate application. Depending on the expected emergency operation, the possibility of having to re-bed the patient during the operation must be considered. Even under time pressure, a minimum level of perioperative safeguards should always be provided, to prevent the patient from falling off the table, to avoid further damage from pressure sores, etc.

Management is defined by the operating surgeon, who stipulates the scope and sequence of the surgical procedure in consultation with other disciplines (e.g. anaesthetist) even under time pressure. Typical operation preparations are usually carried out parallel to diagnosis, anaesthetic preparations, transport and transfer to the operating table.

Immediately before the operation begins, the operating site is prepared quickly but thoroughly (depilation, washing) while the surgeon disinfects his hands. But it does happen that such measures have to be omitted completely.

9.3 Preparations for open fractures

The patient with an open extremity fracture is usually brought into the operating suite with a lying splint (e.g. air chamber splint). Usually sterile bandages have already been applied to the wound by the emergency doctor (Fig. 9.7).

9.3 · Preparations for open fractures

In the emergency room, the emergency doctor reports about the extent of the injury so that the wound does not have to be uncovered and inspected again here (risk of contamination).

The patient is usually placed under anaesthetic already in the resuscitation room, but at the latest on arrival in the operating theatre; under certain circumstances, this may already take place on the emergency stretcher to save the patient from the pain of transfer.

It is advisable to keep the required materials in a special cabinet or mobile unit which can be positioned at the anaesthesia induction sluice without any problems. It is important that the utensils required to prepare surgery for closed and open fractures are always at the ready.

The washing trolleys we use keep adequate quantities of the following materials at the ready (see also Fig. 9.8):
- non-sterile razors,
- non-sterile disposable gloves,
- non-sterile, absorbent disposable sheets,
- sterile razors,
- sterile gloves,
- sterile absorbent disposable sheets,
- sterile hand brushes,
- sterile bacteriology tubes,
- sterile disposable drapes,
- sterile saline bowls (*separate bowl and washing utensils for every open fracture!*),
- compresses *without* contrasting stripe!
- saline solution in 1-l bottles (also from the warming cabinet),
- washing lotion,
- disinfectant.

After placing the patient under anaesthetic, the fracture splint is removed, the affected extremity is held up under longitudinal tension by an assistant who wears disposable gloves for protection, and the sterile bandage is removed.

After removing the sterile bandage, a first swab is taken from the wound for forensic reasons before cleansing the wound. According to the protocol valid in our institution, an intravenous antibiotic was already administered in the emergency room.

An absorbent disposable sheet (sterile if the extremity is put down in between!) is placed under the injured extremity to soak up any dripping blood and the washing lotion and disinfectant.

If necessary the wound or operating site is shaved as sparsely as possible, dry or wet, with a sterile disposable razor, taking note of the fact that the shaved hairs can only be removed efficiently from the skin with a strip of plaster after a dry shave.

Under continuing longitudinal tension to avoid further damage to the soft tissues, the injured extremity is now washed by an assistant who already wears sterile gloves (Fig. 9.9).

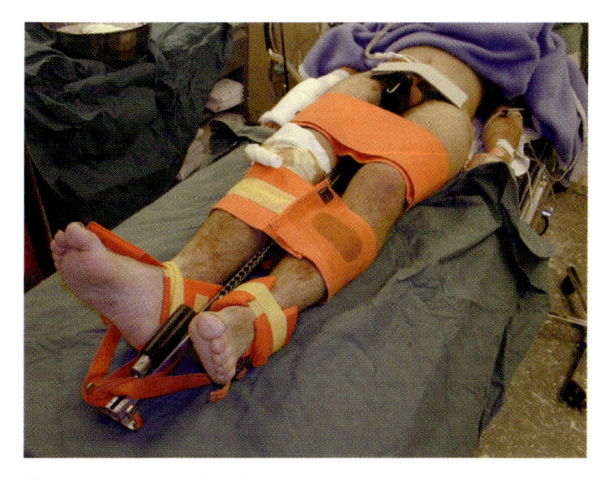

Fig. 9.7. Fracture splints for the lower extremities

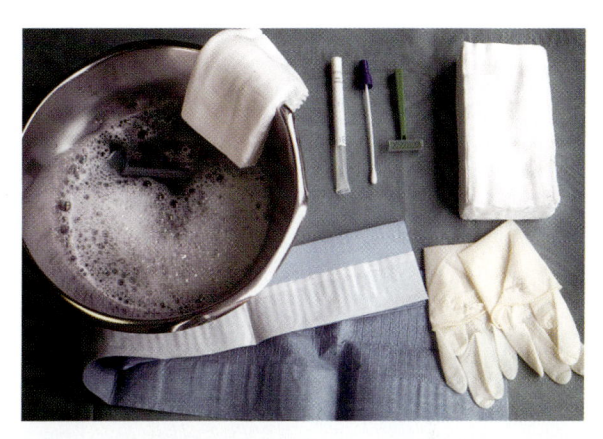

Fig. 9.8. Prepared washing utensils

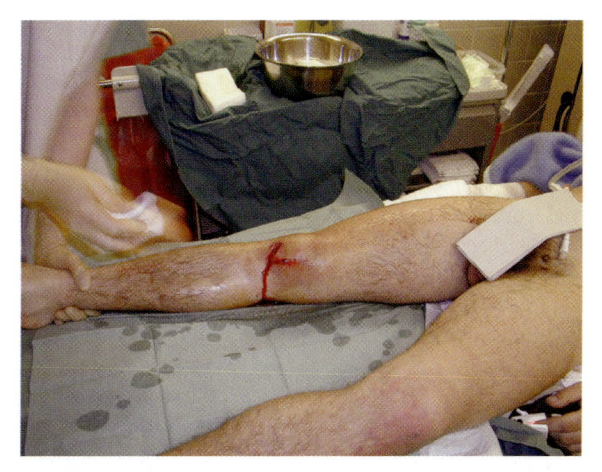

Fig. 9.9. Cleaning the injured extremity

The extremity is lathered thoroughly with sterile compresses and a saline washing solution mixed in a sterile saline bowl. The patient could be shaved with a wet shave at this point, but this is not advisable in our opinion because it is difficult to remove the shaved hair.

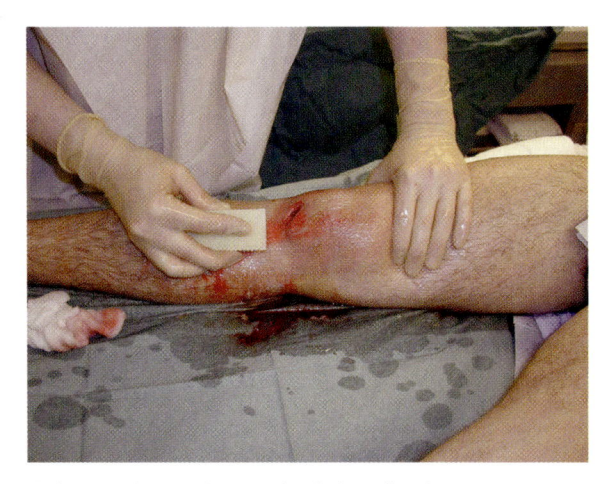

Fig. 9.10. Cleaning the wound with the nailbrush

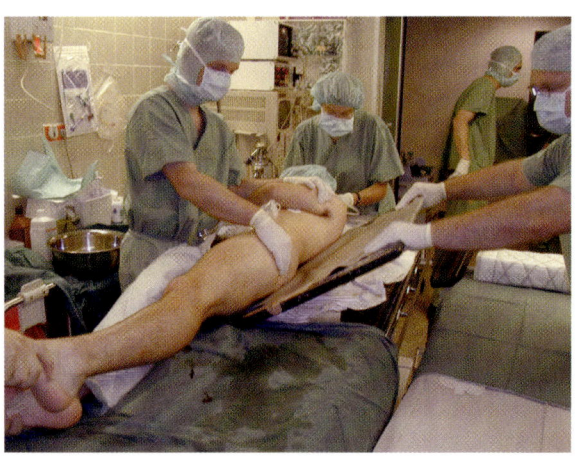

Fig. 9.12. Pushing the roll board under the patient

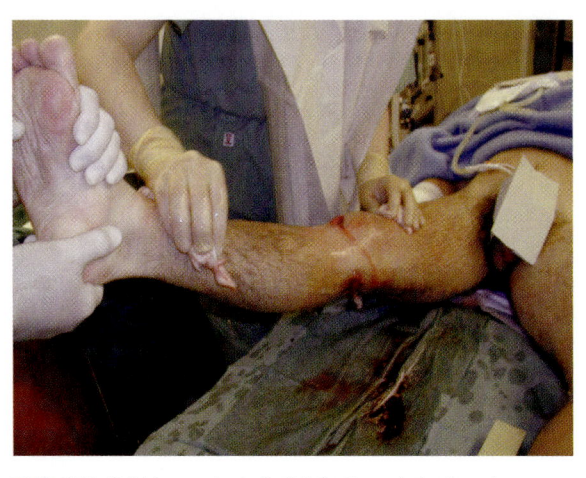

Fig. 9.11. Rubbing an alcoholic disinfection solution into the extremity under longitudinal tension

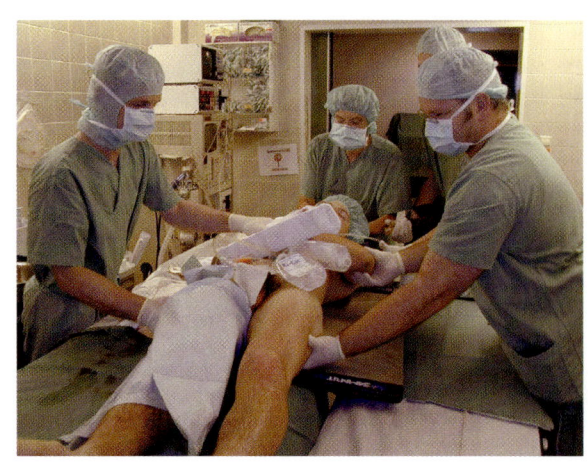

Fig. 9.13. Transferring the patient

The wound is then cleansed firstly by removing any residual coarse dirt. Larger particles are carefully removed from the wound, which is then cleaned with the hand brush to remove any impurities. Any minor bleeding at this stage is irrelevant, because this helps to clean the wound from the inside (Fig. 9.10).

After rinsing the extremity with saline solution again to remove any residual soap, the extremity is dried with sterile compresses.

The extremity is then rubbed with an alcoholic disinfectant around the area of the wound together with the wound itself (Fig. 9.11). Another swab can be taken from the wound at this point in time, with a third following after the operation has begun (Fig. 9.17).

The wound is now covered with sterile compresses and the injured extremity is wrapped in a sterile disposable towel. The patient is now transferred from the transporter to the operating table using a roll board (Figs. 9.12–9.14).

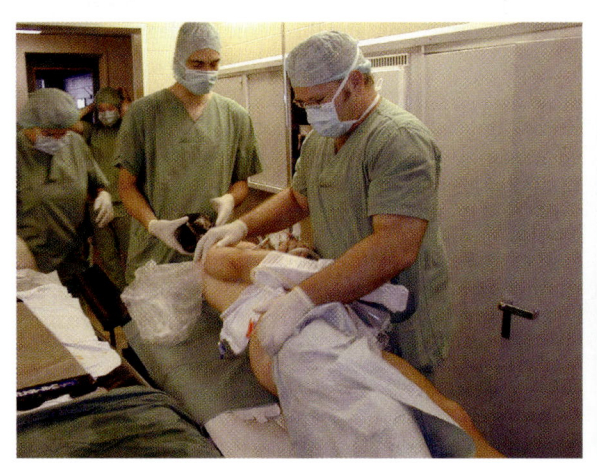

Fig. 9.14. Removing the roll board

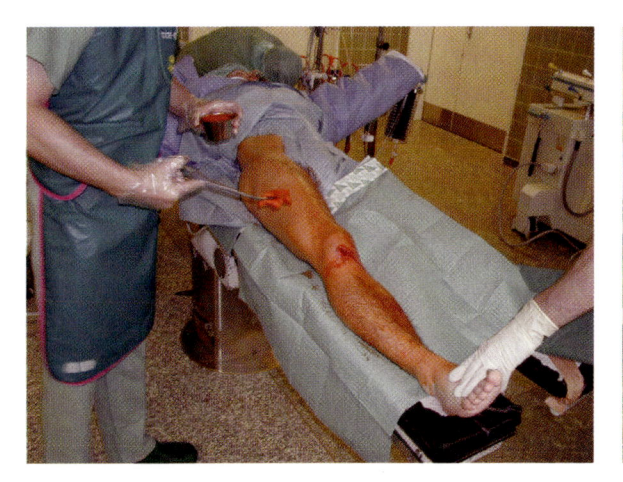

Fig. 9.15. Permanent stabilisation of the fractured extremity

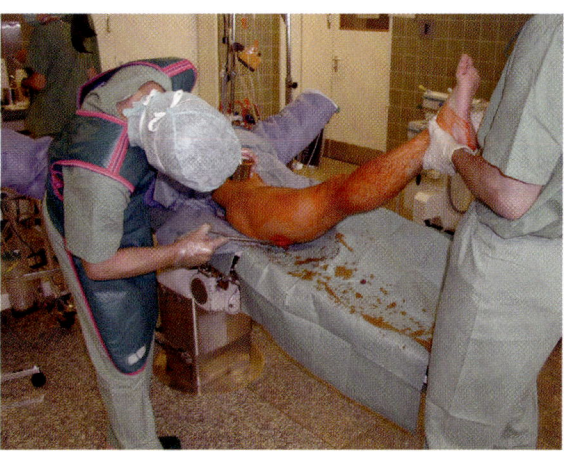

Fig. 9.16. Disinfecting the fractured extremity under longitudinal tension

Practical tip: in the case of several open fractures, each fracture must be treated as described above. However, it is important that the procedure is only performed for one injury at a time, and that completely new cleaning utensils are used after every extremity. Parallel preparations can result in an unwanted exchange of germs between the individual injuries.

As a rule, a tourniquet is not applied in the case of fractures with damaged soft tissues, even for injuries to the distal extremity. After these measures, the patient is brought into the operating theatre. Self-adhesive drapes are applied for preoperative disinfection of the skin. Finally, this is followed by definitive disinfection and sterile covering of the injured extremity (Figs. 9.15–9.17).

To optimise these procedures, the preparations can be carried out by several »teams« depending on human resources. But this is usually only possible in centres. This can help to avoid disadvantages for the patients such as hypothermia and further blood loss.

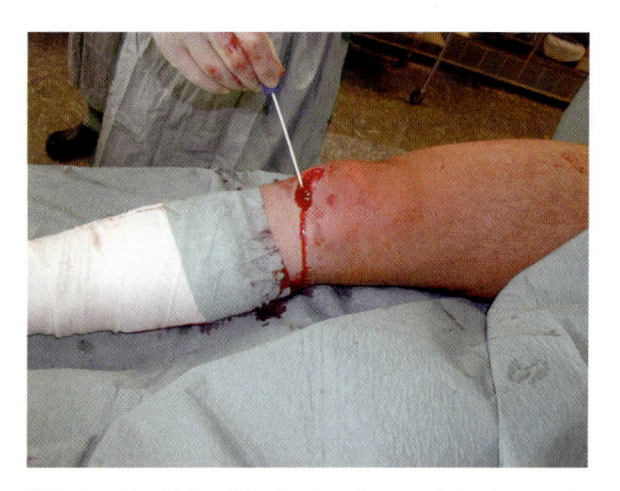

Fig. 9.17. The third swab is taken from the wound after the operation has begun

10 Complications

M. Bund, F. Logemann, H. Müller-Vahl

10.1 Positioning injuries as seen by the anaesthetist – 116
10.1.1 Division of labour between surgeon and anaesthetist – 116
10.1.2 Occurrence of positioning injuries – 116
10.1.2.1 Frequency – 116
10.1.2.2 Kind of injuries – 117
10.1.3 Supine position – 119
10.1.3.1 Struma position – 120
10.1.3.2 Extension table – 120
10.1.3.3 Lithotomy position – 121
10.1.3.4 Head-down position – 121
10.1.4 Lateral position – 121
10.1.5 Prone position – 122
10.1.6 Sitting/half-sitting position – 123
10.1.7 Final remarks – 123

10.2 Positioning the patient under resuscitation conditions – 123
10.2.1 Necessary measures – 124
10.2.2 Positioning injuries following resuscitation – 125

10.3 Positioning injuries as seen by the neurologist – 125
10.3.1 Introduction – 125
10.3.2 Frequency – 125
10.3.3 Pathophysiology – 125
10.3.4 Symptoms – 126
10.3.4.1 Diagnosis and differential diagnosis – 126
10.3.4.2 Therapy and progress – 126
10.3.5 Special nerve injuries – 127
10.3.5.1 Brachial plexus – 127
10.3.5.2 Ulnar nerve – 127
10.3.5.3 Peroneal nerve – 127
10.3.6 Lesions of the lumbosacral plexus and its branches in the lithotomy position – 128
10.3.6.1 Pudendal nerve – 128
10.3.7 Compartment syndrome following surgical positioning – 128

References – 128

10.1 Positioning injuries as seen by the anaesthetist

M. Bund

10.1.1 Division of labour between surgeon and anaesthetist

Shared responsibility

The positioning of the patient on the operating table and monitoring the correct position is a shared task for surgeon and anaesthetist. The shared responsibility and distribution of labour is stipulated in the agreements between the Professional Federation of German Anaesthetists and the Professional Federation of Surgeons or of Orthopaedic Specialists [8–10].

Accordingly, the anaesthetist is responsible for positioning the patient to put him under anaesthetic and for the phase through to starting the actual surgical positioning [74]. The patient is arranged in the operating position once all anaesthesia measures have been completed. This is defined in the responsibility of the surgeon according to the requirements of the specific operation. He monitors the initial positioning of the patient on the operating table and is also responsible for intraoperative repositioning.

During the operation, the anaesthetist is responsible for the positioning of those parts of the body which he must have under his control for the anaesthetic procedure, i.e. primarily the head and the extremities required for monitoring and infusions [11]. He uses suitable measures to secure these areas so as to prevent injuries even when the covering over the patient hinders constant visual control or the position has to be changed during the operation. The anaesthetist must warn the surgeon urgently if a positioning required for a surgical position makes it difficult to monitor the patient or even jeopardises sustaining the vital functions. The same applies if there is a risk of positioning injuries from malpositioning, unintentional changes in position during the operation or from the direct intervention of the surgeons. The benefits and risks of certain positioning are to be weighed up critically. Basically, the positioning of the patient should come as close as possible to the physiologically neutral position of the joints.

The phase of immediate postoperative monitoring through to releasing the patient from the recovery room then sees the anaesthetist with responsibility for positioning again. According to the interdisciplinary agreement, this includes transferring the patient to another bed after the end of the operation, »... unless special circumstances require the surgeon's involvement in patient transfer« [9]. It is also possible for hospitals to reach their own agreements, for example with the fundamental involvement of a surgeon in patient transfer [68].

Preoperative information and documentation

An essential issue in the anaesthetist's visit to the patient before the operation is to detect potential hazards and risks for the patient and take measures to avoid them. This also includes the risk of positioning injuries. Case history, clinical examination and X-rays can draw attention to anatomic anomalies or pathological change, such as arthrosis, cervical rib, endoprostheses or »shunt« arm. These findings are documented and their relevance discussed with the surgeon. If cervical ribs are known, the arms will not be moved out from the body because of the risk of plexus injuries [65]. In the case of neurological deficits or previous conditions, the preoperative status should be examined and documented by a neurologist. Special risks may entail giving the patient specific information about positioning injuries. Otherwise the general reference printed in the information form is adequate, to the effect that it is possible but rare for injuries to the nerves to occur with dysaesthesia and paralysis from pressure or tension in the position required for the operation.

The anaesthetist must document the kind of operative positioning on the anaesthesia protocol. A detailed description and the documentation of routine measures to control the position is not necessary in the case of standard positioning (Federal Supreme Court in its judgement pronounced on 24.01.1984, MedR 1985 p. 221/222). The situation is different if it is necessary to deviate from the standard. It is also advisable to keep a record of any discrepancies between the surgeon's explicit requirement for a certain positioning and the anaesthetist's objections. Increasingly stringent requirements in legal practice also entail stricter requirements for documentation.

During the operation, observant monitoring with repeated controls of the relevant parts of the body can help to detect or prevent unintentional changes in position and new possibilities of injuries (pressure points, incorrect joint positions, etc.).

10.1.2 Occurrence of positioning injuries

10.1.2.1 Frequency

Cases of »anaesthesia paralysis« were already reported more than 100 years ago, which soon transpired to be cases of injuries occurring during and not through anaesthesia [16].

Positioning injuries are said to occur about 50 times per 10,000 anaesthetics, including nerve lesions in 6 to 12 of 10,000 anaesthetics [19]. Other studies [25, 53] also describe the frequency of nerve injuries during an anaesthetic at approx. 0.1% (31/30,000 anaesthetics). In decreasing order, these affected the brachial plexus (11 times), ulnar nerve (8 times), radial nerve (7 times) and peroneal nerve (5 times) [25]. But the specific use of electrophysiological examinations reveals a far higher incidence of postoperative nerve injuries; in the case of heart surgery, the incidence of sensibility or motor neuropathy in the ulnar nerve is said to reach up to 38% [32,75]. But a considerable share of preexisting dysfunctions (up to 30%) must be taken into account, together with the possibility of other injury mechanisms (circulatory problems, microembolism) [75]. A follow-up study of peripheral nerve lesions of iatrogenic cause revealed 226 of 267 cases of nerve injuries (85.4%) in the context of surgical procedures [31]. But in this study, most of the cases had been caused directly by the surgical procedure, with positioning injuries only ascertained in 14 cases.

10.1.2.2 Kind of injuries

The range of positioning injuries extends from harmless surface abrasions through to severe, possibly incapacitating lesions. Isolated lethal cases have occurred, for example following positioning injuries with compartment syndrome in both lower legs with rhabdomyolysis and subsequent multiple organ failure [45]. Structures at risk from positioning injuries are the skin and surface soft tissues, joints and ligaments, brachial plexus and peripheral nerves, blood vessels and the eyes.

Skin and soft tissues

Long immobilisation on the operating table can cause pressure sores in the skin and subcutaneous tissues. Exposed areas such as the heels or buttocks are especially at risk. Patients with poor trophic status or circulation e.g. in the case of diabetes mellitus or arteriosclerosis and older patients are affected more frequently. Local pressure effects are usually also accompanied by more serious factors, particularly poor perfusion resulting from longer phases of hypotension or from cooling down. Together with generous padding of exposed areas (silicon gel and foam pads or padded cuffs for the extremities), formable silicon gel mats with a large support area can be used for risk patients, or multiple water mats where the support surfaces are replaced periodically, to avoid pressure necrosis. Warming mats can help to prevent drops in temperature over the operating table. Indeed, maintaining the patient's normal body temperature is an important measure to counteract peripheral circulation problems and thus pressure injuries to the skin. The influence of hypothermia and hypotension is also illustrated by the occurrence of skin ulcers at the back of the head of HLM patients (heart-lung machine) whose head was not placed on a positioning cushion [39].

Mechanical injuries to the soft tissues or muscles during surgical procedures can be caused by the operating tables and instrument tables or brackets. Soft tissues can get caught between the operating table and attached fittings if the table has to be adjusted during the operation. This can happen for example if the positioning is changed to make it easier to close the wound or if the legs are positioned horizontally from the lithotomy position. However, design features of modern operating tables prevent such complications to a great extent.

Joints and ligaments

Enforced movements to the relaxed body of the patient deprived of protective reflexes and pain reactions can cause injuries to the joints and ligaments. This applies in particular in the case of degenerative or traumatic conditions. In isolated cases it may be appropriate to test the required positioning while the patient is still awake to ask the patient whether the positioning is tolerable. Extremities spread out from the body should always be secured on holders to prevent them from falling. Any changes in position are carried out carefully with an adequate number of experienced helpers.

Nerves

Injuries to the nerves are caused by direct compression, by tension or pressure in unphysiological positions of the joints, and in isolated cases also if tourniquets are applied for too long [61]. In the case of tension and pressure injuries, inadequate blood circulation in the nerves (ischaemia of the vasa nervorum) plays a major role [24]. Blunt application of force which does not destroy the nerve structure will usually see good recovery of the sensory and motor deficits if the pressure injury or ischaemia was only short lived [75]. Exposed nerves of the upper and lower extremities and the brachial plexus are particularly at risk.

If a nerve lesion is ascertained after the operation, other possible causes should be examined as well as positioning injuries, such as direct injuries from the operation, pressure injuries from haematomas or oedemas and anatomic anomalies which can favour injuries. Patients with various conditions will be predisposed to neuropathies, e.g. alcohol abuse, diabetes mellitus, uraemia, vitamin deficiency, malignant tumours [71,75,79]. Two-sided postoperative reduction in the velocity of nerve conduction in particular will probably reveal (subclinical) neuropathy already existing before the operation [23].

Brachial plexus. After leaving the intervertebral foramina of the cervical spine, the brachial plexus runs through the scalene gap and narrow space between the clavicle and first rib to the axilla. The humerus head provides a fixation point here. Injuries are caused either from pressure with further narrowing of the physiological constrictions, or from positioning causing an enlargement of the distance between the named fixation points and thus stretching the plexus. The stretch mechanism impairs circulation to the nerve fibres. Depending on how long the inadequate circulation lasts, hypaesthesia and paraesthesia can be observed, and even irreversible functional loss if ischaemia lasts for several hours [45]. Possible injury mechanisms include [12]:

- shoulder supports fitted too far in the medial direction, jamming the plexus between clavicle and first rib,
- relapse of the shoulder girdle in the anaesthetised, relaxed patient, bringing the clavicle against the first rib,
- hyperextension of the cervical spine with the head turned to the other side.

Abduction and outer rotation of the upper arm can make the humerus head act as a hypomochlion and stretch the plexus in the axilla. Stretching injuries of the brachial plexus can also occur after a sternotomy with use of thorax clamps, and primarily affects the lower roots [23].

People with various anomalies (cervical rib, scalene syndrome, costoclavicular syndrome, hyperabduction syndrome) in the upper thorax outlet (thoracic outlet syndrome) are particularly at risk from injuries to the brachial plexus. Compression of the vessel nerve bundle is common for these anomalies [55].

It is important above all to prevent a relapse of the shoulders, abduction of the upper arm exceeding 90°, extreme outer rotation of the upper arm, dorsal extension and excessive distal tension of the arm.

Ulnar nerve. The ulnar nerve is at risk because of its anatomically exposed position in the medial epicondyle of the humerus and also to a lesser extent at the wrist. The nerve runs in the flat groove of the sulcus of the ulnar nerve at the medial epicondyle of the humerus with inadequate cover from connective tissues or muscles to provide sufficient protection from pressure [31]. Extreme flexion of the elbow and/or pronation of the lower arm increases the exposure and risk of compression for the ulnar nerve [3, 63]. The olecranon offers a certain protection with the lower arm in supination, but up to now there has been no evidence of supination positioning resulting in a lesser incidence of pressure injuries [63]. Injuries were also reported caused by unfavourable cables or infusion leads running in the area of the medial condyle and from blood pressure cuffs pulled too far in the distal direction over the elbow from too frequent blood pressure measurements [79].

During the operation, the elbow must be padded from below to prevent pressure lesions. Ekerot recommends careful padding, and positioning with stretched elbow and supinated lower arm, particularly for anatomic anomalies of the ulnar nerve with habitual luxation [27]. Positioning with pronation position of the hand should be avoided, together with greater flexion in the elbow and adduction close to the patient's body.

Radial nerve. The radial nerve runs in a spiral around the humerus. In the proximal section it is at risk if the inside of the upper arm is pressed against the edges of the operating table or rails. The arm must not hang down over the edge of the table! In the middle to distal part of the upper arm, lateral brackets or instrument tables pressing against the upper arm or instrument tables can compress the radial nerve. Stirrups, retractors and the edges of the table must be checked for an adequate distance to the patient's body. The wrist can be injured if fixation cuffs are pulled too tight [22].

Median nerve. Intraoperative injuries to the median nerve are rare and usually caused by a direct surgical trauma (e.g. in the area of the carpal tunnel). As far as anaesthesia is concerned, injuries are most likely from paravenous injections in the elbow [12], which is one reason why anaesthetists usually prefer distal access to the vessels. The arm must not be fixed in the area of the elbow with blood pressure cuffs or similar.

Nerves of the lower extremities. Bending and outer rotation in the hips can stretch the sciatic nerve. In the proximal calf, the peroneal nerve is at risk from its exposed position beneath the fibular head, and in the medial calf the saphenous nerve below the medial condyle of the tibia is at risk from compression [65].

Vessels

Complications occur from massive compression to blood vessels in exposed places or if extreme positioning kinks the blood vessels. In the prone position, congestion in the veins of the lower extremities is possible from compression of the inferior vena cava if positioning pads are put too far in the cranial direction, or the arterial circulation in the legs can be affected if positioning aids are put too far in the distal direction in the groin. Patients with peripheral occlusive vascular disease are at risk from ischaemia if the lower extremities are positioned up high and/or bent (lithotomy position). Capillary injuries caused by long-lasting tissue hypoxia can cause a reperfusion oedema after reperfusion with development of a compartment syndrome [46]. Compartment syndrome caused by positioning has been described for the lower leg, lower arm and shoulder [45]. The symptoms can also occur several hours after the operation [36, 45].

Circulatory problems caused by positioning for certain syndromes can be ascertained by provocation tests. In the case of thoracic outlet syndrome, a backwards tilt of the head while turning the chin sideways to the affected side (Adson's manoeuvre) not only causes sensibility problems but also compression of the subclavian artery with diminished radial pulse [55]. Similar symptoms can be triggered by raising the arm above the horizontal in the case of hyperabduction syndrome. This would prohibit any »over-head« positioning of the patient's arm. But these tests are not performed during routine preoperative examinations, nor are they demanded by law because of the rarity of thoracic outlet syndrome, for example [68]. If during an operation doubts occur with regard to circulation of the extremities, pulse oximetry at the corresponding extremity can provide initial indications of circulatory problems.

Depending on cuff pressure and length of time used, tourniquets can conceal the risk of ischaemic injuries to the tissue (nerve lesions, myasthenia, rhabdomyolysis, compartment syndrome). Arterial vascular occlusions occur, the frequency of deep vein thrombosis is not increased [6, 28]. Cuff pressure of 100–150 mmHg above the systolic blood pressure is considered adequate, and the tourniquet time should not exceed 2 h [76].

»Shunt« arms are wrapped up well in cotton wool, loosely fixed and protected with arm positioning rails against exerted pressures.

Eyes

Lacking eyelid closure at the same time as a decrease in lacrimation while under anaesthetic can cause erosion of the cornea. Lacking eyelid closure increases the risk of direct injuries to the cornea, e.g. from face masks, fingernails, catheters or adhesive drapes. High persistent pressure on the orbita and bulbus can cause a fatal reduction in vision through to irreversible loss of sight. Irreversible loss of sight has been observed after being exposed to pressure for just 10 min in the prone position [22]. This is caused by ischaemia of the optic nerve and retina as a result of compression. Hypotension and anaemia can cause the ischaemic injuries and loss of sight [14]. The blood flow through the optic nerve and choroid is essentially passive from the arterial blood pressure, with only very slight autoregulation mechanisms [67]. According to Wolfe [78], unexpected bradyarrhythmia can be a warning sign of increased intraocular pressure.

Although impaired vision has been described for various positionings, specific significance is attributed to the prone position with the use of headrests. In rare cases, the use of face masks with a hard bead can cause pressure injuries to the optic nerve when the mask is unsuitably held. To avoid injuries of this kind, while under anaesthetic the patient's eyelids are closed without any pressure on the eyeball and complete orbital region. If the eyes cannot be seen during the operation, the eyelids must always be held closed with a plaster.

In the case of loss of vision after heart surgery, consideration must always also be given to the possibility of an embolism with occlusion of the central retinal artery [77].

10.1.3 Supine position

Head and neck

The patient's head is positioned on a pillow or head ring so that the cervical spine is in the middle position. When the patient is relaxed, turning the head suddenly to the side can cause pain in the muscles and joints after the operation and even cause irritation to the branches of the cervical plexus. Turning the head with an extreme movement can stretch the brachial plexus on the contralateral side. In the case of bone disease in the cervical spine, the posture assumed by the patient while still awake is retained. Special care is required when operating a patient with a cervical fracture. These patients are brought into the operating theatre with a halo extension. They are intubated with fibre-optic intubation in bed without changing the position of the head and cervical spine.

A strong turn of the cervical spine interrupts the flow of blood in the arteries to the brain. Turning the head 90° to the side must be expected to completely interrupt the flow of blood in the contralateral vertebral artery [66]. In the case of stenosis of the carotid artery, interference with the collateral flow can cause deleterious ischemia in the brain stem and cerebellum [61]. Venous drainage is also best with the head in the middle position.

In the supine position, the eyes are free. The only routine measure entails ensuring that the eyes are closed to prevent them from drying out.

Suitable devices must be provided to neutralise any tension or pressure on the tubus, e.g. from respiratory tubes or measuring sensors.

Arms

In the supine position, the arms can be basically positioned at the body, spread out on an arm support or one arm is raised on the anaesthesia stirrup. All kinds of arm positioning require special protection for the brachial plexus, for the radial nerve in its progress along the humerus and for the ulnar nerve in the medial elbow. Principle mechanisms causing injuries have already been discussed (▶ see Sect. 10.1.2.2, Nerves).

Arms at the body. To relieve the brachial plexus, the clavicle is raised from the first rib with a stationary pad under the shoulder when the arm is positioned at the body. This is particularly important for example if tension is applied to the arms with strips of sticky plaster when the cervical vertebrae are blocked, because otherwise there is a risk of the plexus getting caught between the clavicle and first rib.

If the upper arm protrudes beyond the edge of the table, there is a risk of pressure injuries to the radial nerve. Not even a pad between the arm and operating table will withstand the pressure if an assistant leans against it! Further in the distal direction, the radial nerve can be compressed on the outside of the humerus and injured if the upper arm is jammed between the thorax and various holders fastened to the operating table.

The ulnar nerve is at risk from the pressure of the edge of the table in the area of the medial epicondyle of the humerus, particularly if the arm is not fixed adequately, for example just at the wrist. The risk is increased by flexion in the elbow and pronation of the lower arm, for example when positioning and fixing the lower arms at the body. These risks are frequently caused by the arm not having enough space next to the body on the operating table. They can be avoided by widening the table with a metal or plastic support device and laying the arm in a padded cuff (Aschemann arm positioning support, see Figs. 8.15 and 8.16). A rare cause for pressure injuries to the ulnar nerve can come from infusion leads or cables along the inside of the arm.

Spreading the arms out away from the body. If the arms are spread out away from the body, the brachial plexus can be injured by overstretching the arm in the shoulder joint, because the humerus head acts as a hypomochlion on the nerve bundles of the brachial plexus. In fact, abduction of the upper arm through more than 90° is the most frequently mentioned kind of positioning mistake causing plexus injuries [48]. But even keeping to an angle under 90° in the shoulder joint cannot always prevent intraoperative injuries to the plexus, because with the patient relaxed under the anaesthetic, the shoulder can fall back onto the table surface and clamp the plexus between the clavicle and first rib.

Effective prophylaxis consists of raising the arm above the level of the shoulder joint and padding under the shoulder, thus enlarging the distance between the clavicle and the first rib. The arm is extended from the body on a padded support. The upper arm is slightly rotated inwards in the shoulder joint and abducted by maximum 90°, the elbow is slightly bent (about 150°) and the back of the hand is pronated. Turning the head slightly to the side of the extended arm also takes the tension from the brachial plexus.

Even if the arm is correctly extended at first, during the operation it is not rare for critical changes to take place if the position of this arm is changed because of space requirements at the operating table or an assistant leaning against it. It is therefore vital for the arm to be fixed to the arm rest by suitable means such as a tape or non-compressive plaster so that it cannot fall down, because if the relaxed arm falls down, this can cause luxation of the shoulder and/or acute overstretching of the brachial plexus with a loss of functions. The arm itself, in particular the medial elbow, must not rest on the edge of the arm support.

Raising one arm. Pads must be used at the raised arm to prevent pressure injuries from the metal structure [65]. No tension must be exerted to the shoulder joint and brachial plexus.

Spinal column

About 30% of all patients claim »backache« after an operation, regardless of the anaesthetic procedure [38]. This is caused primarily by negating the lordosis in the lumbar spine and coccyx on the hard operating table so that the ligaments are stretched. Patients with »backache« should be allowed to dictate their own position on the operating table, indicating the painful area and using positioning cushions to improve the situation.

On the other hand, hyperlordosis of the lumbar spine as is common practice for some abdominal, gynaecological and urological operations, can also cause postoperative discomfort. Particularly in the case of predisposed patients with degenerative change in the spinal column, there is evidence of postoperative injuries to the vertebral joints caused by subluxation, microfractures and haematomas [40]. In the case of a patient with stenosis of the vertebral canal, hyperlordosis during an extended urological operation caused spinal infarction at L2/3 [4].

Lower extremities

As far as possible, the hips and knees are arranged in a physiological position, i.e. with a slight bend. The legs must not be crossed.

At the fibular head, the exposed peroneal nerve is at risk from support structures for drapes or operating tables and from incorrectly positioned tourniquets. In particular when the table is tilted, attention must be paid to a compression-free area. The Achilles tendon and heel must not protrude beyond the operating table and are secured from pressure.

10.1.3.1 Struma position

In patients with arthrotic conditions, extreme extension of the cervical spine, as required for example to expose the goitre, can cause pain and blockages. The head must never be allowed to »float freely« in extension.

Together with hyperextension of the cervical spine, the main risk in this position consists of the poor access and restricted possibilities for controlling the tracheal tubus and eyes because of the vicinity of the operating site and sterile covered operating area [65]. An eye ointment should therefore be administered as prophylaxis and both eyes covered.

10.1.3.2 Extension table

The extension table is required for reposition and osteosynthesis of fractures to the femur head and per/subtrochanteric fractures of the femur. A brace is positioned at the perineum to support the pelvis. In male patients, com-

10.1.3.3 Lithotomy position

The lithotomy position with raised legs bent at the hips and knees causes considerable changes to respiration and circulation. Movement of the diaphragm is limited. Raising the legs results in autotransfusion of up to 600 ml of blood with a corresponding increase in the intrathoracic blood volume [41]. This change in position must be brought about with particular care in patients with cardiac insufficiency. Similarly, moving the patient back out of this position results in a sudden drop in volume with a decrease in venous return and consecutive fall in blood pressure. This risk of hypotension is increased even further in spinal or peridural anaesthesia because the sympathetic nervous system is blocked.

The lithotomy position poses problems for nerve supply and circulation of the lower extremities, with descriptions of injuries to the sciatic nerve and compartment syndrome on both sides [61]. The sciatic nerve is stretched by bending and outer rotation in the hips. The leg support can cause pressure to the lateral peroneal nerve (caught between the support and head of the fibula) and compression of the medial saphenous nerve (caught between the support and tibia) [65]. This is why the largest possible contact surface and padding is important. The bend in the hips must be produced carefully and adjusted to the existing mobility of the patient.

Extreme flexion in the hips can prevent venous drainage, cause stasis and finally thrombosis. At an angle >90°, this can result in arterial vascular compression through to occlusion of the inguinal vessels. The leg support can cause compression in the back of the knee and to the calf. Patients with peripheral arterial vascular disease are at risk from ischaemia from the raised position and kinking of the lower extremities. Stretching injuries to the sciatic nerve are aggravated further by inadequate blood flow. Ischaemia of the lower extremities on both sides with compartment syndrome in the calves has been described after a gynaecological operation lasting several hours in the lithotomy position [43].

With the arms positioned at the body, there is a risk of injuring the patient's fingers when the legs are returned to their normal position after the operation.

10.1.3.4 Head-down position

The so-called Trendelenburg position is used for example for laparoscopic procedures and urological operations, as well as for treating shock.

The head-down position should not be so extreme that shoulder supports have to be used to prevent the patient sliding down. The pressure on the costoclavicular space then poses a risk of injuries to the plexus. Otherwise in positioning terms, there are no major differences to the neutral supine position.

But the Trendelenburg position does have a major effect on respiration (cranial displacement of the diaphragm, diminished functional residual capacity and long compliance) and circulation (increase in cardiac filling pressure, increase in cardiac output, but in the case of left ventricular failure also the risk of a lung oedema caused by positioning) [22, 42]. There is also an increase in intracranial pressure [36] and there are reports about possible retinal detachment in the context of the Trendelenburg position [36].

To prevent any drop in blood pressure, the patient should be returned to the neutral position slowly and after correcting any hypovolaemia.

10.1.4 Lateral position

The patient is turned into the side position in a co-ordinated procedure with several helpers, ensuring that the head, shoulders, pelvis and legs are all turned along the axis. Bearing supports are then put in place.

Head

The head is supported with pads so that the cervical spine forms a straight line with the thoracic spine (neutral position). Extension and flexion are avoided because too great a deviation from the neutral position poses the same risks for cervical spine, brachial plexus and cerebral circulation as already described for the supine position. The head padding must not bend or crush the lower ear. The eyes must be freely accessible and protected from pressure caused by padding, cables, tubes and the assistant's elbows. Stretching of the cervical sympathetic chain can cause Horner's syndrome [35].

Shoulders and arms

The lateral position endangers the brachial plexus when the weight of the upper body rests on the lower axle. To relieve the shoulder and vessel nerve bundle, a roll is placed in the caudal direction from the axilla under the upper chest. This support roll must fulfil the following requirements [45]:
— It must be so thick that the thorax is raised from the operating table to such an extent that the lower shoulder is relieved. Easily compressible materials are therefore not suitable.
— The roll must be so wide that the contact pressure is distributed across several ribs.
— The complete anterior-posterior depth of the thorax must be supported.

(pression of the genitals must be avoided [65]. Image converters are used to check reposition and osteosynthesis. Care must be taken to ensure that adjustment of the C-arm does not clamp or cause pressure injuries to any parts of the patient's body.)

- The roll must not be positioned too high under the axilla because it can then compress the vessel nerve bundle. A position in the distal direction from the sixth rib has a negative effect on respiratory excursion. The shoulder is pulled forwards with the lower arm to move the clavicle away from the first rib.

If the lateral position is extended beyond 90° towards the prone position, the lower arm should be positioned backwards parallel to the body. It is helpful to check the radial pulse after positioning.

The upper arm is spread out on a support in accordance with the function. The arm is to be positioned in such a way that it is spread out horizontally from the body, certainly not at an acute angle to the head. Tension in particular can cause injuries to the brachial plexus. The operating site must never be exposed by force from tension to the arm.

Pelvis and legs

The operating table must be bent for kidney operations in such a way that the pivotal point is on the level of the iliac blade. A higher pivotal point in the side or lower ribs increases intra-abdominal pressure and restricts respiration. Even a case of obstruction of the inferior vena cava has been described [36]. The joints are arranged in a neutral position (slight bend). The lower leg must be protected from the pressure of the upper leg by suitable positioning and padding, e.g. cushions between the two knees. Pads must prevent the head of the fibula and thus the peroneal nerve from being squashed against the operating table. Belts, plasters etc. must not hinder the blood flow.

10.1.5 Prone position

Numerous orthopaedic, neurosurgical and trauma surgery procedures are performed in the prone position as a matter of routine. Together with the problems resulting from changing the patient's position, the main interest is focussed on positioning of the head and arms with free mobility for thorax and abdomen.

Changing the position

Changing the position of the anaesthetised patient from the supine to the prone position is a critical phase. Successful procedures without complications depend on the quality and number of experienced helpers. When the patient is relaxed under anaesthetic, the natural protective functions of the muscles and ligaments do not apply, so that in particular the head, vertebral column and joints of the extremities are at risk. Specific anaesthesia-related complications include the unintended disconnection or dislocation of the tube and infusion leads, and interruption of the monitoring system.

In practice, the anaesthetist stands at the patient's head during repositioning and secures the head and endotracheal tube. Any monitor and infusion leads which are not vital are disconnected. But there must not be a longer interruption in the monitoring procedure. The tube is also briefly disconnected from the respirator to reliably prevent dislocation under tension. A controlled, step-by-step procedure is vital. In the case of patients with instable circulation or respiration, the fundamental question of feasibility should be discussed with the surgeon before starting to change the patient's position. In the case of injuries to the cervical spine, the surgeon is responsible for the patient's head and corresponding positioning.

Head

Longer low positioning of the head below the heart can cause blepharoedema or swelling in the face, and possibly also an increase in brain pressure. The neck must remain free so as not to prevent venous drainage from the head. Pressure on the carotid sinus can cause cardiac irregularity and a drop in blood pressure. Turning the head sideways from the median position can impair the blood flow in the vessels supplying the brain [66]. This matters when impending carotid stenosis makes it necessary to establish a collateral circulation using the circulus arteriosus Willisii.

When positioning the head in U-shaped headrests, foam blocks with C-shaped cut-outs or gel pillows for the prone position, the eyeballs must be reliably protected from pressure to prevent impaired vision or even loss of vision. Eye ointment can be administered and the eyelids closed with plasters to prevent erosion to the cornea. Correct positioning of the eyes free of pressure must be checked from time to time by inspecting and palpating the complete orbita. Nor should there by any infusion leads, tubes and cables anywhere near the eyes.

In addition to being fixed by plaster to the patient's head, the tubus is secured so as to prevent extubation from tension on the tubus and tubes even if the plaster works loose from saliva flowing out of the patient's mouth. It must be possible to detect any changes in the position of the headrests or any twisting of the head out of the support or headrest.

Shoulders and arms

The shoulders should hang down to the front; the arms are also guided forwards and slightly downwards and positioned on a padded support with bent elbow. If necessary, the arms can be positioned slightly bent at the body. Elevation or extreme abduction of the arms can cause compression of the vessel nerve bundle in the area of the scalene gap or costoclavicular space. In extreme abduction, the head of the humerus can also compress the vessel nerve bundle.

Thorax and abdomen

In the prone position, the weight of the spinal column and back muscles rests on the thorax, and impairs respiration and restricts the mobility of the abdominal wall. The maximum of expandable lung sections is preserved if the thorax is supported with padding from under the jugular to the sixth rib. Padding positioned too far in the cranial direction can compress the plexus between the clavicle and first rib. [61]. The abdominal wall must always remain free, because otherwise this places extreme restrictions on the mobility of the diaphragm as a result of increased intra-abdominal pressure. There must not be any pressure on the inferior vena cava. Compression of the inferior vena cava during operations to the spinal column causes increased blood loss, because this results in bypass circulation through epidural venous plexus.

Pelvis and legs

The iliac blades act as distal support point for the body. Positioning padding located too far down under the groin causes severe restrictions in the blood flow to the legs. If in any doubt about an adequate blood supply to the lower extremities, it helps to check the pulses of the popliteal artery, posterior tibial artery and dorsalis pedis artery of the foot, and to do a plethysmograph curve at a toe.

The genitals must be checked and penis and scrotum protected from pressure injuries. The bladder catheter must be protected from getting crushed and from tension.

The legs must be positioned so that venous reflux is not impeded by gravity. Pressure bandages are obligatory, but they must be checked to ensure that they are not displaced and cannot cause any constriction. The nerves and tendons of the back of the foot are protected by padding to prevent them being squashed against the operating table.

10.1.6 Sitting/half-sitting position

The sitting position in neurosurgery entails known risks, particularly those of a drop in blood pressure and embolism, which shall not be considered in any greater detail at this point. These problems can also be encountered to a lesser extent in beach-chair positioning, which is used above all for surgery to the shoulders.

Raising the patient from the supine position must be carried out step-by-step. Skull clamp or headrests are fixed carefully and secured to prevent unintentional displacement. Tracheal tubes and respiratory tubes are fastened without any tension and secured to prevent disconnection.

The patient's head is fixed in the middle position to avoid any negative effects on the cervical spine, cervical plexus and vessels. If the head is anteflected too much so that the chin comes closer to the thorax, this can impair venous and lymphatic drainage and cause an increase in intracranial pressure. This position can also cause overstretching of the cervical medulla with a decrease in spinal perfusion. Position-induced tetraplegic injuries have been described as a consequence [21]. The bulbus of the eye must be protected from pressure and the conjunctiva protected from drying out.

Stretching the shoulder to obtain better surgical exposure can cause stretching of the brachial plexus when combined with an extension of the cervical spine and turning the head to the opposite side. A Horner's syndrome from stretching the nerve fibres in the stellate ganglion has also been described in this context [59].

Strong flexion in the hip and extension in the knee causes overstretching of the sciatic nerve [36]. In cachectic patients, the sciatic nerve can be injured directly by pressure in the absence of padding [36].

10.1.7 Final remarks

Knowledge of possible injury mechanisms and a correspondingly planned and cautious approach to positioning the patient should clearly reduce the risk of positioning injuries. Even then they cannot be avoided completely. Positioning procedures with a high risk of complications must be given due consideration, weighing up the possible advantages for the surgical procedure against the risks of injuries to the patient. After the procedure, exposed parts of the body (joints, nerves, circulatory system) must be checked critically.

After the operation, there should be an increased awareness for possible positioning injuries already in the recovery room, if the surgical or anaesthetic procedure does not explain any swelling, pain or sensibility and movement problems. This must be followed immediately by exact diagnosis and therapy where possible. If nerve injury is presumed, arrangements are made for a clinical and electrophysiological examination by a neurologist. It is not rare for anatomic anomalies or previously existent neuropathies to be ascertained in retrospect as being partly responsible for the injuries [31, 55].

10.2 Positioning the patient under resuscitation conditions

F. Logemann

In many hospital areas, routine procedures have to be left behind in situations requiring resuscitation. Together with the emergency room, the operating theatre is particularly frequently affected. The positioning of the patient must support the resuscitation measures in all key aspects.

Examples for surgical interventions for resuscitation of patients:

Staunching acute bleeding	Lesions of the aorta Polytrauma
Connection to the heart-lung machine	Cardiac problems Pulmonary embolism Hypothermia
Revision because of surgical complications	

10.2.1 Necessary measures

Individual circumstances can differ greatly. But experience indicates that the following situations occur with particular frequency:

The patient comes into the operating suite in a hospital bed under resuscitation conditions

Depending on the situation, the patient is positioned for surgery in the hospital bed (acute bleeding) or is transferred to the operating table (if absolutely necessary).

Arguments in favour of positioning the patient in the hospital bed instead of on the operating table include the time factor until surgery can begin, reduced manpower requirements, better space conditions for heart massage and less manipulation of the patient. These advantages have to be weighed up against the major drawbacks such as poorer intraoperative handling, poorer hygiene and pressure sores in the dorsal parts of the body (resuscitation board). Consideration should certainly be given to the fact that particularly for obese patients, adequate heart massage is not possible under transport conditions on the operating table.

If the decision is taken to use an operating table, preferably all materials should be ready at the table before the patient arrives in the operating suite to prevent any unnecessary delays.

The patient is transferred from the hospital bed to the operating table under the following conditions:
Do not interrupt the resuscitation measures.
Any time lost by measures such as
- exact positioning on the operating table,
- padding the extremities,
- shaving,
- keeping the dorsal parts of the body dry during skin disinfection

can have a marked negative effect on the resuscitation measures.

Procedures in these circumstances should rather concentrate on elementary measures such as positioning and fixing the extremities to be used for measuring blood pressure, securing infusion and signal leads, and positioning and fixing the head and extremities for puncture procedures.

Rapid patient transfer can be assisted by using a simple transfer aid in the form of a roll board, prefixed arm extension and infusion and perfusor supports fitted to the operating table. A trolley should be ready with medication and respirator.

The patient needs resuscitation during the transfer process

The causes for resuscitation in surgical patients are manifold and rarely calculable. An indispensable prerequisite for providing adequate patient care under these conditions is to ensure that qualified, trained staff are present during the transfer process. The staff should be capable of detecting when the patient is in a critical condition and taking the necessary immediate measures. Depending on the individual situation, here again the decision has to be taken whether to resuscitate the patient, including surgical components, in the hospital bed or on the operating table. Furthermore, immediate availability of several qualified assistants and aids (e.g. board for heart massage in the hospital bed, defibrillator, mobile cardiovascular monitor) must also be guaranteed in the patient transfer section of the operating suite.

Transferring the patient from the operating table to the hospital bed after the operation constitutes a typical danger particularly for patients with an instable cardiovascular system. This is why adequate resources must be provided in advance, and the corresponding operating table with all its padding and special anaesthesia/surgical features not dismantled until the patient has left the operating suite.

Intraoperative resuscitation

Generally the various requirements for positioning the patient come from the specific surgical procedures and are only extremely rarely influenced by the probable need for perioperative resuscitation.

But ideally in an emergency, priority should be given to positioning for resuscitation over optimum positioning for the operation.

As a rule, the anaesthetist co-ordinates the necessary measures. He is also responsible for deciding before the operation to reduce the ideal positioning for the surgical procedure to the maximum tolerable positioning. In certain cases, it would appear to be quite justified to reject a prone or lateral positioning under certain circumstances because of the anticipated need for resuscitation, because heart massage can in fact only be performed effectively in the supine position.

If the need for resuscitation occurs in the prone position, the patient should be turned into the supine position immediately. Under these conditions, all surgical counter-indications can only be relative. Under certain circumstances it can be a great help to have a second operating table at the ready. This allows for rapid patient transfer with only a few assistants by rolling the patient onto the parallel operating table.

Transfer from the lateral to the supine position is possible without problems in most cases without any considerable delay to starting heart massage.

But thorax surgery can often pose an absolute counter-indication to changing the patient's position, if resuscitation should become necessary with the patient in the lateral position, because as a rule direct manual compression of the heart is given preference in the case of an open thorax.

10.2.2 Positioning injuries following resuscitation

In principle there is an increased incidence of positioning injuries in patients who had to undergo resuscitation. While fractures to the ribs and sternum can be caused by heart massage and also occur regularly even with optimum positioning, typical positioning injuries such as nerve lesions, pressure sores, burns and eye injuries are far more rare. They frequently result from the relatively slight relevance of prophylactic measures under resuscitation conditions. Every resuscitation attempt proceeds along its own dynamic lines so that it is difficult to give general recommendations as to when the prophylactic measures should have been implemented. Even so, responsible assistants should keep adequate records of their careful working procedures, because even following successful resuscitation, legal disputes are not rare in the case of suspected positioning injuries.

10.3 Positioning injuries as seen by the neurologist

H. Müller-Vahl

10.3.1 Introduction

Nerve injuries are one of the complications feared after surgery. They have a considerable negative effect on postoperative rehabilitation and cause lasting handicaps in many cases. Most iatrogenic nerve injuries are caused directly by the surgical procedure. But they can also result from other medical measures, including positioning during or after an operation.

While many cases of surgical nerve injuries also occur under optimum procedures, position-induced nerve injuries can be avoided as a rule [13, 26, 52, 53]. The basic principles in the pathogenesis of position-induced nerve lesions have been clarified for a long time. Prevention of such lesions entails all doctors and nursing staff responsible for positioning being acquainted with these principles and being capable of recognising which positioning endangers the peripheral nerves.

10.3.2 Frequency

The frequency of position-induced nerve injuries is only known approximately. Most injuries of this kind recede rapidly and are in many cases not featured in the patient's records. In older retrospective studies, the frequency of position-induced nerve injuries amounts to about 0.05–0.3% [25, 53]. This has scarcely changed in the meanwhile. Cooper et al. [20] recorded 3 cases of position-induced arm plexus paralysis after 15,000 general anaesthetics. Following total hip replacement surgery, Posta et al. [56] observed nerve injuries in the arm with a frequency of 0.22%. The most frequent injuries are to the arm plexus, the ulnar nerve and the peroneal nerve [25]. In a group of altogether 134 doctor liability processes because of position-induced nerve injuries observed in recent years in our hospital, these nerves were affected in 46, 41 and 29 cases, respectively.

10.3.3 Pathophysiology

Position-induced nerve injuries are caused by pressure or tension. In addition, in very rare cases nerve injuries can be caused during long operations in the framework of a compartment syndrome.

The severity of nerve injuries caused by pressure depends on the corresponding extent and duration [49]. Brief, moderate pressure can cause a line blockage which is reversible within a few minutes, probably as an expression of a metabolic disorder following compression of intraneural microvessels. If the pressure persists, this can result in an intraneural oedema. The endoneural pressure increases. It can take a few days or weeks for the paralysis to recede. Even greater pressure causes histologically verifiable injuries to the myelin sheath of the nerve fibres. The axons remain intact (neurapraxy according to Seddon). Large-calibre myelinised nerve fibres suffer earlier and greater injuries from pressure than non-myelinised fibres. Regeneration of the injured myelin sheaths can take several weeks, in rare cases a few months. Even greater pressure injures the axis cylinders (axonotmesis). This leads to wallerian degeneration of the distal axons in the lesion site, marked in neurophysiological terms by the occurrence of pathological spontaneous activity in the electromyogram. Regeneration entails regrowth of the axons in a distal direction from the lesion site. This happens at a rate of approx. 1 – 2 mm per day. Position-induced pressure only causes little change to the inner structure of the nerves so that there are good conditions for successful regeneration.

All physiological movements subject the peripheral nerves to a certain stretching load. Their histological structure prepares them well for such load. Sustained, extreme stretching load can cause nerve paralysis. When a critical stretching limit is exceeded, this causes occlusion of the intraneural blood vessels, initially the venules, then also the arterioles and capillaries. Greater stretching causes histologically verifiable changes to the myelin sheaths, axons and connective tissues. The extent of structural injuries depends on the strength and duration of stretching. Abrupt extreme stretching is not well tolerated. The most severe positioning injuries are caused when an arm or leg falls from a support during repositioning.

The risk of position-induced nerve injuries increases with the length of the operation. But positioning injuries can also not be ruled out during short operations. For example, Mitterschiffthaler et al. [48] described severe paralysis of the arm plexus after an operation lasting only 20 min. Position-induced nerve injuries occur preferably at anatomically predisposed places. Thin patients are at greater risk from pressure injuries than obese patients. The risk during the anaesthetic is related to the reduction in muscular tone (particularly when using muscle relaxants) and to eliminating the physiological protection reflexes. If a patient were awake he would automatically correct his position after a few minutes because of paraesthesia and pain. A special predisposition can result from anatomic anomalies (for example lower arm plexus paralysis in cases of cervical rib). The tolerance of peripheral nerves to pressure or tension is reduced in cases of latent or manifest polyneuropathies (most frequently with diabetes or alcoholism). Finally, arterial hypotension and hypothermia are also discussed as disadvantageous factors. But it is not possible to verify any predisposition factors in the large majority of patients with position-induced nerve damage.

10.3.4 Symptoms

An external sign of pressure being applied can include a pressure mark on the skin. In cases of pressure ulcers, these indicate extensive damage of the inner nerve structure, with a less positive prognosis.

Nerve injuries involve motor and sensory deficits to differing extents, together with vegetative malfunctions corresponding to the supply area of the damaged nerve. The motor malfunctions are generally greater than the sensory deficits. Position-induced compartment syndromes are accompanied by the classical local clinical symptoms, occasionally also with the consequences of rhabdomyolysis (crushed kidney, electrolyte disorders).

Table 10.1. Differential diagnosis of nerve injuries ascertained after operations

No causal context with medical procedures	Injuries already existed Injuries occurred after the operation
Causal context with	Injection Positioning Operation Tourniquet Regional anaesthetic

10.3.4.1 Diagnosis and differential diagnosis

As a rule, position-induced nerve injuries are to be diagnosed in a binding fashion on the basis of a careful study of the case history together with clinical and possibly neurophysiological examinations. In any case, due consideration must be given to possible causes independent of the surgical procedure and also other iatrogenic causes (Table 10.1).

Differential diagnosis requires a good knowledge of the pathogenesis and symptoms of peripheral nerve injuries, because otherwise there is a risk of confusion. Medical literature repeatedly classified nerve injuries following heart operations with median sternotomy as position-induced injuries because it was not known that arm plexus paralysis is frequently inevitably caused by this surgical procedure itself.

It is advisable to consult a neurologist familiar with the problems in every suspected case. Failure to clarify the cause of the nerve injuries at an early point in time can often have a negative effect for the doctors in the case of open questions during a later dispute.

10.3.4.2 Therapy and progress

Position-induced nerve injuries are not treated any differently from other paralysis. As a rule, conservative therapy is required with active and passive movement exercises, and suitable measures to prevent secondary complications. Whether electrotherapy is effective is a subject for controversial discussion. The administration of so-called neurotropic vitamins can be considered useless.

The prognosis for position-induced nerve injuries is generally favourable. In Parks' cases [53], the paralysis receded completely within 6 weeks in 52% of the cases and within 6 months for another 40%. Only 8% of the patients still suffered from major deficits even after 12 months.

10.3.5 Special nerve injuries

10.3.5.1 Brachial plexus

The emergence of position-induced arm plexus paralysis is explained well in scientific terms following many clinical examinations and examinations of corpses [34, 37]. During operations in the supine position with the operating table in a horizontal position, the nerve injuries occur in the arm spread out [13, 20, 64]. The arm nerve plexus is fixed at the cervical spine and in the axilla. All movements enlarging the distances between the fixed points cause a more or less large stretching load on the arm plexus. The injury is usually caused by overstretching as a result of abducting the arm too far. The stretching effect is reinforced if the arm is retroverted, turned outside and/or supined at the same time, and also if the head is turned to the opposite side. Simultaneous abduction of both arms is problematical.

In the case of arm plexus paralysis in the Trendelenburg position with the head lowered, various different mechanisms are discussed. Some authors presume that the shoulder supports aiming to prevent the patient from sliding off the operating table can cause direct pressure injuries to the arm plexus if positioned too far in a medial direction. Stöhr [64] on the other hand presumes for various reasons that in this position too, the cause is probably overstretching by moving the body and head against the fixed shoulders or arms.

In most cases the injuries consist of upper arm plexus paralysis with paresis of the movements in the shoulders and upper brachial muscle. Sensory deficits are frequently limited to the outside of the arm, but can also reach right down to the thumb. As a rule, there is no significant pain.

Where position-induced lower arm plexus paralysis is concerned, consideration must always be given to anomalies in the cervicothoracic transitional area. A hyperplastic transverse process C7 with fibrous ligament from here to the first rib is probably more dangerous than a fully formed cervical rib. The worst injuries can be caused if the arm falls off the operating table, particularly because tension forces are transferred to the nerves in full force with the muscles in relaxed state [64].

With regard to differential diagnosis, it is important to differentiate position-induced arm plexus paralysis from postoperative neuralgic shoulder myatrophy (time interval between anaesthetic and the onset of neurological symptoms, sharp pain, other distribution of the neurological deficits [44]). It is very rare for the positioning of central vein catheters to cause arm plexus lesions.

10.3.5.2 Ulnar nerve

The large frequency of position-induced paralysis of the ulnar nerve results from its exposed position at the back of the elbow. Here the nerve runs under the surface in a bone furrow (ulnar nerve sulcus) so that it cannot evade influences from the outside. Its histological structure (nerve fibres in just a few fascicles, little epineurium) is also not very beneficial. The nerve is most frequently injured by pressure from the outside, for example as a result of inadequate padding. If the elbow is held very bent for a longer period of time, this can cause endogenous compression through aponeurosis of the flexor carpi ulnaris muscle [62].

The main symptoms of an ulnar lesion include paraesthesia and sensory deficits in the fourth and fifth rays in the hand (typical restriction in the middle of the ring finger) and weaker movements in the hands and fingers, expressed particularly in clumsiness.

There are considerable differences of opinion about how ulnar paralysis occurs and can be avoided in the direct time context of an operation – referred to in literature as perioperative ulnar paresis. Some opinions claim that perioperative paralysis of the ulnar nerve constitutes a special case and cannot be avoided [18, 63]. An appropriate appraisal requires a thorough differentiation of position-induced ulnar paralysis from nerve injuries caused by other means with similar symptoms, particularly impending ulnar paralysis, lower arm plexus paralysis (typical consequence of heart surgery) and ulnar paralysis caused after the operation while the patient is confined to bed and repeatedly supports himself on his elbows [51, 69, 73].

10.3.5.3 Peroneal nerve

The special susceptibility of the peroneal nerve comes, like that of the ulnar nerve, from its exposed position near to the surface behind the fibular head, together with a disadvantageous histological structure. In a typical case, compression is caused in the lateral or half-lateral position as a result of inadequate padding on the operating table, in the supine position from a lack of leg holders [64]. In the supine position, nerve injuries can also be caused by pressure, if the legs are positioned with extreme outer rotation, for example as part of removing the long saphenous vein during vascular surgery [30].

A lesion of the peroneal nerve is expressed in paralysis of the foot and toe elevator muscle and the elevator muscle for the outer edge of the foot (drop foot). The sensory deficit is apparent on the medial back of the foot and front outside of the distal lower leg.

Paralysis of the peroneal nerve must be differentiated from lesions of the sciatic nerve with a peroneal emphasis or lesions of corresponding branches of the lumbosacral plexus, as can occur for example during operations in the lithotomy position (▶ see below).

10.3.6 Lesions of the lumbosacral plexus and its branches in the lithotomy position

The various forms of the lithotomy position are a relatively problematical kind of positioning with regard to peripheral nerve injuries. Why lesions occur to parts of the lumbosacral plexus has still not been completely clarified. Pathogenetic mechanisms involved here can include pressure, overstretching and also ischaemia [70].

The best explanations are given for injuries to the femoral nerve following gynaecological operations. Experiments on corpses have verified that excessive flexion and outer rotation of the legs press the femoral nerve against the unyielding inguinal ligament [2, 33, 57, 64]. This causes paralysis of the knee extensor muscle and impaired sensitivity at the front inner side of the thigh and calf. In isolated cases, involvement of the hip flexor and obturator nerve has been verified, indicating a stretching effect at the same time. Occasionally isolated obturator lesions are also caused [54].

The lithotomy position can also cause overstretching of the sciatic nerve, usually affecting its peroneal part [7, 17, 47]. The sciatic nerve is fixed in the area of the major sciatic foramen and in the knee and is stretched by bending and outer rotation in the hip joint. This is particularly disadvantageous when the knee is stretched at the same time.

Injuries to the branches of the lumbosacral plexus must always be differentiated from more distal lesions of the leg nerves.

10.3.6.1 Pudendal nerve

Operations on the extension table apply pressure to the perineal region and thus to the pudendal nerve against the rod of the table. This is an example for injury to a nerve which has to be accepted to a certain extent in order to bring the operation to its required conclusion. According to studies by Brumback et al. [15], pudendal lesions can be expected in about 10%. This results in sensory deficits in the perineal region and genitals, with erection and ejaculation disorders in men. The principles for preventing such nerve injuries consist of distributing the pressure to the largest possible area of soft tissue (wide counter bar between genitals and uninjured leg), with a restriction on the duration and intensity of traction to the leg.

10.3.7 Compartment syndrome following operation positioning

During longer operations, compartment syndrome can be caused by the positioning. Most relevant publications refer to the lithotomy position [29, 50, 60] or the semi-lateral lithotomy position [1]. This major complication also occurs very rarely in operations in the knee-elbow position [5] or in the lateral position [58]. Most cases involve the compartments of the lower leg. The mean operating time in the published cases was about 7 h. All age groups can be affected.

The crucial increase in pressure in the compartments for the development of compartment syndrome and the corresponding drop in the arteriovenous pressure gradients is caused on the one hand by persistent pressure from the body weight. In addition, in the lithotomy position the raised position of the legs and possibly additional position-induced compression of arteries and veins can result in additional impairments to the circulation. A general drop in blood pressure during the operation can be just as disadvantageous as impending arteriosclerosis.

In contrast to position-induced isolated nerve injuries, the earliest possible detection of the development of compartment syndrome is crucial with regard to the necessary therapy (fasciotomy) in order to prevent permanent injuries.

References

1. Adler L. M., Heppenstall R. B., Eserhai L. L. (1997) Compartment syndrome in the leg: a complication of hemilithotomy position. Tech Orthop 12: 133–135
2. Al Hakim M., Katirji B. (1993) Femoral mononeuropathy induced by the lithotomy position: a report of 5 cases with review of -literature. Muscle Nerve 16: 891–895
3. Alvine F. G., Schurrer M. E. (1987) Postoperative ulnar-nerve palsy. Are there predisposing factors? J Bone Joint Surg Am 69: 255–259
4. Amoiridis G., Wöhrle J. C., Langkafel M., Maiwurm D., Przuntek H. (1996) Spinal cord infarction after surgery in a patient in the -hyperlordotic position. Anesthesiology 84: 228–230
5. Aschoff A., Steiner-Milz H., Steiner H. H. (1990) Lower limb compartment syndrome following lumbar discectomy in the knee-chest position. Neurosurg Rev 13: 155–159
6. Bailey M. K. (1994) Use of the tourniquet in orthopedic surgery. In: Conroy J. M., Dorman B. H. (eds) Anesthesia for orthopedic surgery. Raven Press, New York, Chapter 5, pp 79–88
7. Batres F., Barclay D. L. (1983) Sciatic nerve injury during gynecologic procedures using the lithotomy position. Obstet Gynecol 62: 92–94
8. Berufsverband Deutscher Anästhesisten und Berufsverband der Deutschen Chirurgen (1982) Vereinbarung über die Zusammenarbeit bei der operativen Patientenversorgung. Anästh Intensivmed 23: 403–405
9. Berufsverband Deutscher Anästhesisten und Berufsverband der Deutschen Chirurgen (1987) Vereinbarung für die prä-, intra- und postoperative Lagerung des Patienten. Anästh Intensivmed 28: 65
10. Berufsverband Deutscher Anästhesisten und Ärzte für Orthopädie (1984) Vereinbarung über die Zusammenarbeit bei der operativen Patientenversorgung. Anästh Intensivmed 25: 464–466
11. Biermann E. (1997) Medico-legale Aspekte in Anästhesie und Intensivmedizin. Anästhesiol Intensivmed Notfallmed Schmerzther 32: 175–193
12. Britt B. A., Gordon R. A. (1964) Peripheral nerve injuries associated with anaesthesia. Can Anaesth Soc J 11: 514–536

References

13. Britt B. A., Joy N., Mackay M. B. (1983) Positioning Trauma In: Orkin F. K., Cooperman LH (ed) Complications in anesthesiology. Lippincott, Philadelphia London pp 646–670
14. Brown R. H., Schauble J. F., Miller N. R. (1994) Anemia and hypotension as contributors to perioperative loss of vision. Anesthesiology 80: 222–226
15. Brumback R. J., Ellison T. S., Molligan H., Molligan D. J., Mahaffey S., Schmidhauser C. (1992) Pudendal nerve palsy complicating intramedullary nailing of the femur. J Bone Joint Surg Am 74: 1450–1455
16. Budinger K. (1894) Über Lähmungen nach Chloroformnarkosen. Arch Klin Chir 47: 121
17. Burkhart F. L., Daly J. W. (1966) Sciatic and peroneal nerve injury: a complication of vaginal operations. Obstet Gynecol 28: 99–102
18. Cheney F. W., Domino K. B., Caplan R. A., Posner K. L. (1999) Nerve injury associated with anesthesia: a closed claims analysis. Anesthesiology 90: 1062–1069
19. Cohen M. M., Duncan P. G., Pope W. D. B., Wolkenstein C. (1986) A survey of 112.000 anaesthetics at one teaching hospital (1975–83). -Canad Anaesth Soc J 33: 22–31
20. Cooper D. E., Jenkins R. S., Bready L., Rockwood C. A. (1988) The prevention of injuries of the brachial plexus secondary to malposition of the patient during surgery. Clin Orthop 228: 33–41
21. Cottrell J. E., Hassan N. F., Hartung J., Cracco R. Q., Capuano C., Bendo A. (1985) Hyperflexion and quadriplegia in the seated position. -Anesthesiol Rev 12: 34
22. Dalton E. M., Bowe E. A. Patient positioning. 1994. In: Conroy JM, - Dorman B. H (eds). Anesthesia for orthopedic surgery. Raven Press, New York Chapter 2, pp 14–20
23. Dawson D. M., Krarup C. (1989) Perioperative nerve lesions. Arch Neurol 46: 1355–1360
24. Denny-Brown D., Brenner C. (1944) Paralysis of nerve induced by direct pressure and by tourniquet. Arch Neurol Psychiatry 51: 1
25. Dhuner KG (1950) Nerve injuries following operations: a survey of cases occuring during a six-year period. Anesthesiology 11: 289–293
26. Dornette W. H. L. (1986) Compression neuropathies: medical aspects and legal implications. Int Anaesthesiol Clin 24: 201–229
27. Ekerot L. (1977) Postanesthetic ulnar neuropathy at the elbow. Scand J Plast Reconstr Surg 11: 225–229
28. Fahmy N. R., Patel D. G. (1981) Hemostatic changes and postoperative deep-vein thrombosis associated with use of a pneumatic tourniquet. J Bone Joint Surg Am 63: 461–465
29. Goldsmith A. L., McCallum M. I. D. (1996) Compartment syndrome as a complication of the prolonged use of the Lloyd-Davies position. Anaesthesia 51: 1048–1052
30. Hatano Y., Arai A., Iida H., Soneda A. (1988) Common peroneal nerve palsy. A complication of coronary artery bypass surgery. Anaesthesia 43: 568–569
31. Haupt W. F. (1989) Intraoperative Lagerungsschäden des N. ulnaris bei anatomischen Varianten. Dtsch med Wochenschr 114: 1789–1792
32. Hickey C., Gugino L. D., Aglio L. S., Mark J. B., Son S. L., Maddi R. (1993) Intra-operative somatosensory evoked potential monitoring predicts peripheral nerve injury during cardiac surgery. Anesthesiology 78: 29–35
33. Hopper C. L., Baker J. B. (1968) Bilateral femoral neuropathy complicating vaginal hysterectomy. Analysis of contributing factors in 3 patients. Obstet Gynecol 32: 543–547
34. Jackson L., Keats A. S. (1965) Mechanism of brachial plexus palsy following anesthesia. Anesthesiology 26: 190–194
35. Jaffe T. B., McLeskey C. H. (1982) Position-induced Horner' syndrome. Anesthesiology 56: 49–50
36. Kienzle F., Ullrich W., Krier C. (1997) Lagerungsschäden in Anästhesie und operativer Intensivmedizin (Teil 2). Anästhesiol Intensivmed Notfallmed Schmerzther 32: 72–86
37. Kwaan J. H. M., Rappaport I. (1970) Postoperative brachial plexus palsy. A study on the mechanism. Arch Surg 101: 612–615
38. Larsen R. Lagerung des Patienten zur Operation (1999) In: Anästhesie, 6. Aufl. Urban & Fischer, München, S 603–608
39. Lwason N. W., Mills N. L., Ochsner J. L. (1976) Occipital alopecia following cardiopulmonary bypass. J Thorac Cardiovasc Surg 71: 342–347
40. Lincoln J. R., Sawyer H. P. (1961) Complications related to body positions during surgical procedures. Anesthesiology 22: 800–809
41. Little D. M. Posture and anaesthesia (1960) Can Anaesth Soc J 7: 2–15
42. London G. M., Levenson J. A., Safar M. E. et al. (1983) Hemodynamic effects of head-down tilt in normal subjects and sustained hypertensive patients. Am J Physiol 245: H194–202
43. Lydon J. C., Spielman F. J. (1984) Bilateral compartment syndrome following prolonged surgery in the lithotomy position. Anesthesiology 60: 236–238
44. Malamut R. I., Marques W., England J. D., Sumner A. J. (1994) Postsurgical idiopathic brachial neuritis. Muscle Nerve 17: 320–324
45. Martin J. T. (1992) Compartment syndromes: Concepts and perspectives for the anesthesiologist. Anesth Analg 75: 275–283
46. Matsen F. A. (1980) Compartmental syndromes. Grune & Stratton, New York
47. McQuarrie H. G., Harris J. W., Ellsworth H. S., Stone R. A., Anderson A. E. (1972) Sciatic neuropathy complicating vaginal hysterectomy. Am J Obstet Gynecol 113: 223–232
48. Mitterschiffthaler G., Theiner A., Posch G., Jäger-Lackner E., Fuith L. C. (1987) Läsionen des Plexus brachialis, verursacht durch fehlerhafte Operationslagerungen. Anästh Intensivther Notfallmed 22: 177–180
49. Müller-Vahl H. (1998) Grundsätzliches zu den pathogenetischen Mechanismen und zur Ätiologie peripherer Nervenläsionen. In: Mumenthaler H, Schliack H, Stöhr M (Hrsg) Läsionen peripherer Nerven und radikuläre Syndrome, 7. Aufl. Thieme, Stuttgart New York S 99–118
50. Mullhall JP, Drezner AD (1993) Postoperative compartment syndrome and the lithotomy position: a report of three cases and analysis of potential risk factors. Conn Med 57: 129–133
51. Mumenthaler M. (1961) Die Ulnarisparesen. Thieme Stuttgart
52. Opderbecke W. (1978) Anästhesie und ärztliche Sorgfaltspflicht. Springer, Berlin Heidelberg New York, S 63–65
53. Parks B. J. (1973) Postoperative peripheral neuropathies. Surgery 74: 348–357
54. Pellegrino M. J., Johnson E. W. (1988) Bilateral obturator nerve-injuries during urologic surgery. Arch Phys Med Rehabil 69: 46–47
55. Peterson T., Wissing H. (1995) Lagerungsschäden beim Patienten mit unbekanntem »thoracic outlet syndrome«. Anästhesiol Intensivmed Notfallmed Schmerzther 30: 516–518
56. Posta A. G. Jr., Allen A. A., Nercessian O. A. (1997) Neurologic injury in the upper extremity after total hip arthroplasty. Clin Orthop 345: 181–186
57. Räber G., Schneider H. P. G. (1993) Femoralisparese nach vaginaler Hysterektomie und ihre forensische Bedeutung. Zentralbl Gynäkol 115: 273–278
58. Rommel F. M., Kabler R. L., Mowad J. J. (1986) The crush syndrome: a complication of urological surgery. J Urol 135: 809–811
59. Saady A. (1981) Brachial plexus palsy after anaesthesia in the -sitting position. Anaesthesia 36: 194–195
60. Scott J. R., Daneker G., Lumsden A. B. (1997) Prevention of compartment syndrome associated with the dorsal lithotomy position. Am Surg 63: 801–806
61. Staender S. (1995) Lagerungsschäden. Swiss Surg 1: 152–155
62. Stewart J. D. (2000) Focal peripheral neuropathies. 3rd edn. -Lippincott, Williams & Wilkens, Philadelphia
63. Stoelting R. K. (1993) Postoperative ulnar nerve palsy – is it a preventable complication? Anesth Analg 76: 7–9

64. Stöhr M. (1996) Iatrogene Nervenläsionen. 2. Aufl. Thieme, Stuttgart New York
65. Strauss H. (1990) Vermeidung von Lagerungsschäden. Klin Anaesthesiol Intensivther 38: 101–120
66. Toole J. F. (1968) Effects of change of head, limb and body position on cephalic circulation. N Engl J Med 279: 307–311
67. Tsamparlakis J., Casey T. A., Howell W., Edridge A. (1980) Dependence of intraocular pressure on induced hypotension and posture -during surgical anaesthesia. Trans Ophtalmol Soc UK 100: 521–526
68. Ullrich W., Biermann E., Kienzle F., Krier C. (1997) Lagerungsschäden in Anästhesie und operativer Medizin (Teil 1). Anästhesiol Intensivmed Notfallmed Schmerzther 32: 4–20
69. Vahl C. F., Carl I., Müller-Vahl H., Struck E. (1991) Brachial plexus injury after cardiac surgery. The role of internal mammary artery preparation: a prospective study on 1000 consecutive patients. J Thorac Cardiovasc Surg 102: 724–729
70. Warner M. A., Martin J. T., Schroeder D. R., Offord K. P., Chute C. G. (1994) Lower extremity motor neuropathic associated with surgery -performed on patients in lithotomy position. Anesthesiology 81: 6–12
71. Warner M. A., Warner M. E., Martin J. T. (1994) Ulnar neuropathy. Incidence, outcome, and risk factors in sedated or anesthetized patients. Anesthesiology 81: 1332–1340
72. Warner M. A., Warner D. O., Matsumoto J. Y., Harper C. M., Schroeder D. R., Maxson P. M. (1999) Ulnar neuropathy in surgical patients. Anesthesiology 90: 54–59
73. Warner M. A., Warner D. O., Harper C. M., Schroeder D. R., Maxson P. M. (2000) Ulnar neuropathy in medical patients. Anesthesiology 92: 613–615
74. Weißauer W. (1987) Verantwortung für die Lagerung des -Patienten. Zur Vereinbarung der Berufsverbände Deutscher Anästhesisten und der Deutschen Chirurgen. Anästh Intensivmed 28: 66–67
75. Wey J. M., Guinn G. A. (1985) Ulnar nerve injury with open heart surgery. Ann Thorac Surg 39: 358–360
76. Wilgis E. F. (1971) Observations on the effects of tourniquet -ischemia. J Bone Joint Surg Am 53: 1343–1346
77. Williams E. L., Hart W. M., Tempelhoff R. (1995) Postoperative ischemic optic neuropathy. Anesth Analg 80: 1018–1029
78. Wolfe S. W., Lospinuso M. F., Burke S. W. (1992) Unilateral blindness as a complication of patient positioning for spinal surgery. Spine 17: 600–605
79. Zylicz A., Nuyten F. J., Nutermans S. L., Koene R. A. (1984) Postoperative ulnar neuropathy after kidney transplantation. Anaesthesia 39: 1117–1120

II Special section

*D. Aschemann, C. Krettek, A. Becker, A. Gänsslen, T. Hüfner,
D. Kendoff, T. Kofidis, J. Leonhardt, L. Mahlke, G. Scheumann,
U. Schmidt, B. Ure*

*(Illustrations and picture processing: D. Aschemann, W. Mayrhofer,
A. Lang, P. Lang, K. Adam; Models: M. Prüser, U. Gerber)*

11 Thorax and heart surgery

11.1 Median thoracotomy (sternotomy) – 134
11.1.1 Supine position – 134

11.2 Bilateral thoracotomy – 36
11.2.1 Supine position – 136

11.3 Lateral thoracotomy – 138
11.3.1 Lateral position – 138
11.3.2 Modified lateral position – 140

11.4 Anterolateral thoracotomy – 142
11.4.1 Supine position – 142

11.5 Others – 144
11.5.1 Modified supine position – 144
11.5.2 Supine position – 146

11.1 Median thoracotomy

11.1.1 Supine position

■ Figs. 11.1–11.4.

Indications

Sternotomy for coronary surgery (ACVB, OBCAP), valve surgery (mitral/aortic valve replacement), HTX and type A dissection.

Preparations
- Arm positioning devices
- Padded arm protection

Positioning
- Standard operating table position 1, position 2 or universal operating table
- Anaesthetic preparation and induction in supine position with 2 adapted arm positioning devices
- Normal positioning of the operating table in the theatre
- When positioning the patient, take appropriate measures to prevent decubitus at areas which are subjected to pressure
- Position both arms at the body with arm protection, forearm slings, clips or other positioning aids
- Radial artery removal: position the arm in supination position with 90° abduction on the arm positioning device. An arm protection can be adapted on this side to make it easier to move the arm back to the body again later on
- Apply the neutral electrode and connect to the HF surgery device
- Arrange absorbent drapes or self-adhesive covers for preoperative skin disinfection
- Position the operating lights
- Connect the water mat/patient warming system

11.1 · Median thoracotomy

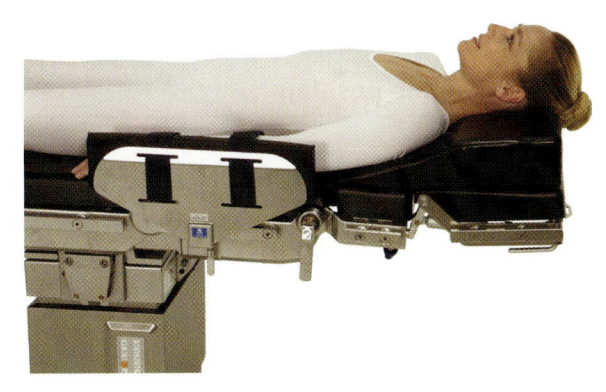

Fig. 11.1. Supine position for sternotomy with arms positioned at the body

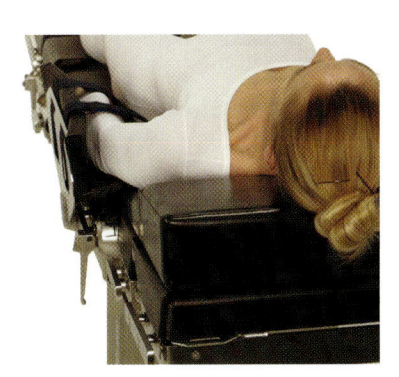

Fig. 11.2. Arms positioned at the body with arm protection and padding

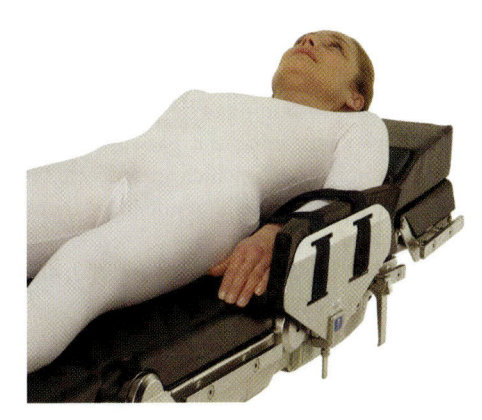

Fig. 11.3. Optimum positioning comfort from the elbow to the hand

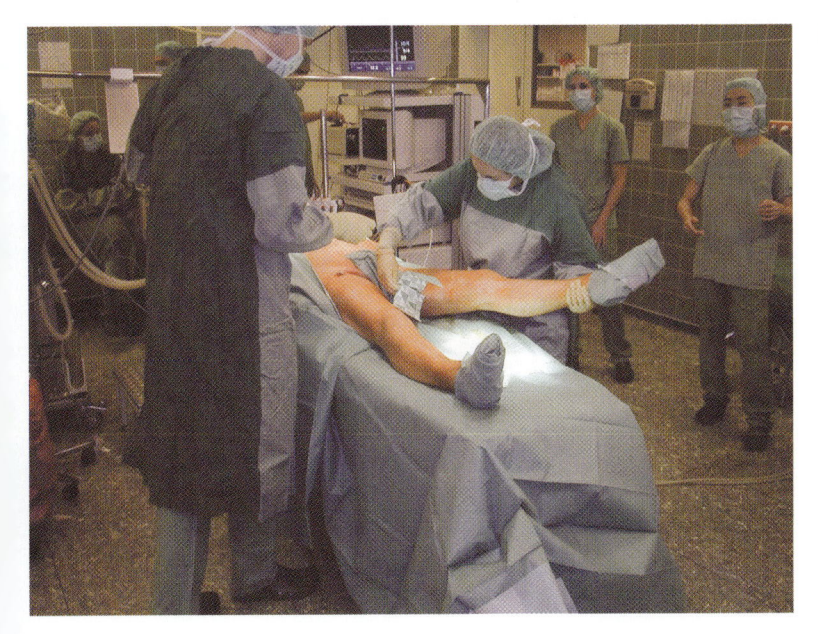

Fig. 11.4. Legs uncovered for free movement

11.2 Bilateral thoracotomy

11.2.1 Supine position

◘ Figs. 11.5–11.7.

Indications
Bilateral access for double lung transplantation (DLuTX).

Preparations
- Arm positioning devices
- Padded arm protection
- Padded cushions

Positioning
- Standard operating table position 1, position 2 or universal operating table
- Anaesthetic preparation and induction in supine position with 2 adapted arm positioning devices
- Normal positioning of the operating table in the theatre
- When positioning the patient, take appropriate measures to prevent decubitus at areas which are subjected to pressure
- Place a padded cushion under the thoracic vertebrae along the body axis (to raise the thorax)
- Position both arms at the body with arm protection, forearm slings, clips or other positioning aids
- Apply the neutral electrode and connect to the HF surgery device
- Arrange absorbent drapes or self-adhesive covers for preoperative skin disinfection
- Position the operating lights
- Connect the water mat/patient warming system

11.2 · Bilateral thoracotomy

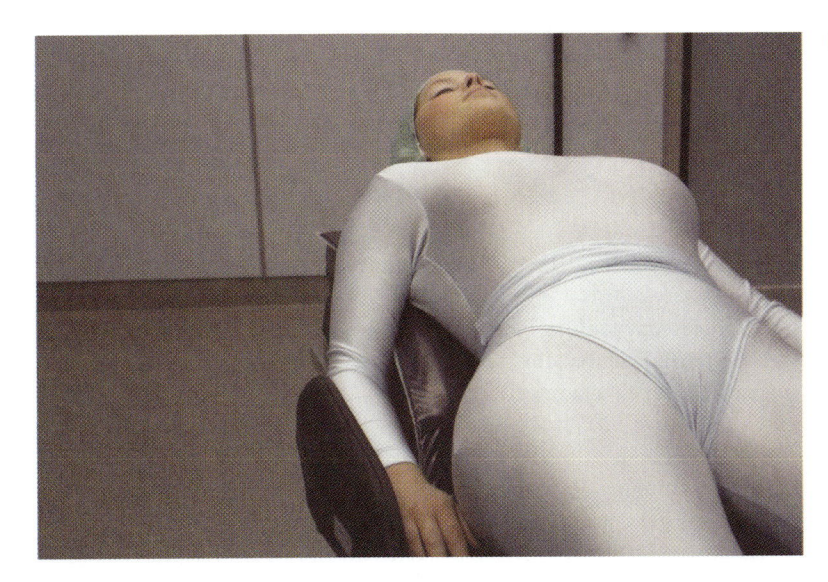

Fig. 11.5. Supine position for bilateral access

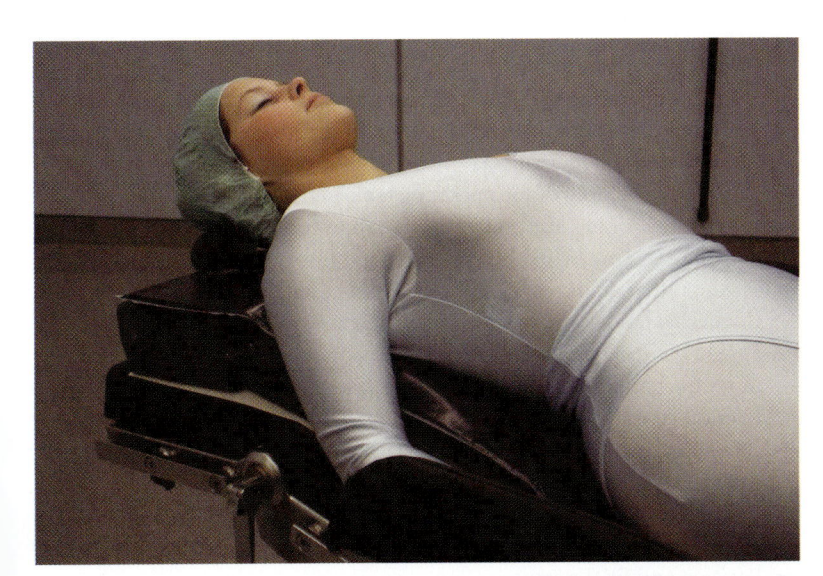

Fig. 11.6. Raised thorax and lowered positioning of the arms

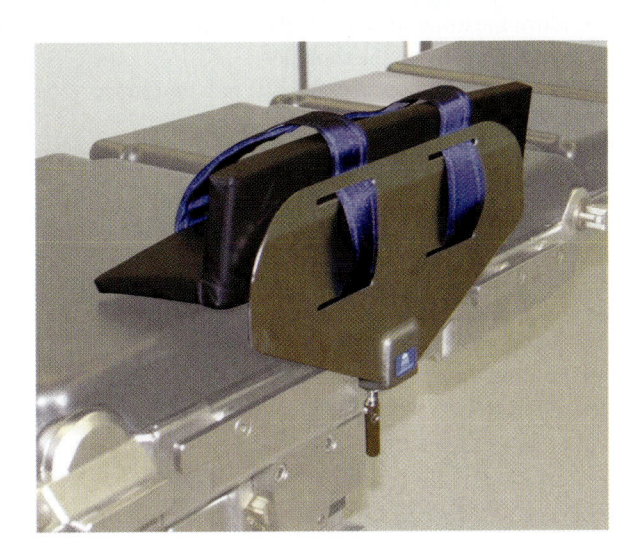

Fig. 11.7. Arm protection 1002.25A0

11.3 Lateral thoracotomy

11.3.1 Lateral position

◘ Figs. 11.8–11.10.

Indications

Lateral access for lung transplantation (LuTX), lung segment resection and lobectomy.

Thoracoscopy for lung biopsy, pleural biopsy, pleural effusion, pericardial effusion, partial pleurectomy, resection of peripheral pulmonary nodules and tangential parenchyma resection.

Preparations
- Arm positioning devices
- Gel ring, gel cushion, Goepel leg holder, body support, radial adjusting clamps, padded cushions (normal and flat) and wedge cushions or tunnel cushions, body belts

Positioning
- Standard operating table position 1 or universal operating table
- Anaesthetic preparation and induction in supine position with 2 adapted arm positioning devices
- Normal positioning of the operating table in the theatre
- When positioning the patient, take appropriate measures to prevent decubitus at areas which are subjected to pressure
- Fit the radial adjusting clamp to the rail of the head plate, position the Goepel leg holder and place a gel padded mat on the operating table
- Spread out the arm on the side not being operated in max. 90° abduction
- Move the patient onto the healthy side, with the back near the edge of the operating table
- Open the operating table step by step by lowering the pelvic and back plate (operating table in roof position)
- Raise the head plate and position the head on a padded cushion with gel ring to leave the ear free
- Position and fix the arms
- Move the lower arm forwards so that the weight of the upper body does not lie directly on the shoulder
- Fit the body supports to the side rails and support the body at the level of the sacrum and symphysis
- **1st possibility:** position the legs with the padded cushions (normal and flat) and possibly wedge cushions
- Fix the lower leg and the positioning aids with the body belts
- **2nd possibility:** position the legs with the tunnel cushion
- Apply the neutral electrode and connect to the HF surgery device
- Arrange absorbent drapes or self-adhesive covers for preoperative skin disinfection
- Position the operating lights
- Connect the water mat/patient warming system

11.3 · Lateral thoracotomy

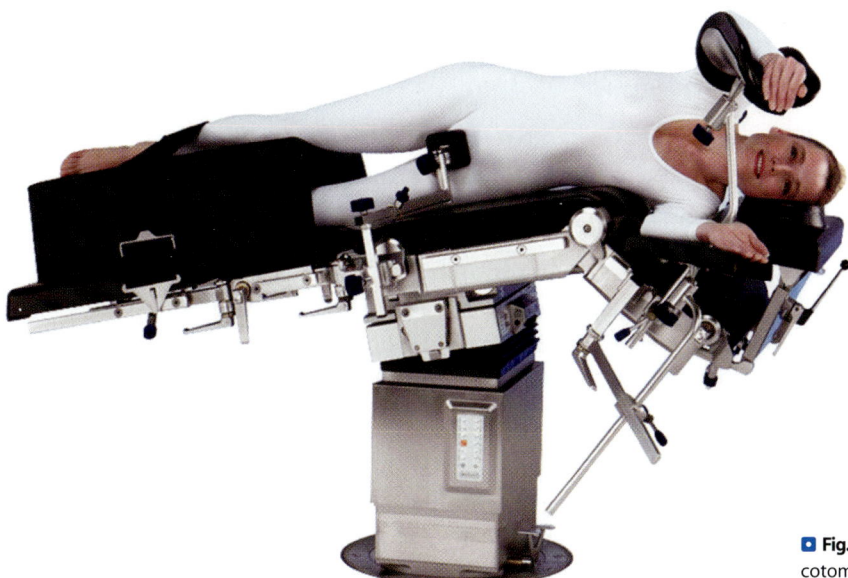

Fig. 11.8. Lateral position for lateral thoracotomy

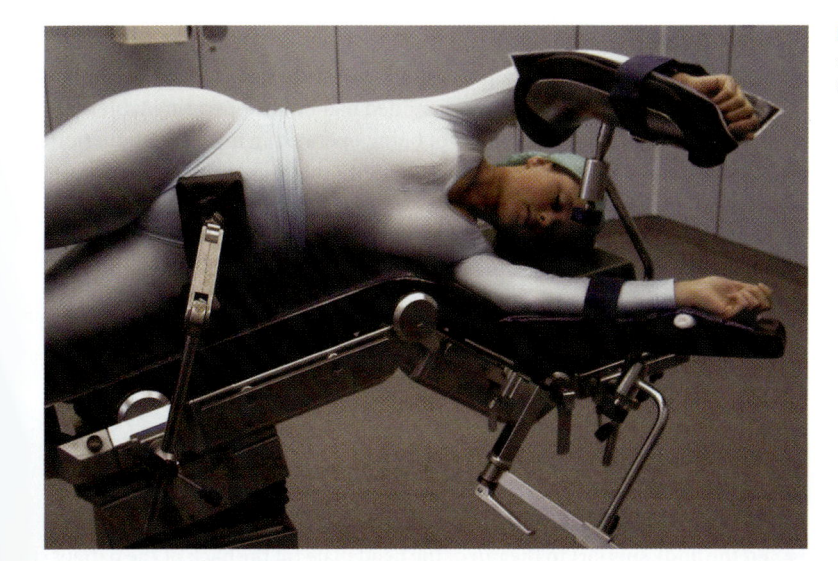

Fig. 11.9. Operation table in flex position and maximum longitudinal displacement toward the head

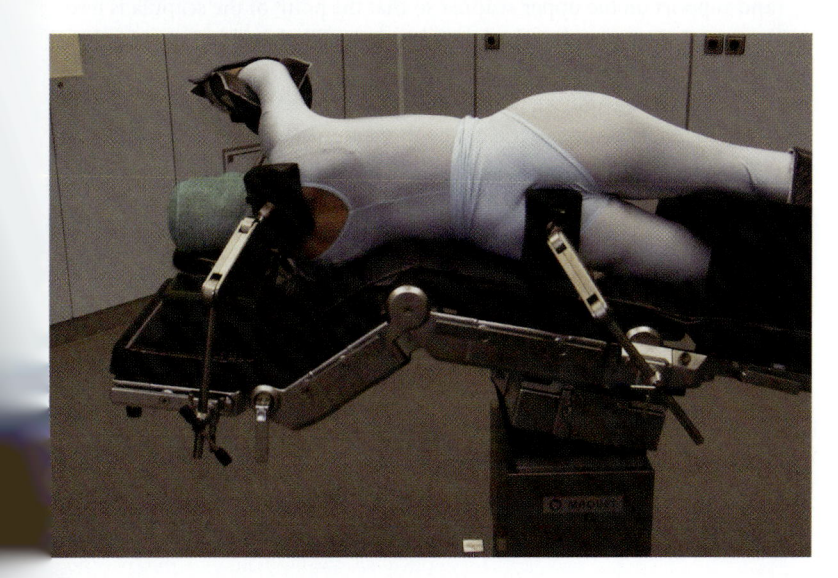

Fig. 11.10. Cervical spine in middle position, tip of the scapula is free with a dorsal thorax support

11.3.2 Modified lateral position

◘ Figs. 11.11–11.13.

Indications
Lateral access for descending aorta replacement and thoracoabdominal aorta replacement.

Preparations
- Arm positioning devices
- Gel ring, gel cushion, Goepel leg holder, body support, radial adjusting clamps, padded cushions (normal and flat) and wedge cushions or tunnel cushions, body belts

Positioning
- Standard operating table position 1 or universal operating table
- Anaesthetic preparation and induction in supine position with 2 adapted arm positioning devices
- Normal positioning of the operating table in the theatre
- When positioning the patient, take appropriate measures to prevent decubitus at areas which are subjected to pressure
- Fit the radial adjusting clamp to the side rail of the head plate, position the Goepel leg holder and place a gel padded mat on the operating table
- Spread out the arm on the side not being operated in max. 90° abduction
- Move the patient onto the healthy side, with the back near the edge of the operating table
- Open the operating table step by step by lowering the pelvic and back plate (operating table in roof position)
- Raise the head plate and position the head on a padded cushion with gel ring to leave the ear free
- Position and fix the arms
- Move the lower arm forwards so that the weight of the upper body does not lie directly on the shoulder
- Thorax 90° position, pelvis 45° position
- Fit the body supports to the side rails and support the body at the level of the sacrum and symphysis
- Fit the body support to the rail of the head plate (at the back of the patient) and support on the upper scapula so that the point of the scapula is free
- **1st possibility:** position the legs with the padded cushions (normal and flat) and possibly wedge cushions
- Fix the lower leg and the positioning aids with the body belts
- **2nd possibility:** position the legs with the tunnel cushion
- Position the upper leg in external rotation
- Apply the neutral electrode and connection to the HF surgery device
- Arrange absorbent drapes or self-adhesive covers for preoperative skin disinfection
- Position the operating lights
- Connect the water mat/patient warming system

11.3 · Modified lateral position

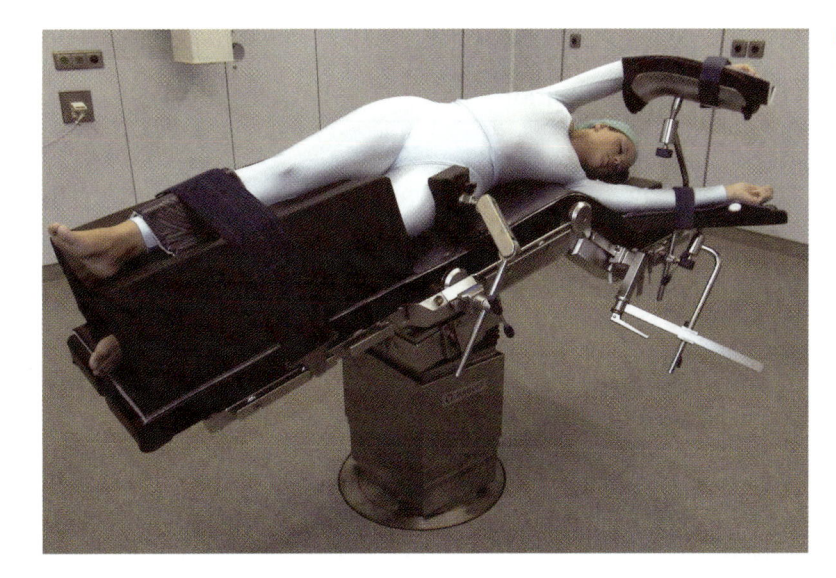

Fig. 11.11. Modified lateral position for thoracoabdominal access

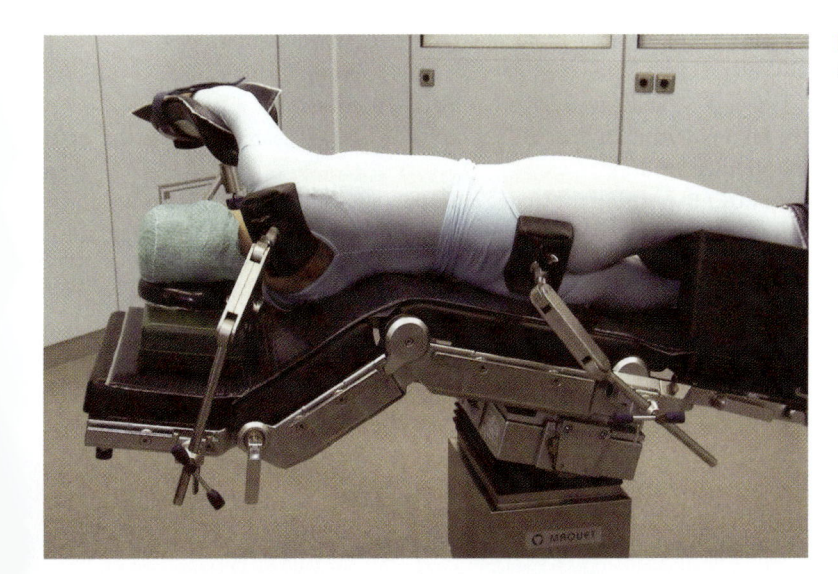

Fig. 11.12. Support for the shoulder and for the pelvis tilted approx. 30–40° backwards

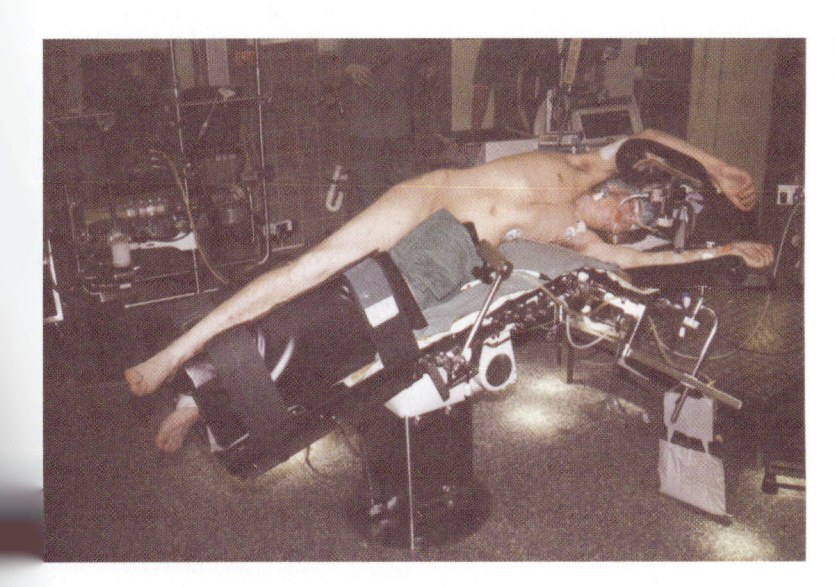

Fig. 11.13. Positioning with freely moving leg

11.4 Anterolateral thoracotomy

11.4.1 Supine position

◘ Figs. 11.14, 11.15.

Indications
Anterolateral access for MIDCAB and minimally invasive ASD.

Preparations
- Arm positioning devices
- Padded arm protection
- Small wedge cushion

Positioning
- Standard operating table position 1, position 2 or universal operating table
- Anaesthetic preparation and induction in supine position with 2 adapted arm positioning devices
- Normal positioning of the operating table in the theatre
- When positioning the patient, take appropriate measures to prevent decubitus at areas which are subjected to pressure
- Minimally invasive ASD: position the wedge cushion under the right shoulder/thorax
- MIDCAB: position the wedge cushion under the left shoulder/thorax
- Position both arms at the body with arm protection, forearm slings, clips or other positioning aids
- Apply the neutral electrode and connect to the HF surgery device
- Arrange absorbent drapes or self-adhesive covers for preoperative skin disinfection
- Position the operating lights
- Connect the water mat/patient warming system

11.4 · Anterolateral thoracotomy

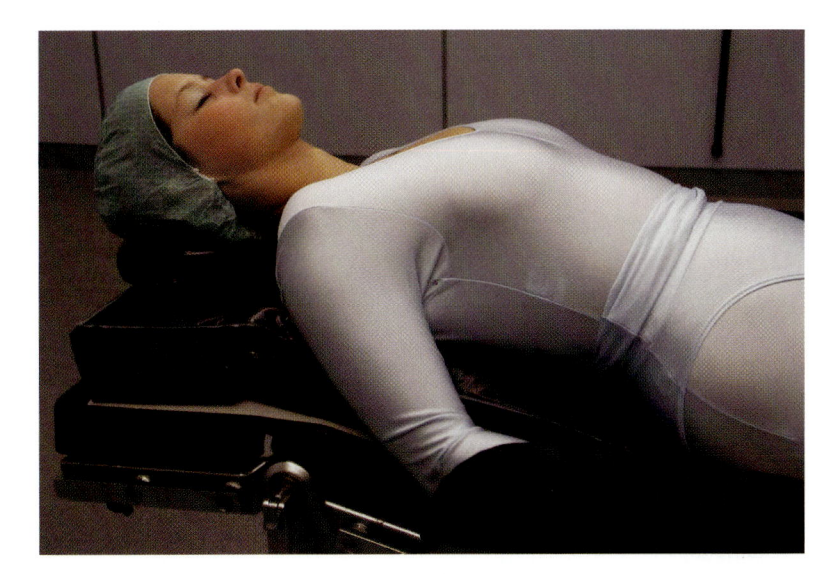

Fig. 11.14. Supine position with wedge cushion under the right shoulder/thoracic side

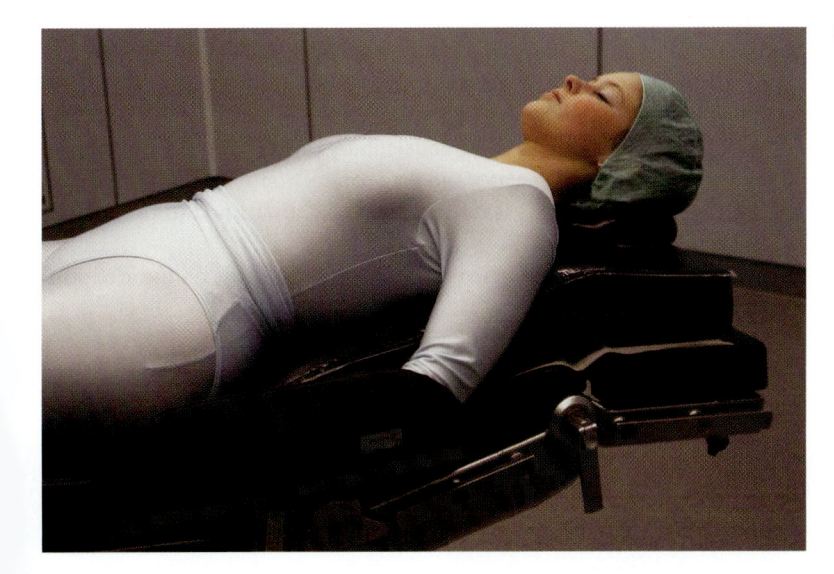

Fig. 11.15. Supine position with wedge cushion under the left shoulder/thoracic side

11.5 Others

11.5.1 Modified supine position

◧ Figs. 11.16, 11.17.

Indications

Mediastinoscopy.

Preparations
- Arm positioning devices
- Padded arm protection
- Gel ring, possibly flat padded cushion

Positioning
- Standard operating table position 1, position 2 or universal operating table top
- Anaesthetic preparation and induction in supine position with 2 adapted arm positioning devices
- Crosswise positioning of the operating table in the theatre
- When positioning the patient, take appropriate measures to prevent decubitus at areas which are subjected to pressure
- Possibly pad the shoulders with a flat padded cushion
- Tilt the operating table in the Trendelenburg position, raise the back plate by 20–30°, lower the leg plates and the head section
- Position the head on a gel ring, possibly slightly turned to the left and reclined
- Position the left infusion arm on the anaesthetist's side on the arm positioning device
- Position the right arm at the body with arm protection, forearm slings, clips or other positioning aids
- Apply the neutral electrode and connect to the HF surgery device
- Arrange absorbent drapes or self-adhesive covers for preoperative skin disinfection
- Position the operating lights
- Patient warming system

11.5 · Others

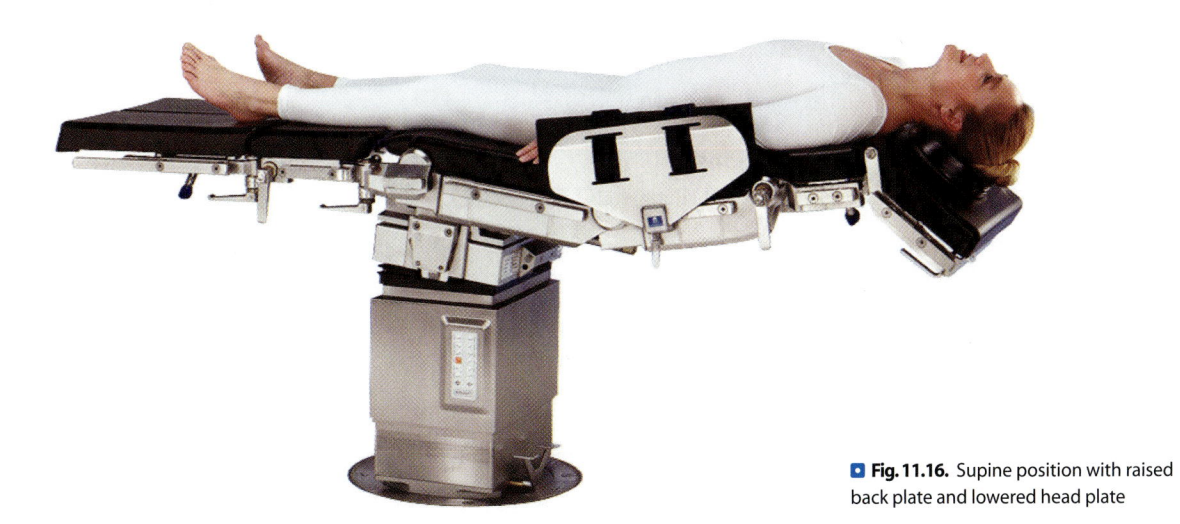

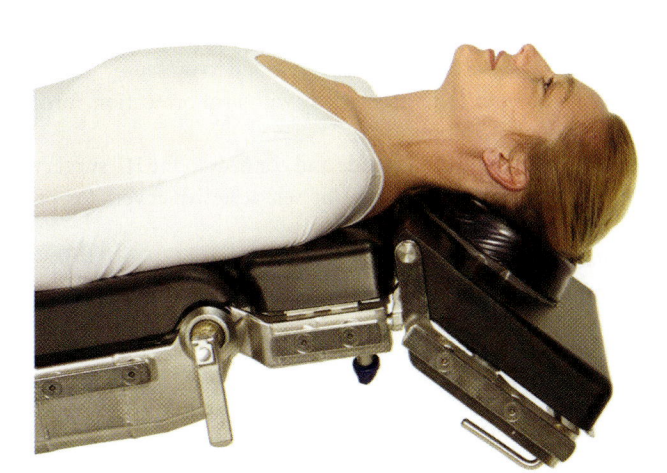

Fig. 11.16. Supine position with raised back plate and lowered head plate

Fig. 11.17. The head is reclined and held in a stable position with a gel ring

11.5.2 Supine position

◘ Figs. 11.18–11.20.

Indications
AICD (defibrillator) and pacemaker.

Preparations
- Arm positioning devices
- Padded arm protection
- C-arm and monitor trolley, X-ray protection

Positioning
- Standard operating table position 1 or universal operating table with X-ray protection
- Anaesthetic preparation and induction in supine position with 2 adapted arm positioning devices
- Normal positioning of the operating table in the theatre
- When positioning the patient, take appropriate measures to prevent decubitus at areas which are subjected to pressure
- Position both arms at the body with arm protection, forearm slings, clips or other positioning aids
- Apply the neutral electrode and connect to the HF surgery device
- Arrange absorbent drapes or self-adhesive covers for preoperative skin disinfection
- Position the operating lights
- Patient warming system

11.5 · Others

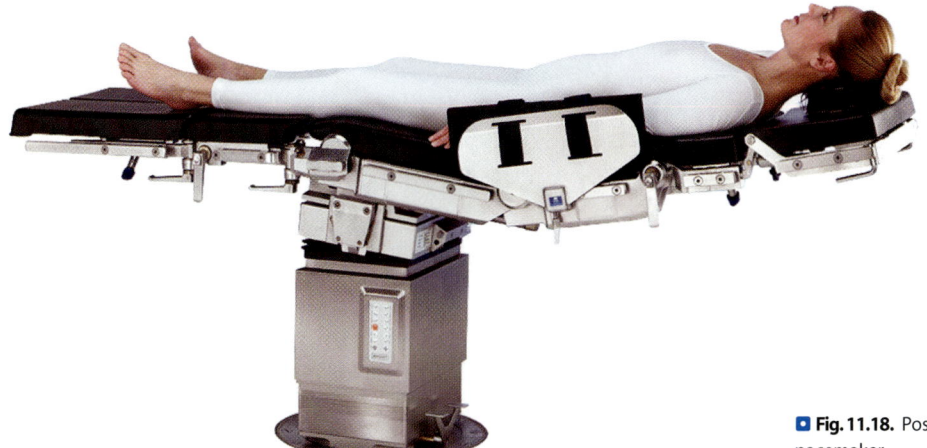

Fig. 11.18. Positioning for implantation of a pacemaker

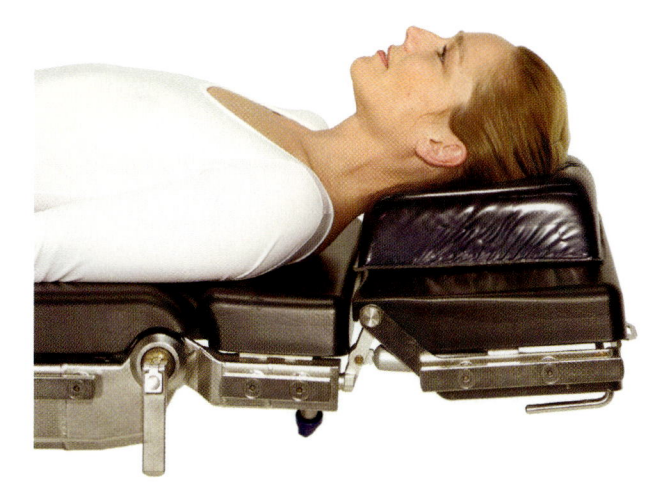

Fig. 11.19. Stable positioning of the head with a gel cushion

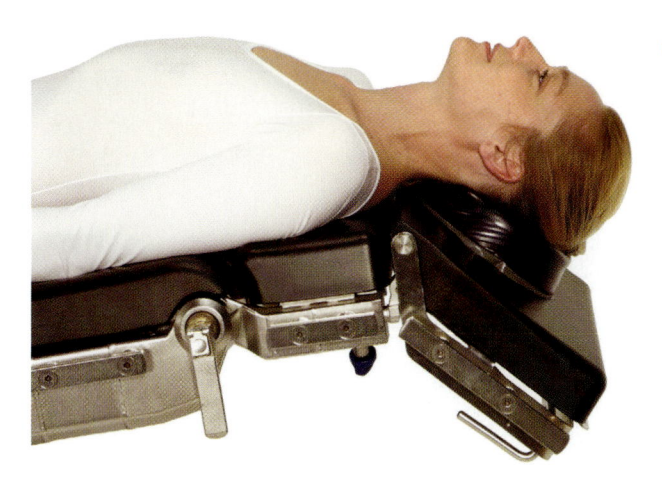

Fig. 11.20. The head can also be reclined and held in a stable position with a gel ring

12 Vascular surgery

12.1 Neck – 150
12.1.1 Supine position – 150

12.2 Upper extremities – 152
12.2.1 Supine position – 152

12.3 Lower extremities – 154
12.3.1 Supine position – 154

12.1 Neck

12.1.1 Supine position

◘ Figs. 12.1–12.4.

Indications

Operation to the carotis: carotid patch, carotid shunt, carotid TEA; *tumour operations* to vessels (glomus tumour).

Preparations
- Arm positioning devices
- Padded arm protection
- Gel ring

Positioning
- Standard operating table position 1, position 2 or universal operating table
- Anaesthetic preparation and induction in supine position with 2 adapted arm positioning devices
- Normal positioning of the operating table in the theatre
- When positioning the patient, take appropriate measures to prevent decubitus at areas which are subjected to pressure
- Possibly pad the shoulders with a flat padded cushion
- Tilt the operating table in the Trendelenburg position, raise the back plate by 20–30°, lower the leg plates and the head section by hand
- Position the head on a gel ring, possibly slightly turned to the side and reclined
- Position both arms at the body with arm protection, forearm slings, clips or other positioning aids or the infusion arm in the supination position with max. 90° abduction on an arm positioning device
- Apply the neutral electrode and connect to the HF surgery device
- Arrange absorbent drapes or self-adhesive covers for preoperative skin disinfection
- Position the operating lights
- Patient warming system

12.1 · Neck

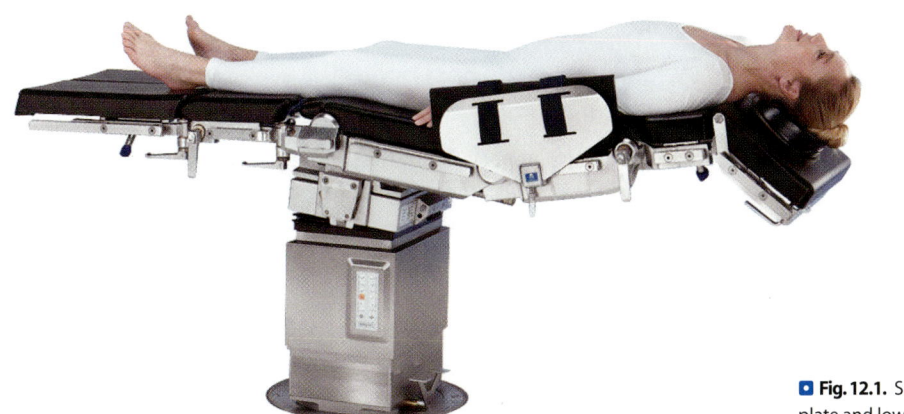

Fig. 12.1. Supine position with raised back plate and lowered head plate

Fig. 12.2. Supine position with raised back plate, adapted connection bar, fastening piece and one-piece horseshoe-shaped headrest

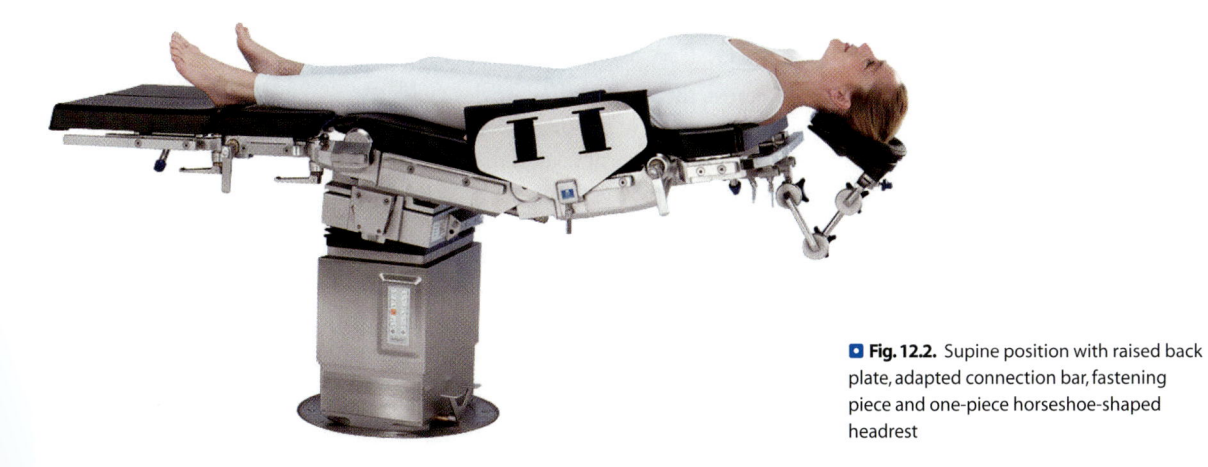

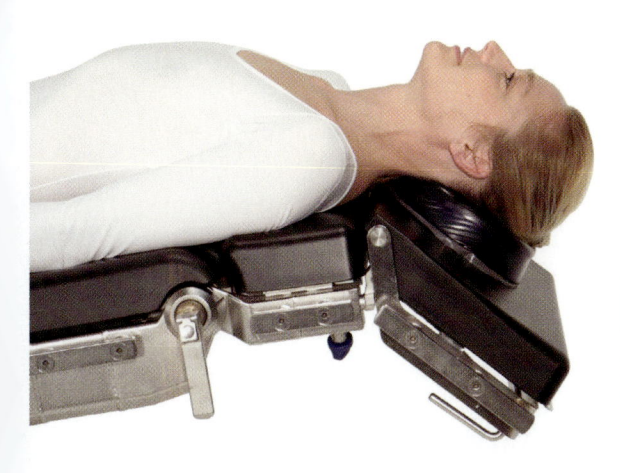

Fig. 12.3. The head is reclined and held in a stable position with a gel ring

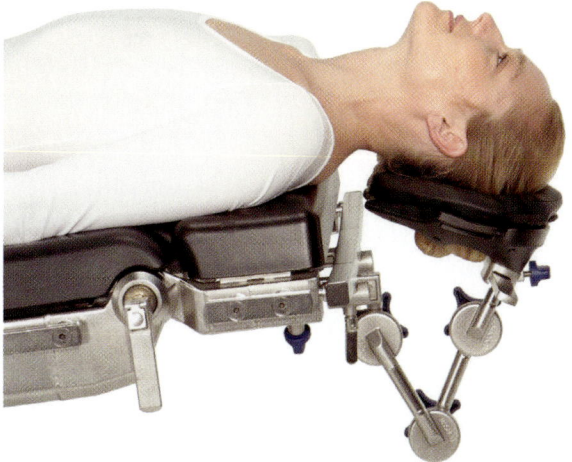

Fig. 12.4. The head is reclined and held in a stable position with a one-piece horseshoe-shaped headrest

12.2 Upper extremities

12.2.1 Supine position

◘ Figs. 12.5, 12.6.

Indications

Embolectomies of the upper extremities; *shunt placement*, (Cimino shunt), shunt revisions; *shunt connections*, e.g. axillofemoral bypass.

Preparations
- Arm positioning devices
- Large arm table

Positioning
- Standard operating table position 1, position 2 or universal operating table
- Anaesthetic preparation and induction in supine position with 2 adapted arm positioning devices
- Crosswise positioning of the operating table top in the theatre
- When positioning the patient, take appropriate measures to prevent decubitus at areas which are subjected to pressure
- Remove the arm positioning device on the operating side and attach the large arm rest to the side rail of the back plate
- Position the patient near to the edge of the table
- Standard supine position, position the infusion arm on the arm positioning device
- Apply the neutral electrode and connect to the HF surgery device
- Arrange self-adhesive covers for preoperative skin disinfection
- Position the operating lights
- Patient warming system

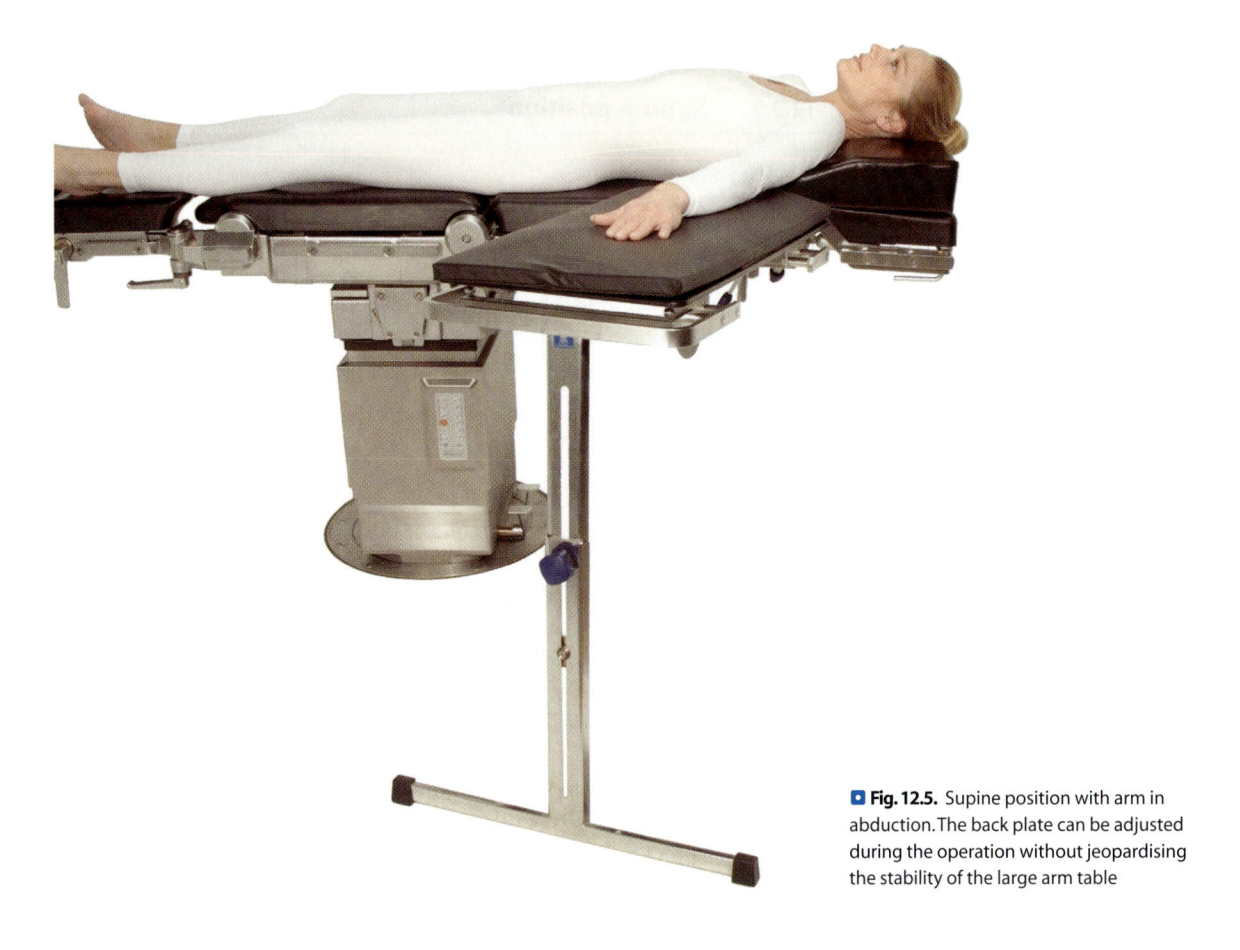

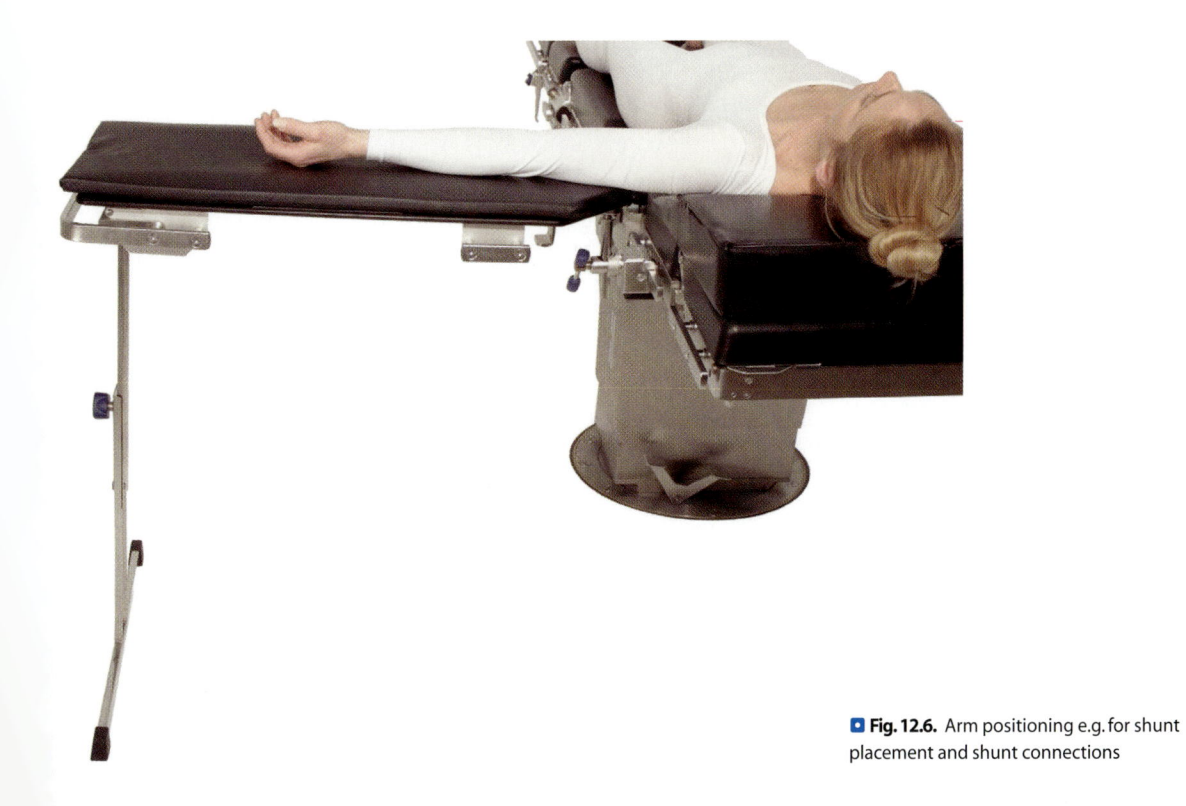

12.2 · Upper extremities

Fig. 12.5. Supine position with arm in abduction. The back plate can be adjusted during the operation without jeopardising the stability of the large arm table

Fig. 12.6. Arm positioning e.g. for shunt placement and shunt connections

12.3 Lower extremities

12.3.1 Supine position

◘ Figs. 12.7–12.9.

Indications

Angioplasty procedures, e.g. profundaplasty, patch graft; *shunts,* e.g. Y-shunt; *aneurysms,* e.g. abdominal aortic aneurysm, embolectomies to the lower extremities; *prosthesis connections, e.g. axillofemoral bypass.*

Preparations
- Arm positioning devices

Positioning
- Standard operating table position 1, position 2 or universal operating table
- Anaesthetic preparation and induction in supine position with 2 adapted arm positioning devices
- Normal positioning of the operating table in the theatre
- When positioning the patient, take appropriate measures to prevent decubitus at areas which are subjected to pressure
- Spread out and pad both arms on the arm positioning devices
- Apply the neutral electrode and connect to the HF surgery device
- Arrange absorbent drapes or self-adhesive covers for preoperative skin disinfection
- Position the operating lights
- Patient warming system

12.3 · Lower extremities

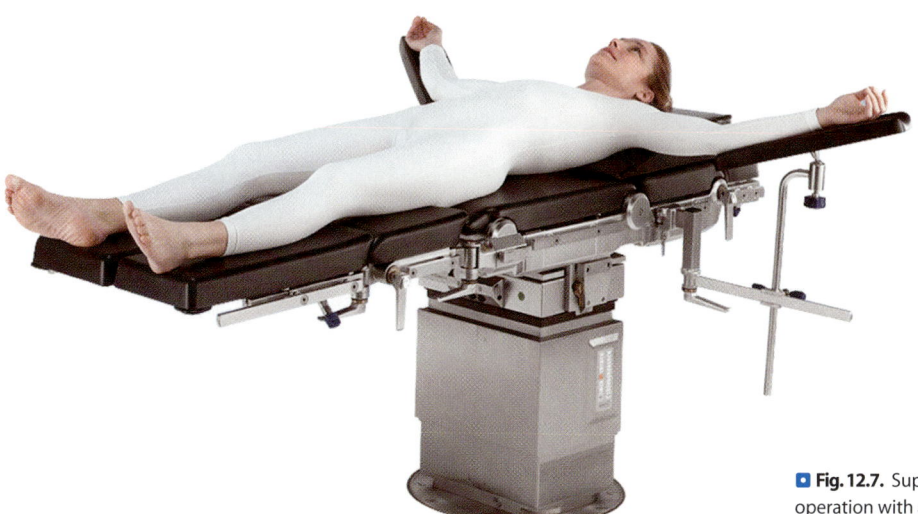

Fig. 12.7. Supine position for Y-shunt operation with arms in abduction

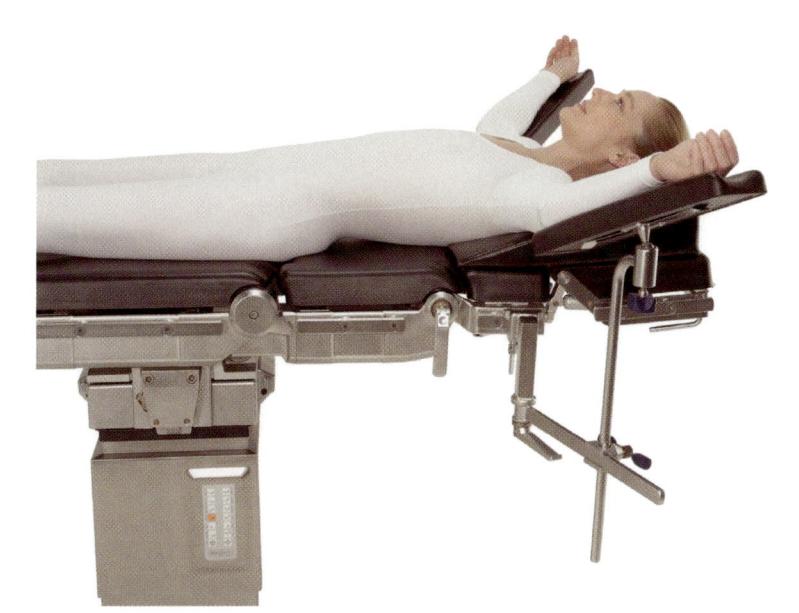

Fig. 12.8. Maximum 90° abduction and supination position of the arms

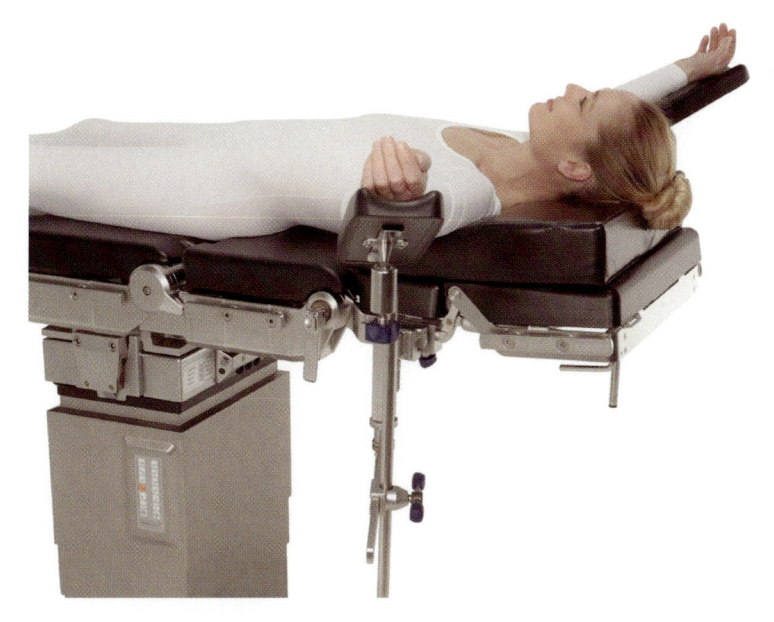

Fig. 12.9. Head positioned on a double wedge cushion

13 Visceral and transplantation surgery

13.1 Neck – 158
13.1.1 Supine position – 158
13.1.2 Supine position, neurosurgical headrest – 160

13.2 Open laparotomy – 162
13.2.1 Supine position (median and transverse laparotomy, incision right or left parallel to the costal margin) – 162
13.2.2 Lithotomy position – 164

13.3 Laparoscopic operations – 166
13.3.1 Supine position – 166

13.4 Heidelberger position (position for Kraske access) – 168
13.4.1 Modified prone position – 168

13.5 Lateral position – 170
13.5.1 Modified lateral position – 170

13.1 Neck

13.1.1 Supine position

◘ Figs. 13.1, 13.2.

Indications

Operations to the thyroid/parathyroid: thyroid operations (e.g. hemithyroidectomy), thyroid operations of tumours with systematic lymphadenectomy (e.g. total thyroidectomy).

Operations to the oesophagus: operations to the oesophagus (e.g. anastomotic connection with stomach pull-up, resection of Zenker's diverticula).

Operations to cysts and embryonal duplications of the oesophagus: e.g. medial or lateral cysts in the neck, cervical oesophagus duplication.

Preparations
- Arm positioning devices
- Gel ring
- Padded arm protection

Positioning
- Standard operating table position 1, position 2 or universal operating table
- Anaesthetic preparation and induction in supine position with 2 adapted arm positioning devices
- Normal positioning of the operating table in the theatre
- When positioning the patient, take appropriate measures to prevent decubitus at areas which are subjected to pressure
- Possibly pad the shoulders with a flat padded cushion
- Tilt the operating table in the Trendelenburg position, raise the back plate by 20–30°, lower the leg plates and head section (by hand)
- Position the head on a gel ring, possibly slightly turned to the side and reclined
- Position both arms at the body with arm protection, forearm slings, clips or other positioning aids or the infusion arm in supination position with 90° abduction on the arm positioning device
- Apply the neutral electrode and connect to the HF surgery device
- Arrange absorbent drapes or self-adhesive covers for preoperative skin disinfection
- Position the operating lights
- Patient warming system

13.1 · Neck

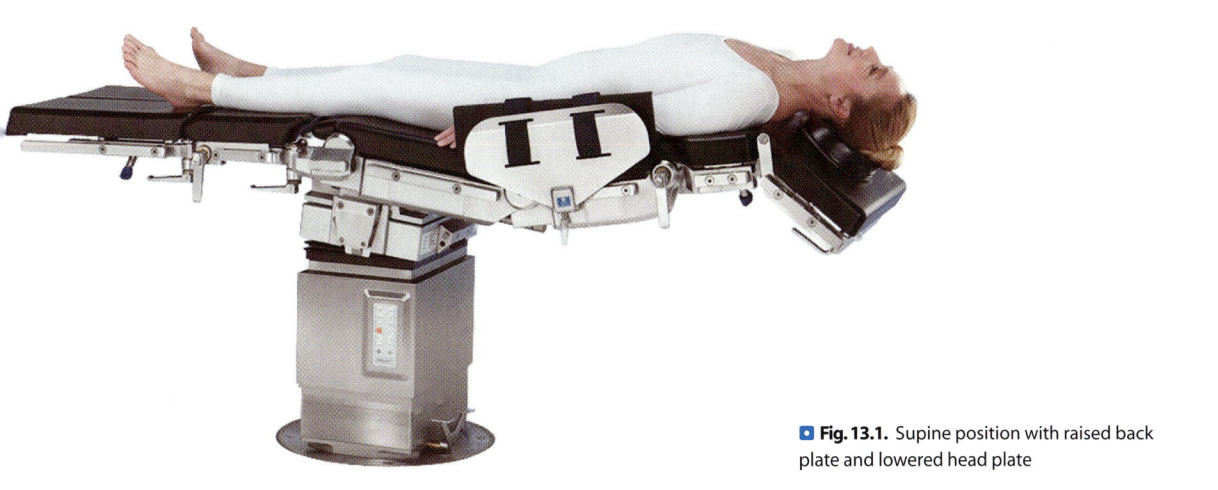

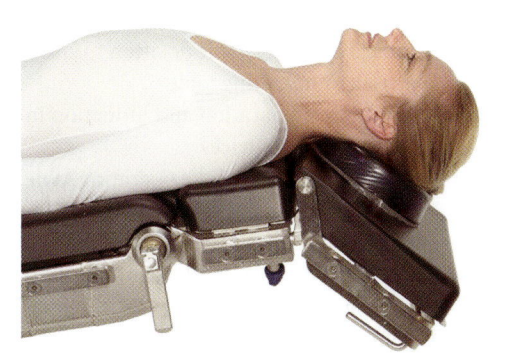

Fig. 13.1. Supine position with raised back plate and lowered head plate

Fig. 13.2. The head is reclined and held in a stable position with a gel ring

13.1.2 Supine position, neurosurgical headrest

◘ Figs. 13.3, 13.4.

Indications

Operations to the thyroid: thyroid operations for tumours with systematic lymphadenectomy, e.g. total thyroidectomy and systematic lymphadenectomy of compartments 2, 3 and 4 (mediastinum via sternotomy).

Operations to cysts and embryonal duplications of the oesophagus: cysts and embryonal duplications of the oesophagus (e.g. medial or lateral cysts in the neck, cervical oesophagus duplication).

Preparations

- Arm positioning devices
- Padded arm protection
- Neurosurgical headrest, wedge cushions, block cushions, knee half roll

Positioning

- Standard operating table position 1, position 2, universal operating table or beach-chair operating table
- Anaesthetic preparation and induction in supine position with 2 adapted arm positioning devices
- Normal positioning of the operating table in the theatre
- When positioning the patient, take appropriate measures to prevent decubitus at areas which are subjected to pressure
- Fasten and pre-position the neurosurgical headrest to the head part of the operating table
- Tilt the operating table in the Trendelenburg position, move the patient towards the head end until the shoulders are flush with the upper edge of the operating table
- Lift the legs and fix the wedge and block cushion under the buttocks and thighs
- Lift the back plate by 20–30°, possibly lower the leg plates
- Position and fix the head in the neurosurgical headrest, possibly slightly turned to the side and reclined
- Position both arms at the body with arm protection, forearm slings, clips or other positioning aids or the infusion arm in supination position with 90° abduction on the arm positioning device
- Apply the neutral electrode to the upper arm and connect to the HF surgery device
- Arrange absorbent drapes or self-adhesive covers for preoperative skin disinfection
- Position the operating lights
- Patient warming system

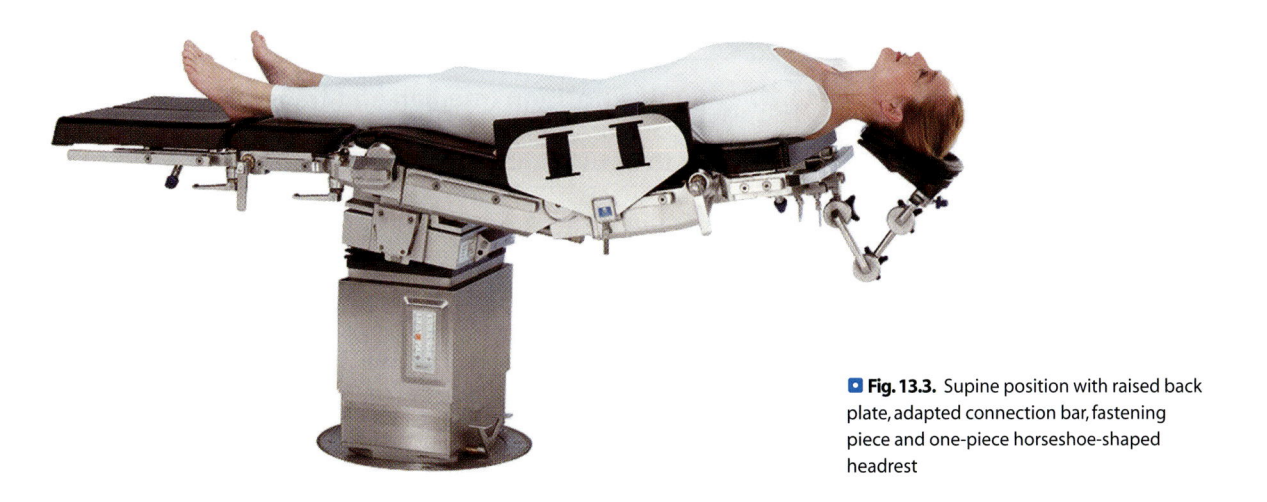

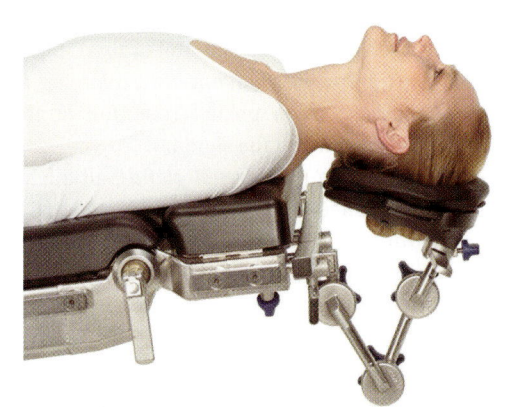

Fig. 13.3. Supine position with raised back plate, adapted connection bar, fastening piece and one-piece horseshoe-shaped headrest

Fig. 13.4. The head is reclined and held in a stable position with a one-piece horseshoe-shaped headrest, thus providing better side access

13.2 Open laparotomy

13.2.1 Supine position (median and transverse laparotomy, incision right or left parallel to the costal margin)

◘ Figs. 13.5–13.9.

Indications

All operations to the ventral abdominal organs and the abdominal wall and for emergency operations such as acute abdomen.

Operations to the distal oesophagus, cardiac orifice and diaphragm, e.g. grafts for achalasia, fundoplication and diaphragm resection.

Operations to the liver and bile ducts, e.g. hemihepatectomy on the right and left, hepatic fork resection, liver transplants.

Operations to the stomach, duodenum, e.g. gastrectomy, total or subtotal, formation of a stomach tube for stomach pull-up.

Operations to the pancreas, spleen, e.g. Whipple's operation, reconstruction of the spleen after injury, subtotal or total splenectomy.

Operations to the small intestine, colon, e.g. resection of the small intestine, appendectomy, colon partial resection of the ascending, transverse and descending colon and the sigma.

Operations to the adrenal glands; all bilateral operations to the adrenal glands, adrenalectomy.

Operations to the abdomen wall/peritoneum, e.g. herniotomy for scar hernias, inguinal hernias and peritonectomy.

Operations for abdominal trauma, traumatic injuries to all abdominal organs.

Operation for organ donation

Operation for organ transplantation, liver transplants, kidney transplants, pancreas/kidney transplants, cluster transplants.

Preparations

— Arm positioning devices

Positioning

— Standard operating table position 1, position 2 or universal operating table
— Anaesthetic preparation and induction in supine position with 2 adapted arm positioning devices
— Normal positioning of the operating table in the theatre
— When positioning the patient, take appropriate measures to prevent decubitus at areas which are subjected to pressure
— Spread out and pad both arms on the arm positioning devices
— Apply the neutral electrode and connect to the HF surgery device
— Arrange absorbent drapes or self-adhesive covers for preoperative skin disinfection
— Position the operating lights
— Patient warming system

13.2 · Open laparotomy

Fig. 13.5. Supine position with arms in abduction

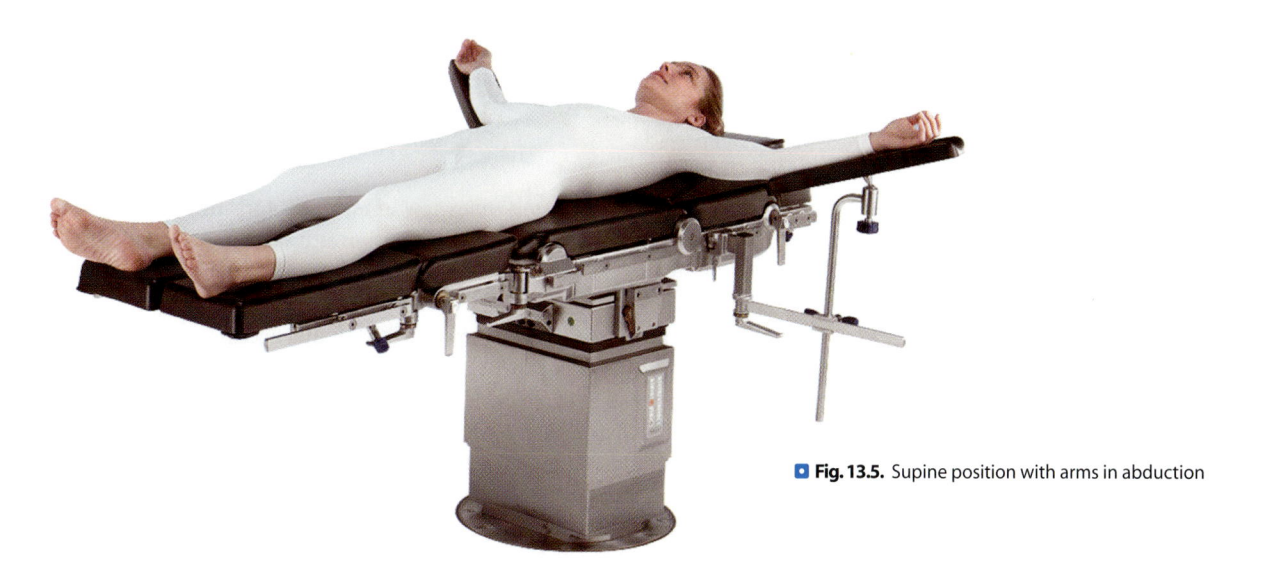

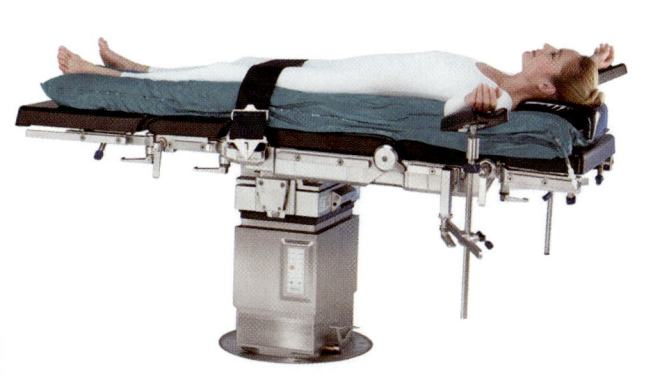

Fig. 13.6. Supine position with vacuum mat and arms in abduction

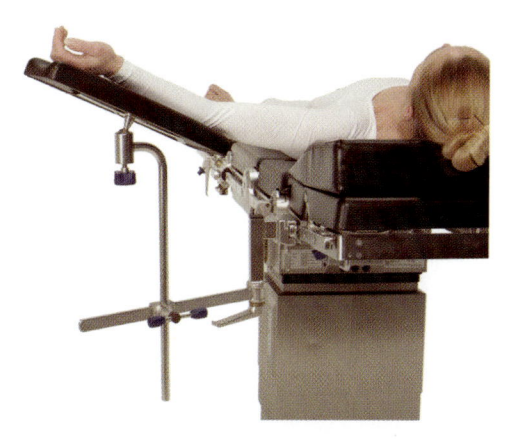

Fig. 13.7. Positioning the head on a double wedge cushion

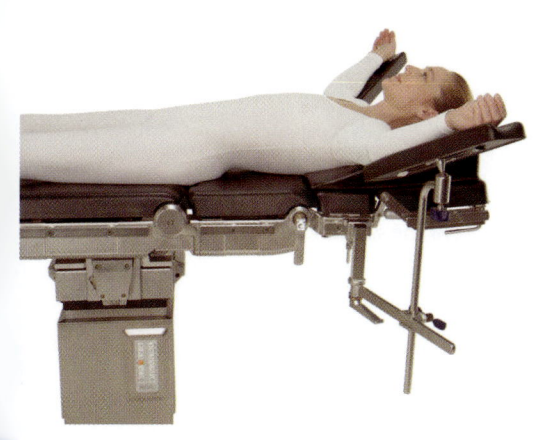

Fig. 13.8. Maximum 90° abduction and supination position of the arms

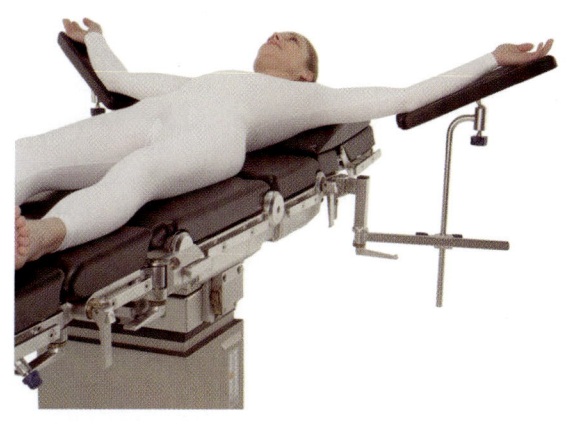

Fig. 13.9. Plexus prophylaxis by raising the shoulders

13.2.2 Lithotomy position

◘ Figs. 13.10–13.13.

Indications

Operations to the rectum and anus: low anterior rectum resection, rectum extirpation, anal resections, pelvic exenteration and sacrum resections.

Transanal operations using retractors (Parks, Gelpi) or using Bues instruments.

The lithotomy position is preferred for transanal access to processes between 3 o'clock and 9 o'clock CRL, i.e. on the back wall and side walls of the anal canal. Processes at 12 o'clock CRL, i.e. on the anal front wall, are accessed preferably in the Heidelberg position (▶ Sect. 13.4) (fistula extirpation and fistulotomy, sphincteroplasty, overlapping sphincteroplasty, perianal thrombectomy, haemorrhoidectomy, abscess incision, transmural adenomectomy, mucosectomy and anastomotic procedures).

Preparations
- Arm positioning devices
- 2 Goepel leg holders or 2 special pneumatic leg holders and 2 adapter pieces
- Gel pads
- Short vacuum mat
- Possibly 2 shoulder supports

Positioning
- Standard operating table position 2 or universal operating table
- Anaesthetic preparation and induction in supine position with 2 adapted arm positioning devices
- Normal or diagonal position of the operating table in the theatre
- When positioning the patient, take appropriate measures to prevent decubitus at areas which are subjected to pressure
- Spread out and pad both arms on the arm positioning devices
- Fit the Goepel leg holders in the corresponding adapter pieces
- Position the legs and remove the leg plates
- Position the pelvis slightly over the edge of the buttocks plate
- Check the leg positioning: lower the still raised legs until the thighs are nearly horizontal
- Possibly position the legs again in this phase and raise them again after the end
- Apply the neutral electrode and connect to the HF surgery device
- Arrange absorbent drapes or self-adhesive covers for preoperative skin disinfection
- Position the operating lights
- Patient warming system

Risks

Risk of pressure sores in the area of the sacrum.

13.2 · Open laparotomy

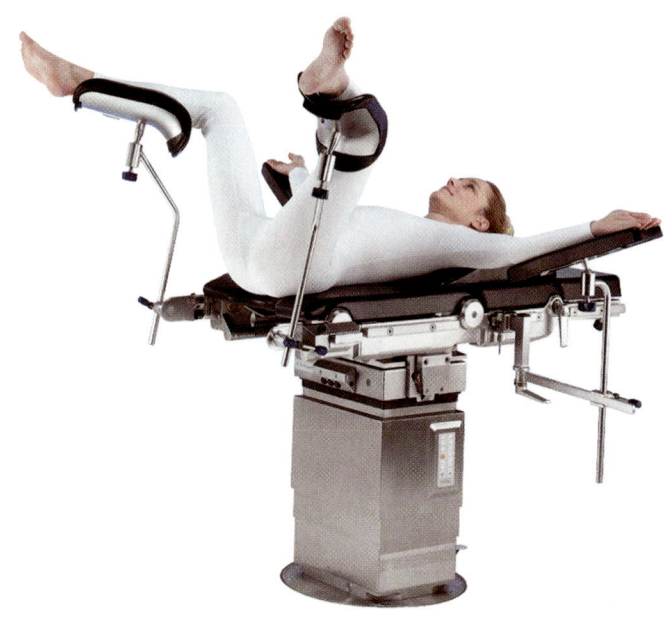

Fig. 13.10. Lithotomy position with Goepel leg holders

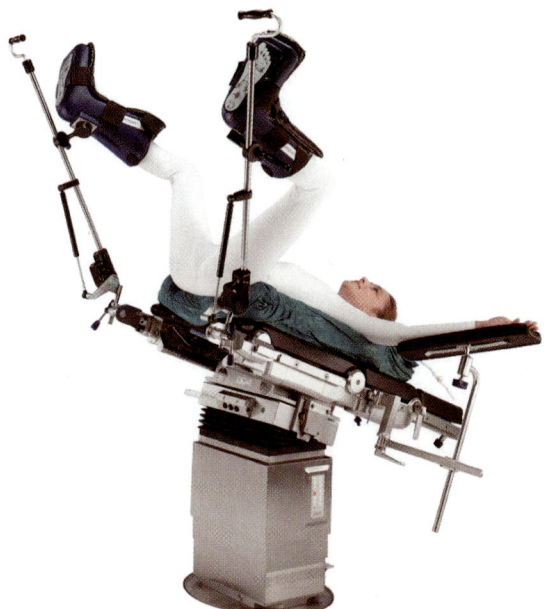

Fig. 13.11. Lithotomy position in Trendelenburg with vacuum mat and leg holders with one-hand operation, good decubitus and plexus prophylaxis

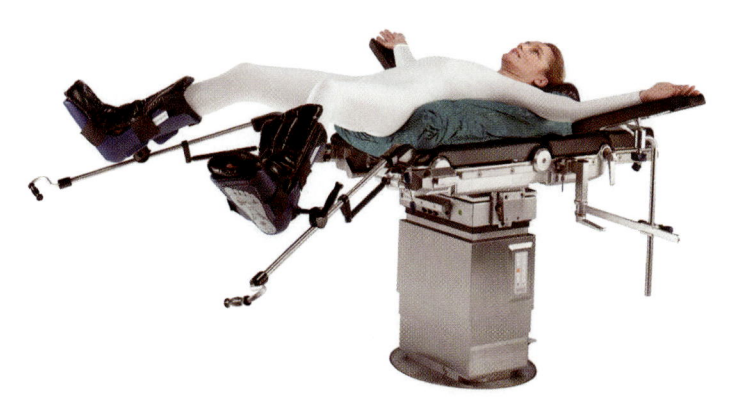

Fig. 13.12. Positioning with lowered leg holders and positioned on vacuum mat

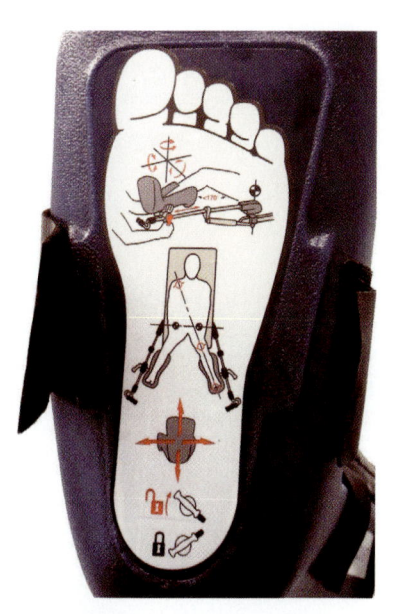

Fig. 13.13. Diagram showing the optimum positioning of the legs in the lithotomy position

13.3 Laparoscopic operations

13.3.1 Supine position

◘ Figs. 13.14–13.17.

Indications

Laparoscopic cholecystectomy, fundoplication, sigma and colon resection, evaluation.

Preparations
- Arm positioning devices
- Short vacuum mat
- Possibly 2 shoulder supports, radial adjusting clamp and body supports

Positioning
- Standard operating table position 2 or universal operating table
- Anaesthetic preparation and induction in supine position with 2 adapted arm positioning devices
- Normal positioning of the operating table in the theatre
- When positioning the patient, take appropriate measures to prevent decubitus at areas which are subjected to pressure
- Spread out and pad both arms on the arm positioning devices
- Spread the leg plates and fix the legs
- Possibly fix the shoulder supports at the side rails of the head plate and support both shoulders
- Possibly fit the radial adjusting clamps on both sides to the side rails of the base plate, and position the body supports at the pelvis
- Apply the neutral electrode and connect to the HF surgery device
- Arrange absorbent drapes or self-adhesive covers for preoperative skin disinfection
- Position the operating lights
- Patient warming system

13.3 · Laparoscopic operations

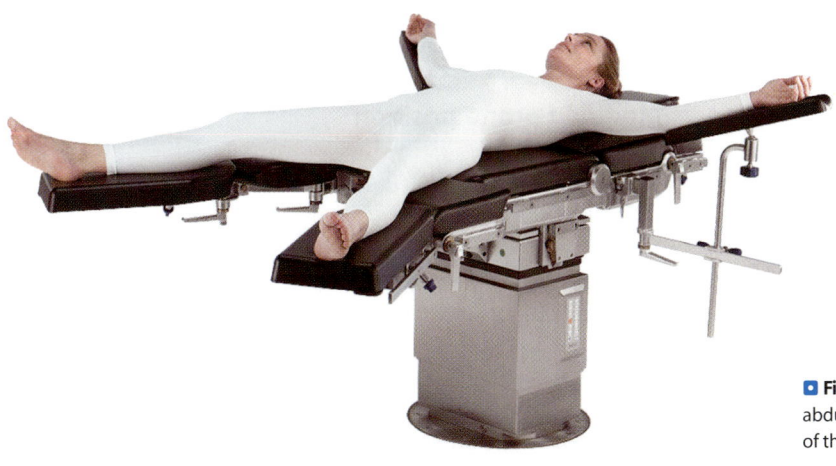

Fig. 13.14. Supine position with legs in abduction and maximum 90° abduction of the arms in supination position

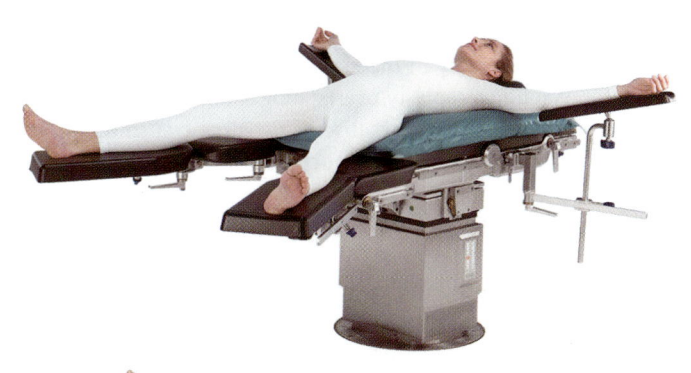

Fig. 13.15. Positioning on short vacuum mat and legs in abduction

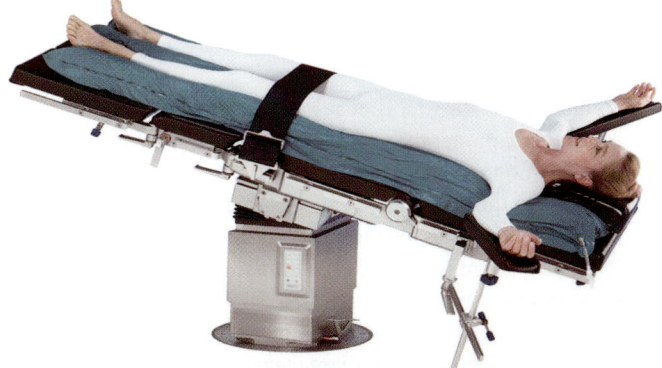

Fig. 13.16. Positioning on vacuum mat, operating table tilted to the left and Trendelenburg position

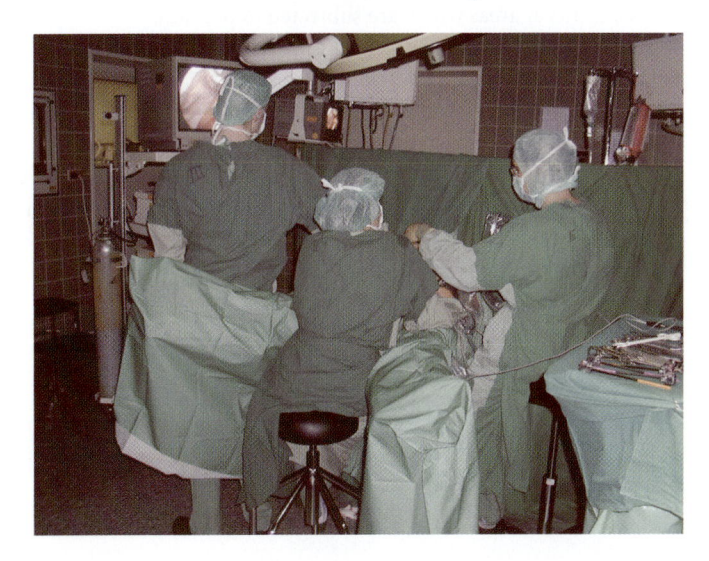

Fig. 13.17. Positioning with in abduction, legs, lateral tilt and Treudelenburg position

13.4 Heidelberg position (position for Kraske access)

13.4.1 Modified prone position

Figs. 13.18, 13.19.

Indications

Operations to the rectum and anus: transmural adenoma resection, fistula extirpation, grafts and tightening operations, pelvic exenteration and sacrum resection

Transanal operations using retractors (Parks, Gelpi) or using Bues instruments.

The lithotomy position is preferred for transanal access to processes between 3 o'clock and 9 o'clock CRL, i.e. on the back wall and side walls of the anal canal (see there). Processes at 12 o'clock CRL, i.e. on the anal front wall, are accessed preferably in the Heidelberg position (fistula extirpation and fistulotomy, sphincteroplasty, overlapping sphincteroplasty, perianal thrombectomy, haemorrhoidectomy, abscess incision, transmural adenomectomy, mucosectomy and anastomotic procedures).

Preparations
- Arm positioning devices
- Special head positioning cushions for the prone position
- Thorax, pelvic and wedge cushions, padded roll
- Possibly special bolster for prone position
- Special leg holder (rectal positioning device)

Positioning
- Standard operating table position 2 or universal operating table
- Anaesthetic preparation and induction in supine position with 2 adapted arm positioning devices
- Transfer to the prepared operating table in the induction room
- Position both tables next to each other, with the prepared table lowered
- Place the patient in prone position on the padded cushion of the operating table and take him into the theatre
- Possibly diagonal positioning of the operating table in the theatre
- When positioning the patient, take appropriate measures to prevent decubitus at areas which are subjected to pressure
- Position the head on the special head positioning cushion
- Position the arms on the arm positioning devices
- Position the knees and lower legs at double right angles, position them in the adapted special leg holders and spread the legs
- Apply the neutral electrode and connect to the HF surgery device
- Arrange self-adhesive covers for preoperative skin disinfection
- Position the operating lights
- Patient warming system

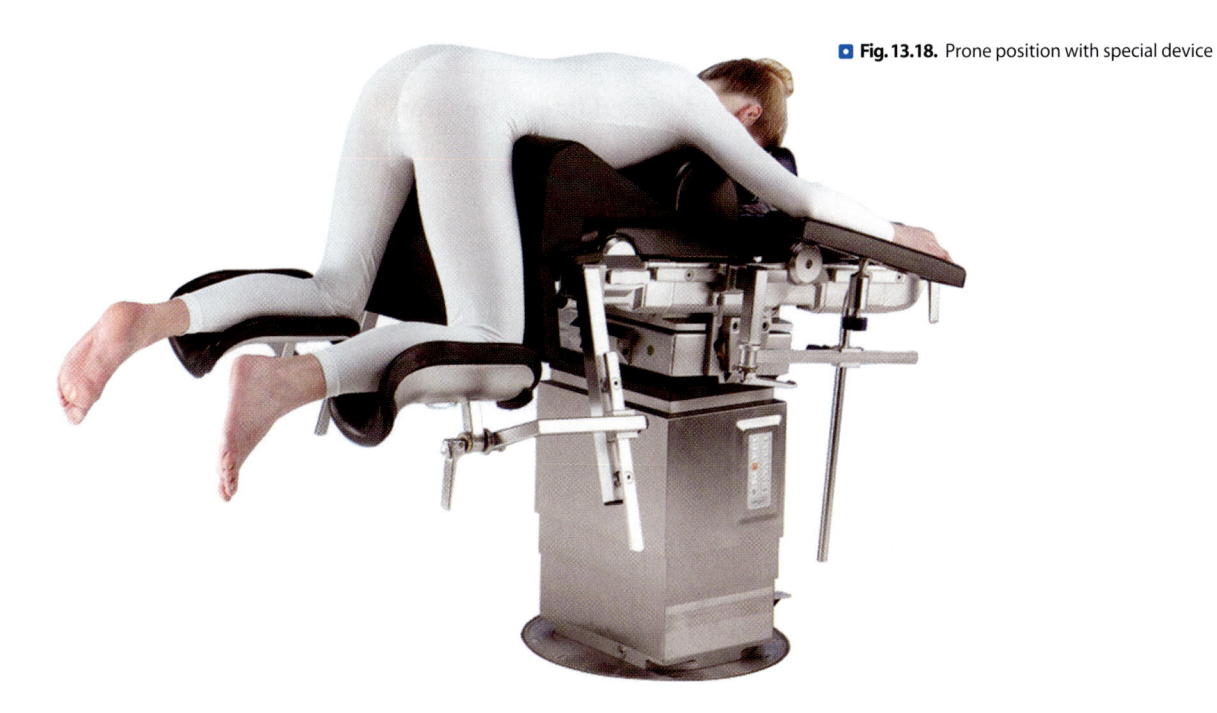

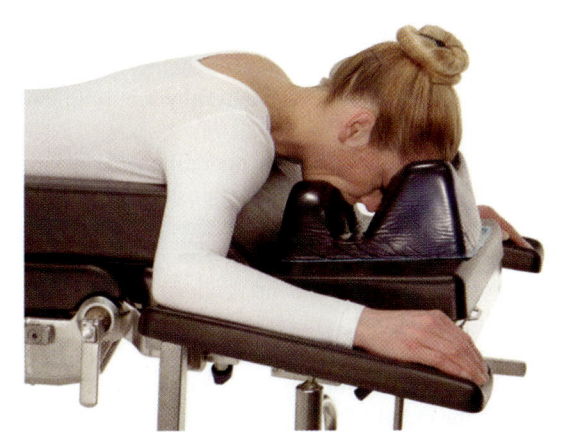

13.4 · Heidelberg position (position for Kraske access)

Fig. 13.18. Prone position with special device

Fig. 13.19. Arm and head positioning in prone position

13.5 Lateral position

13.5.1 Modified lateral position

◨ Figs. 13.20–13.22.

Indications
Stomach pull-up, nephrectomy

Preparations
- Arm positioning devices
- Gel ring, gel cushion, Goepel leg holders, lateral supports, radial adjusting clamp, padded cushions (normal and flat) and wedge cushion or tunnel cushion, body belt

Positioning
- Standard operating table position 1 or universal operating table
- Anaesthetic preparation and induction in supine position with 2 adapted arm positioning devices
- Normal positioning of the operating table in the theatre
- When positioning the patient, take appropriate measures to prevent decubitus at areas which are subjected to pressure
- Fit the radial adjustment clamp at the side rail of the head plate, position the Goepel leg holder and place a gel padded mat on the operating table
- Stretch the arm on the side not being operated
- Move the patient onto the healthy side, with the back near to the edge of the operating table
- Gradually hinge open the operating table by lowering the pelvic and back plate (operating table in roof position)
- Raise the head plate and position the head on a padded cushion with gel ring to leave the ear free
- Position and fix the arms
- Move the lower arm forwards so that the weight of the upper body does not lie directly on the shoulder
- Thorax 90° position, pelvis 45° position
- Fit the radial adjustment clamp to the small side rails of the leg plates and position the body supports at the level of the coccyx and symphysis
- **1st possibility:** position the legs with the padded cushions (normal and flat) and possibly wedge cushions
- Fix the lower leg and the positioning aids with the body belts
- **2nd possibility:** position the legs with the tunnel cushion
- Possibly position the upper leg in outer rotation
- Apply the neutral electrode and connect to the HF surgery device
- Arrange absorbent drapes or self-adhesive covers for preoperative skin disinfection
- Position the operating lights
- Patient warming system

13.5 · Lateral position

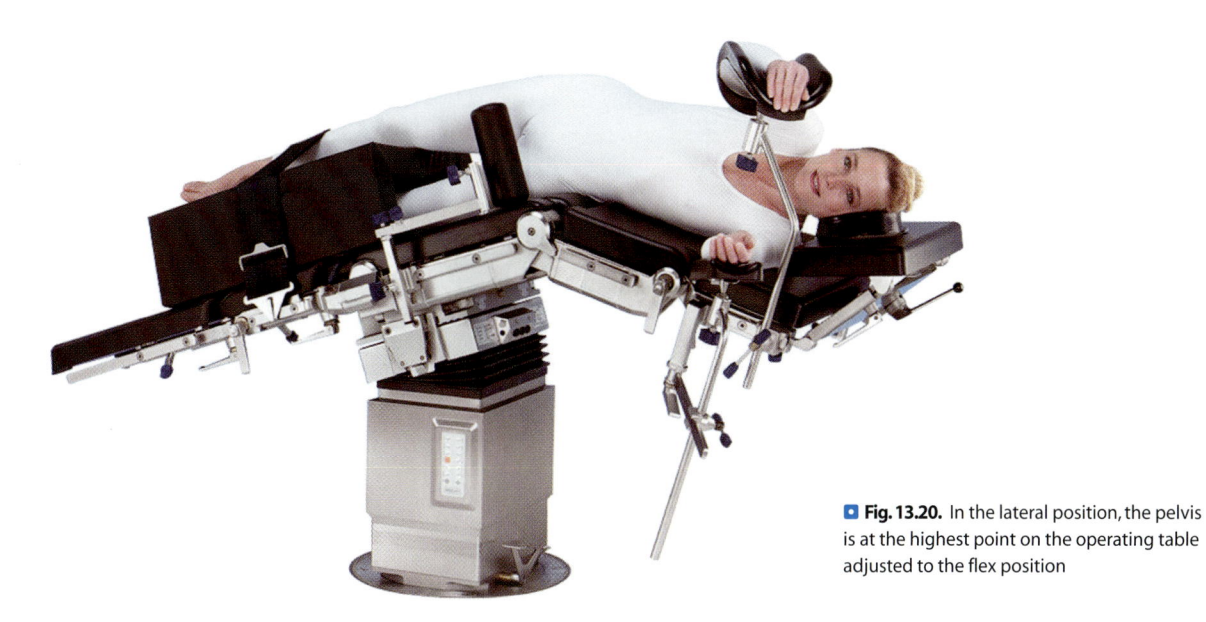

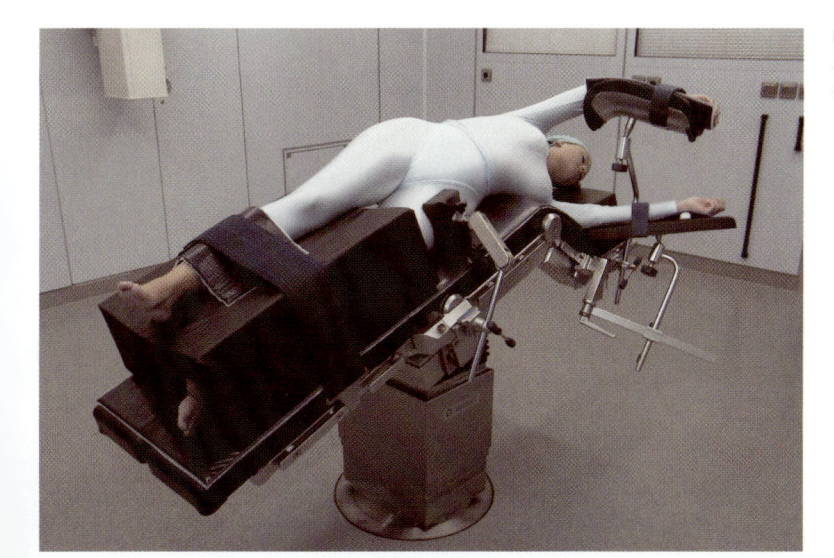

Fig. 13.20. In the lateral position, the pelvis is at the highest point on the operating table adjusted to the flex position

Fig. 13.21. The pelvis is tilted 20–40° back and the legs are positioned with a tunnel cushion

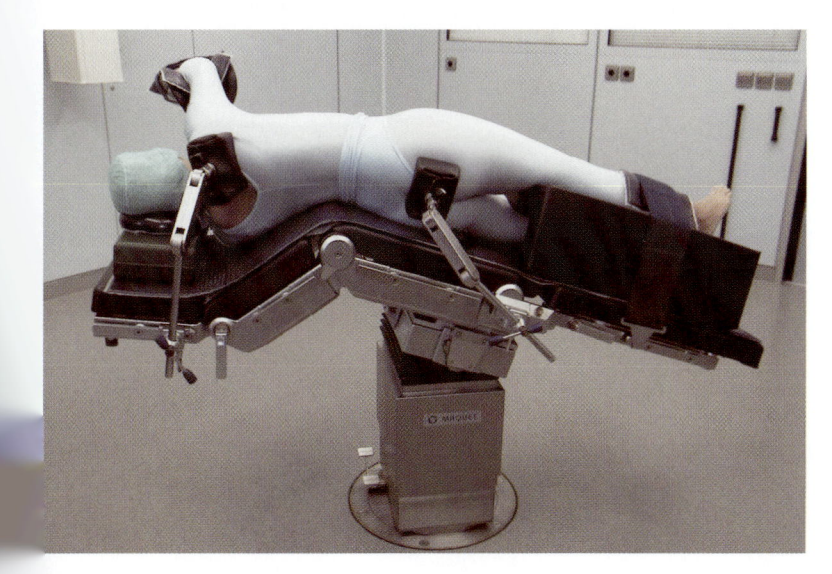

Fig. 13.22. The operating table is moved as far as possible towards the head to allow for an optimum flex position

14 Urology

14.1 Positioning techniques depending on various surgical indications – 174

14.1.1 Supine position – 174
14.1.2 Lithotomy position – 176
14.1.3 Flank position – 178
14.1.4 Modified supine position – 180
14.1.5 Prone position – 182

14.1 Positioning techniques depending on various surgical indications

14.1.1 Supine position

◘ Figs. 14.1–14.3.

Indications

Operations to:

Penis: e.g. penis deviation (Nesbit), hypospadia correction, epispadia correction.

Testicles: e.g. vasectomy, varicocele ligature, vasovasostomy and epididymovasostomy, microepididymal and testicular sperm extraction (MESA and TESE), spermatocelectomy, epididymectomy.

Abdominal operations: e.g. suprapubic cystostomy, retroperitoneal lymphadenectomy, transperitoneal nephrectomy possibly with cavotomy and tumour thrombectomy, intraperitonealisation of the ureters, augmentation of the bladder, ureterocystoneostomy, ureter resection and reconstruction, ureterolithotomy.

Preparations

— Arm positioning devices

Positioning

— Standard operating table position 1, position 2 or universal operating table
— Anaesthetic preparation and induction in supine position with 2 adapted arm positioning devices
— Normal positioning of the operating table in the theatre
— When positioning the patient, take appropriate measures to prevent decubitus at areas which are subjected to pressure
— Spread out both arms on the arm positioning devices
— Apply the neutral electrode and connect to the HF surgery device
— Arrange absorbent drapes or self-adhesive covers for preoperative skin disinfection
— Position the operating lights
— Patient warming system

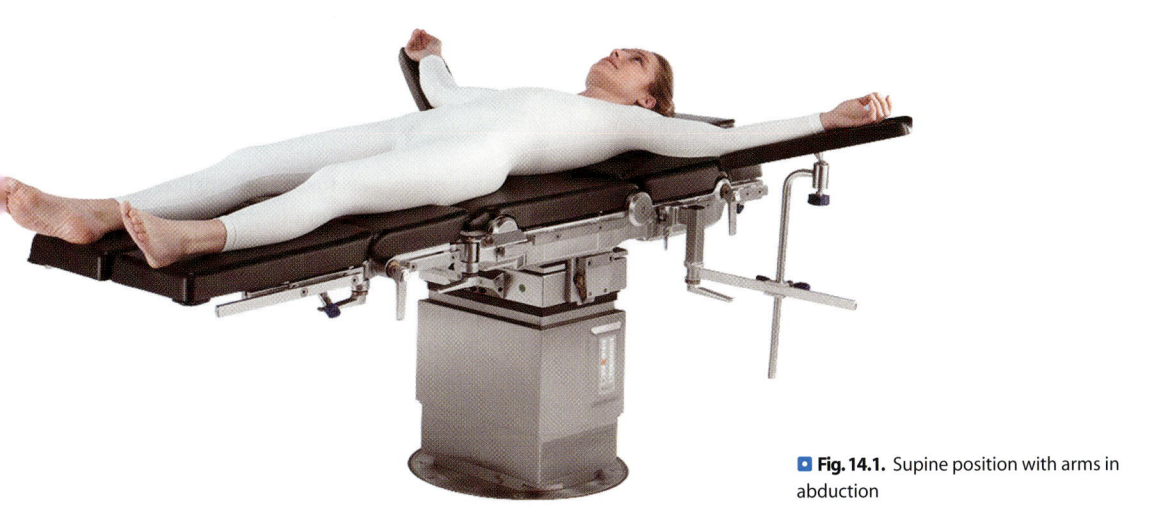

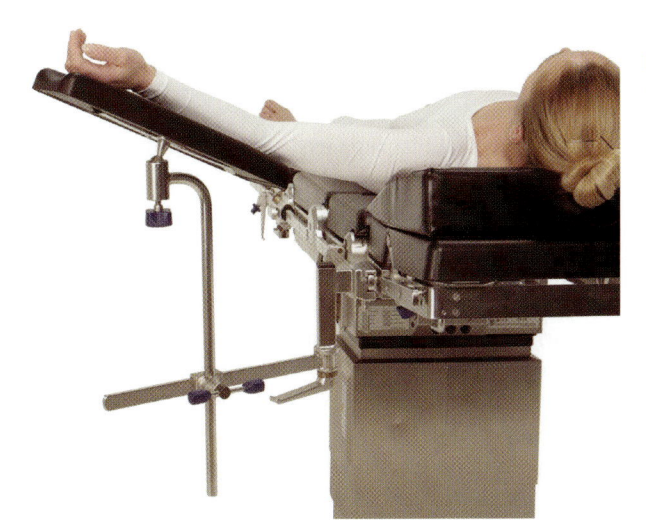

4.1 · Positioning techniques depending on various surgical indications

Fig. 14.1. Supine position with arms in abduction

Fig. 14.2. Positioning the head on a double wedge cushion

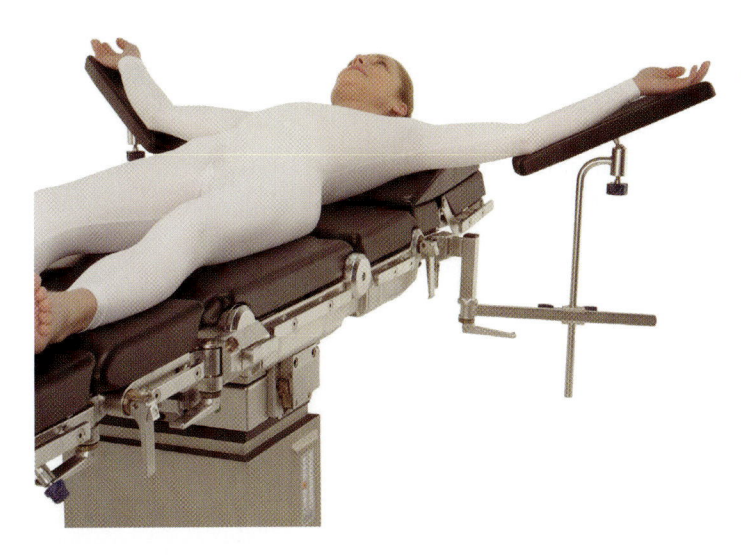

Fig. 14.3. Maximum 90° abduction and supination position of the arms

14.1.2 Lithotomy position

◘ Figs. 14.4–14.7.

Indications

All endourological operations: urethrocystoscopy, transurethral resections (bladder, prostate), punch lithotripsy, retrograde presentation of the upper urinary tract, placement of ureter stent (pigtail), ureter endoscopy (with biopsy and stone extraction).

Penis: total penectomy with placement of the neourethra.

Urethra: open-surgery urethra grafts, excision of urethra diverticula, complete urethrectomy.

Prostate: transvesical adenoma nucleation, pelvic lymphadenectomy and radical prostatectomy.

Bladder: radical cystectomy with continent or incontinent substitute bladder, bladder elevations for stress incontinence, Scott sphincter implantation, vesicovaginal fistula occlusion.

Preparations
- Arm positioning devices
- 2 Goepel leg holders or 2 special pneumatic leg holders and 2 adapter pieces
- Gel pad
- Possibly 2 shoulder supports

Positioning
- Standard operating table position 2 or universal operating table
- Anaesthetic preparation and induction in supine position with 2 adapted arm positioning devices
- Normal or diagonal positioning of the operating table in the theatre
- When positioning the patient, take appropriate measures to prevent decubitus at areas which are subjected to pressure
- Spread out and pad both arms on the arm positioning devices
- Adapt the Goepel leg holders with the provided champs
- Position the legs and remove the leg plates
- Position the pelvis slightly over the edge of the buttocks plate
- Check the leg positioning: lower the still raised legs until the thighs are nearly horizontal
- Possibly position the legs again in this phase and raise them again after the end
- Apply the neutral electrode and connect to the HF surgery device
- Arrange absorbent drapes or self-adhesive covers for preoperative skin disinfection
- Position the operating lights
- Patient warming system

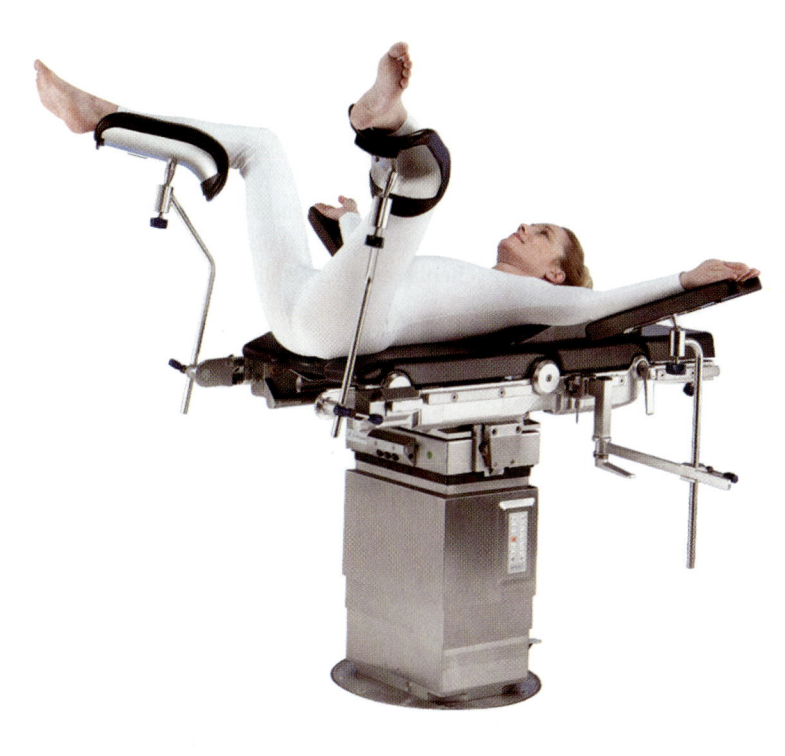

14.1 · Positioning techniques depending on various surgical indications

Fig. 14.4. Lithotomy position with Goepel leg holders

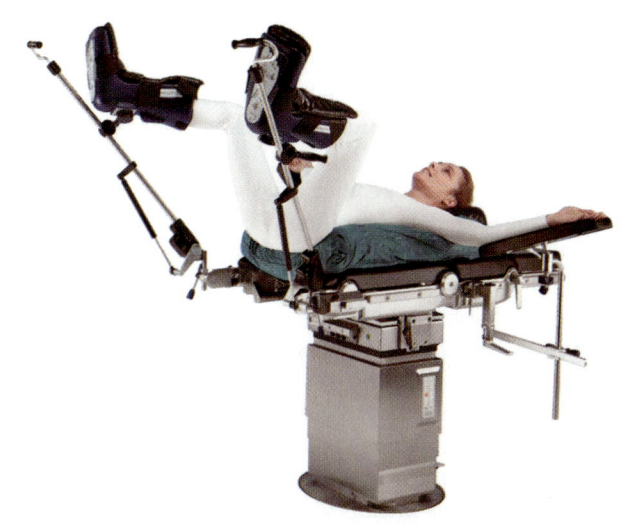

Fig. 14.5. Lithotomy position with vacuum mat and leg holders with one-hand operation

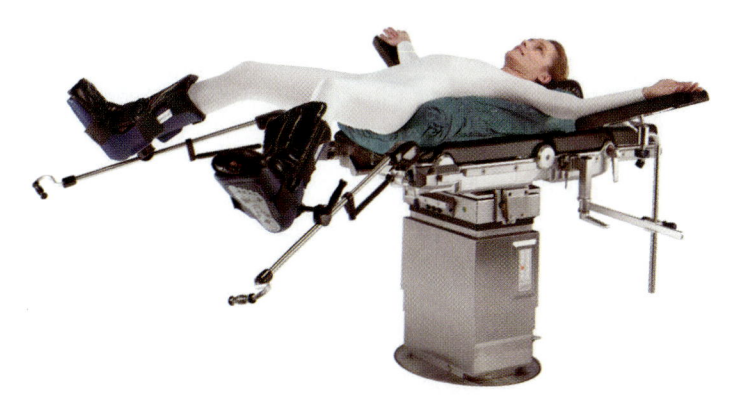

Fig. 14.6. Positioning with lowered leg holders and positioning on vacuum mat

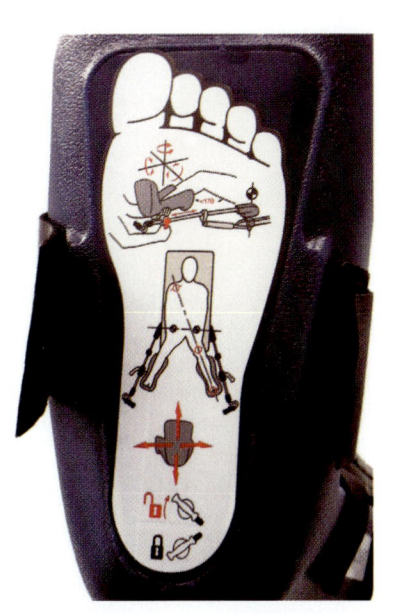

Fig. 14.7. Diagram to show the optimum positioning of the legs in the lithotomy position

14.1.3 Flank position

◩ Figs. 14.8–14.10.

Indications

Kidneys: percutaneous nephrostomy, kidney and kidney cyst puncture possibly with sclerosing, percutaneous nephrolitholapaxy, nephropyeloplasty, tumour nephrectomy, partial nephrectomy, pyelolithotomy, nephrolithotomy, adrenalectomy.

Preparations
- Arm positioning devices
- Gel ring, gel cushion, Goepel leg holder, lateral supports, radial adjusting clamps, padded cushions (normal and flat) and wedge cushions or tunnel cushions, body belts

Positioning
- Standard operating table position 1 or universal operating table
- Anaesthetic preparation and induction in supine position with 2 adapted arm positioning devices
- Normal positioning of the operating table in the theatre
- When positioning the patient, take appropriate measures to prevent decubitus at areas which are subjected to pressure
- Fit the radial adjusting clamp to the side rail of the head plate, position the Goepel leg holder and place a gel padded mat on the operating table
- Spread out the arm on the side not being operated
- Move the patient onto the healthy side, with the back near the edge of the operating table
- Gradually hinge open the operating table by lowering the pelvic and back plate (operating table in roof position)
- Raise the head plate and position the head on a padded cushion with gel ring to leave the ear free
- Position and fix the arms
- Move the lower arm forwards so that the weight of the upper body does not lie directly on the shoulder
- Thorax 90° position, pelvis 45° position
- Fit the radial adjustment clamps to the small side rails of the leg plates and position the body supports on the level of the sacrum and symphysis
- **1st possibility:** position the legs with the padded cushions (normal and flat) and possibly wedge cushions
- Fix the lower leg and positioning aids with the body belts
- **2nd possibility:** position the legs with the tunnel cushions
- Position the upper leg in external rotation
- Apply the neutral electrode and connect to the HF surgery device
- Arrange absorbent drapes or self-adhesive covers for preoperative skin disinfection
- Position the operating lights
- Patient warming system

14.1 · Positioning techniques depending on various surgical indications

Fig. 14.8. In the lateral position, the pelvis is at the highest point on the operating table adjusted to the flex position

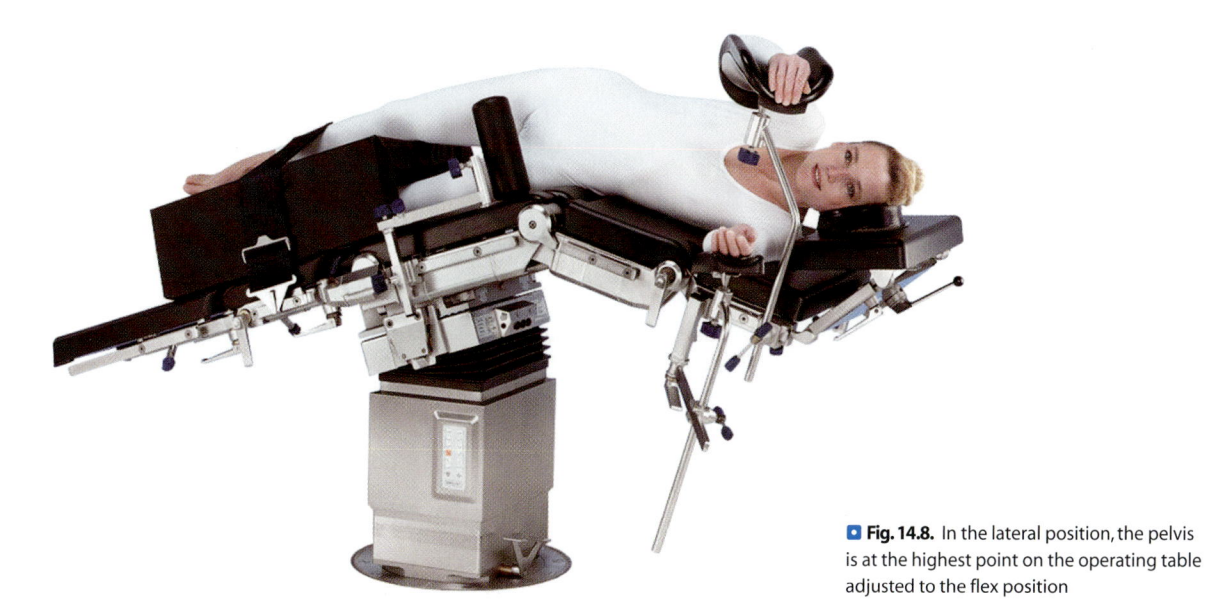

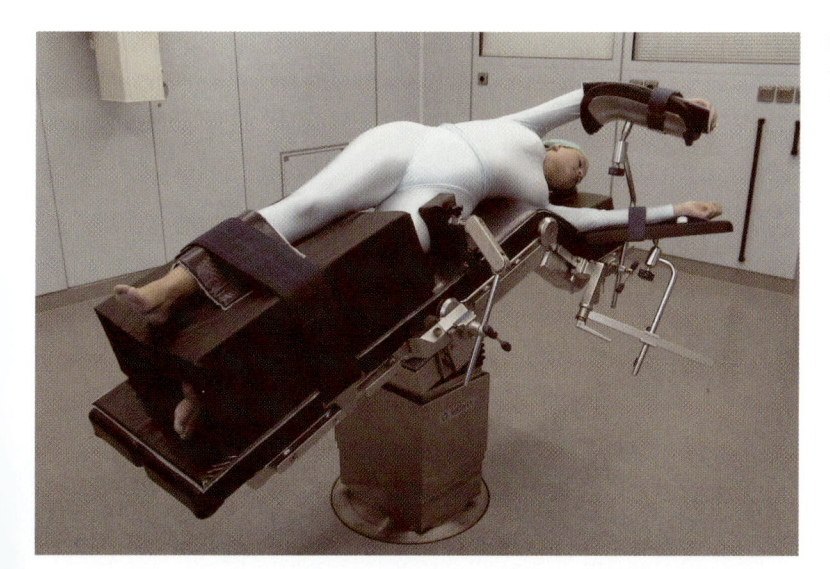

Fig. 14.9. The pelvis is tilted back 20–40° and the legs are positioned with a tunnel cushion

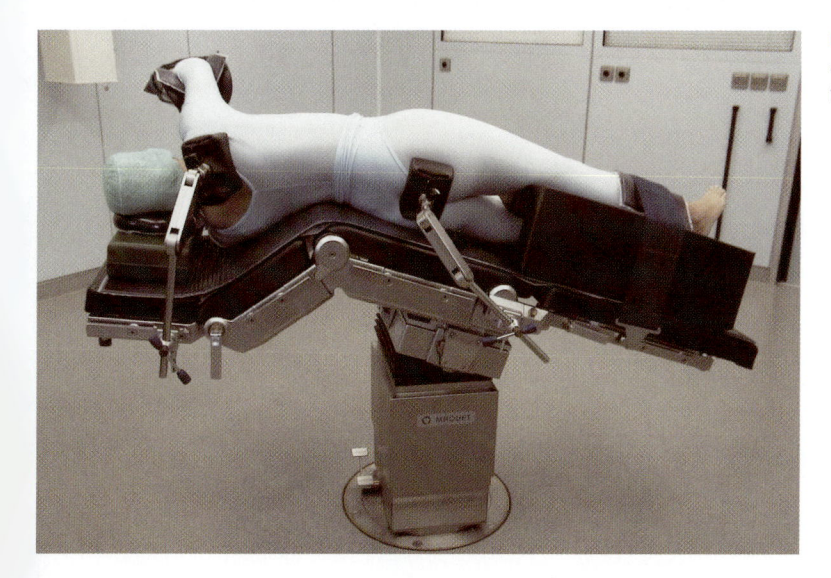

Fig. 14.10. The operating table is moved as far as possible towards the head to allow for an optimum flex position

14.1.4 Modified supine position

◘ Figs. 14.11, 14.12.

Indications
Kidney and ureter: nephroureterectomy, tumour nephrectomy
  Neuromodulation: implanting the neuromodulation stimulator.

Preparations
- Arm positioning devices
- Wedge cushions, radial adjusting clamps, body supports

Positioning
- Standard operating table position 1, position 2 or universal operating table
- Anaesthetic preparation and induction in supine position with 2 adapted arm positioning devices
- Normal positioning of the operating table in the theatre
- When positioning the patient, take appropriate measures to prevent decubitus at areas which are subjected to pressure
- Spread out and pad both arms on the arm positioning devices
- Apply the neutral electrode and connect to the HF surgery device
- Arrange absorbent drapes or self-adhesive covers for preoperative skin disinfection
- Position the operating lights
- Patient warming system

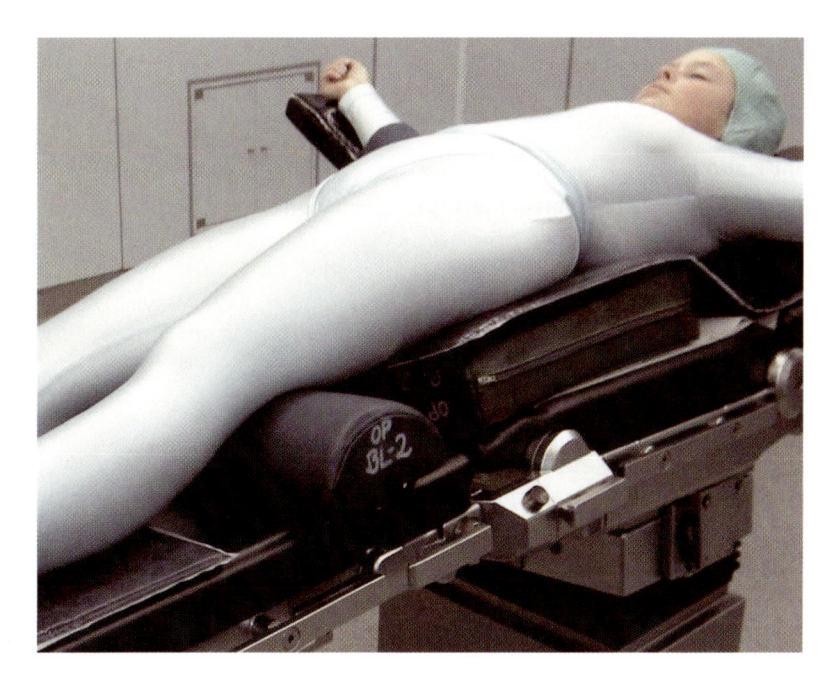

14.1 · Positioning techniques depending on various surgical indications

Fig. 14.11. Positioning with wedge cushions

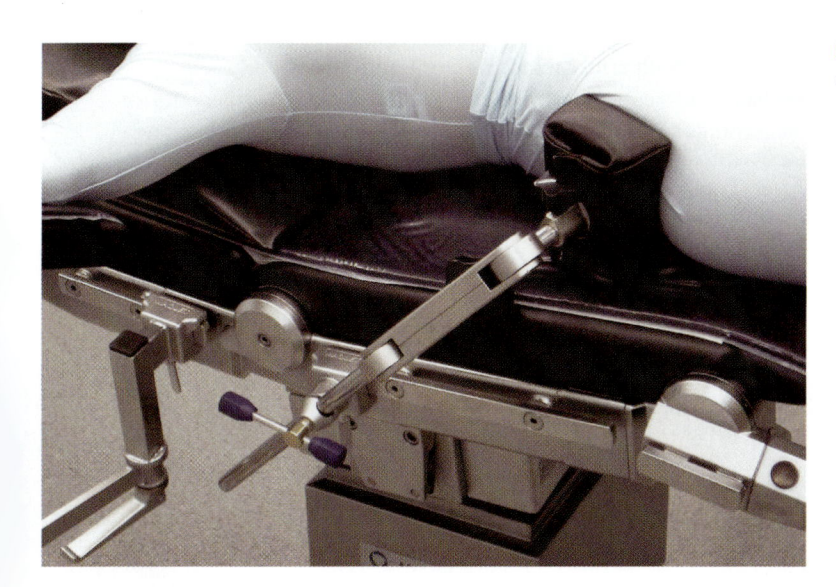

Fig. 14.12. Supported with a body support on the opposite side

14.1.5 Prone position

Figs. 14.13–14.17.

Indications
Neuromodulation: percutaneous neuromodulation testing, implanting the neuromodulation electrodes.

Preparations
- Two arm positioning devices
- Special head positioning cushion for prone position
- Thorax, pelvic and wedge cushion, padded roll

Positioning
- Standard operating table position 1, position 2 or universal operating table
- Anaesthetic preparation and induction in supine position with 2 adapted arm positioning devices
- Transfer to the prepared operating table in the induction room
- Position both tables next to each other, with the prepared table lowered
- Place the patient in prone position on the padded cushion of the prepared operating table and take him into the theatre
- Normal positioning of the operating table in the theatre
- Position the head on the special head positioning cushion
- Position both arms on the arm positioning devices
- Apply the neutral electrode and connect to the HF surgery device
- Arrange self-adhesive covers for preoperative skin disinfection
- Position the operating lights
- Patient warming system

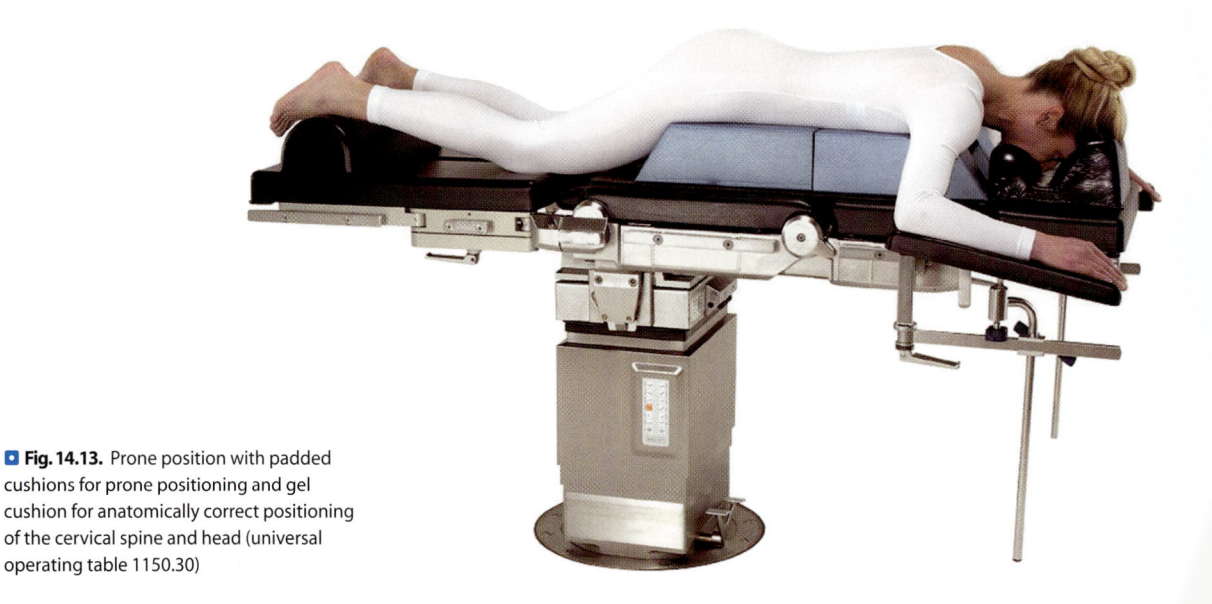

Fig. 14.13. Prone position with padded cushions for prone positioning and gel cushion for anatomically correct positioning of the cervical spine and head (universal operating table 1150.30)

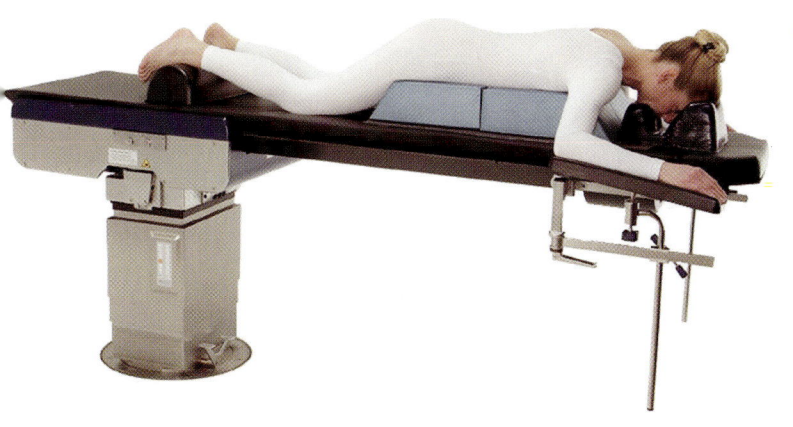

14.1 · Positioning techniques depending on various surgical indications

Fig. 14.14. Prone position with the same positioning aids (CRP operating table 1150.16)

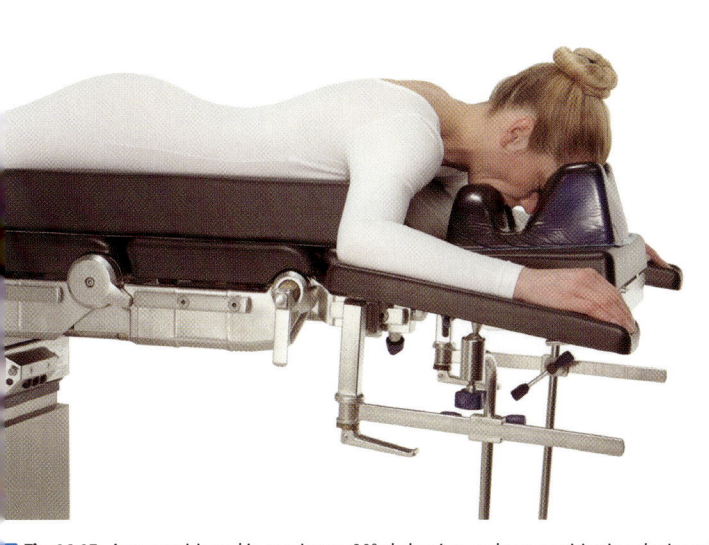

Fig. 14.15. Arms positioned in maximum 90° abduction and arm positioning device adapted at shoulder height

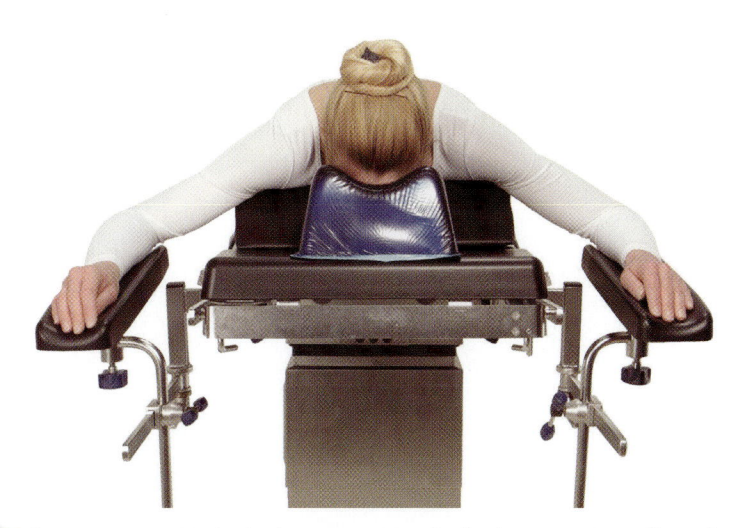

Fig. 14.16. Arm positioning for the prone position: the distal joint is positioned lower than the proximal joint

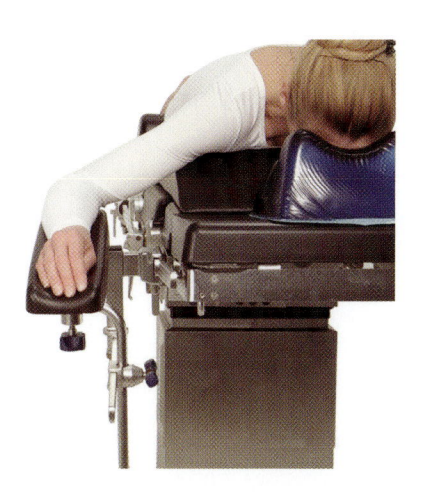

Fig. 14.17. Shoulders and upper arms are free

15 Spine surgery

15.1	Cervical spine	– 186
15.1.1	Supine position/CRP horseshoe-shaped headrest	– 186
15.1.2	Supine position/skull clamp	– 188
15.1.3	Supine position/spine holding unit MAQUET T554.0000	– 190
15.1.4	Prone position/CRP horseshoe-shaped headrest	– 192
15.1.5	Prone position/spine holding unit / skull clamp	– 194
15.2	Thoracic spine, lumbar spine	– 196
15.2.1	Prone position	– 196
15.2.2	Lateral position	– 198
15.2.3	Supine position	– 200

15.1 Cervical spine

15.1.1 Supine position/ CRP horseshoe-shaped headrest

◘ Figs. 15.1, 15.2.

Indications

Ventral access to the upper and lower cervical vertebrae without the possibility of intraoperative, external reposition measures for:
- dens fractures, dens pseudarthrosis
- posttraumatic lesions, misalignment and fractures in the upper and lower cervical vertebrae
- tumours, spondylitis, spondylodiscitis
- degenerative changes of the lower cervical vertebrae

Preparations
- Arm positioning devices
- CRP horseshoe-shaped headrest
- Shaving in the area of the incision and preoperative skin cleansing

Positioning
- Standard operating table position 1, position 2 or universal operating table
- Anaesthetic preparation and induction in supine position with 2 adapted arm positioning devices
- Normal positioning of the operating table in the theatre
- When positioning the patient, take appropriate measures to prevent decubitus at areas which are subjected to pressure
- Fix and pre-position the CRP horseshoe-shaped headrest to the head part of the operating table
- Move the patient towards the head end until the shoulders are at the upper edge of the operating table, scapula still on the table
- Position and fix the head on the CRP horseshoe-shaped headrest
- Position both arms at the body with arm protection or secure the arms, possibly fixing with plasters
- Apply the neutral electrode and connect to the HF surgery device
- Arrange absorbent drapes or self-adhesive covers for preoperative skin disinfection
- Position the operating lights
- Patient warming system

Risks
- Iatrogenic injuries to the eyes and soft tissues (head fixing!)
- Dislocation, reposition loss

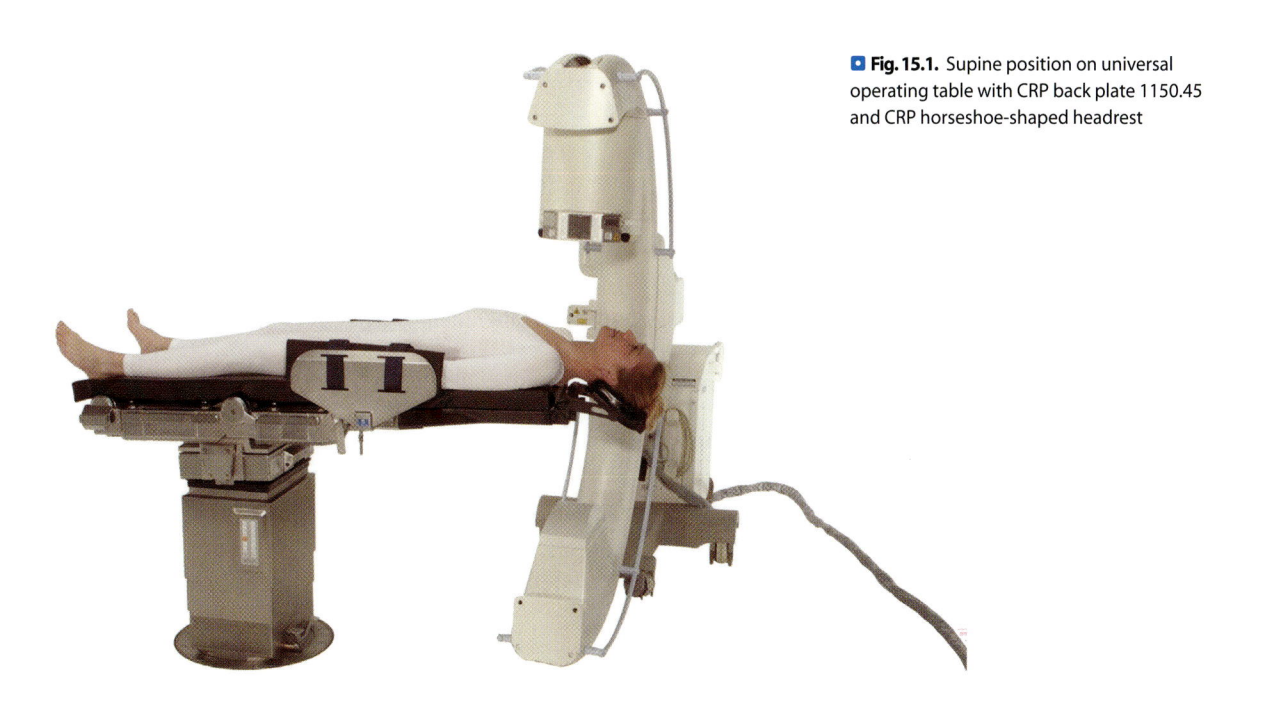

15.1 · Cervical spine

Fig. 15.1. Supine position on universal operating table with CRP back plate 1150.45 and CRP horseshoe-shaped headrest

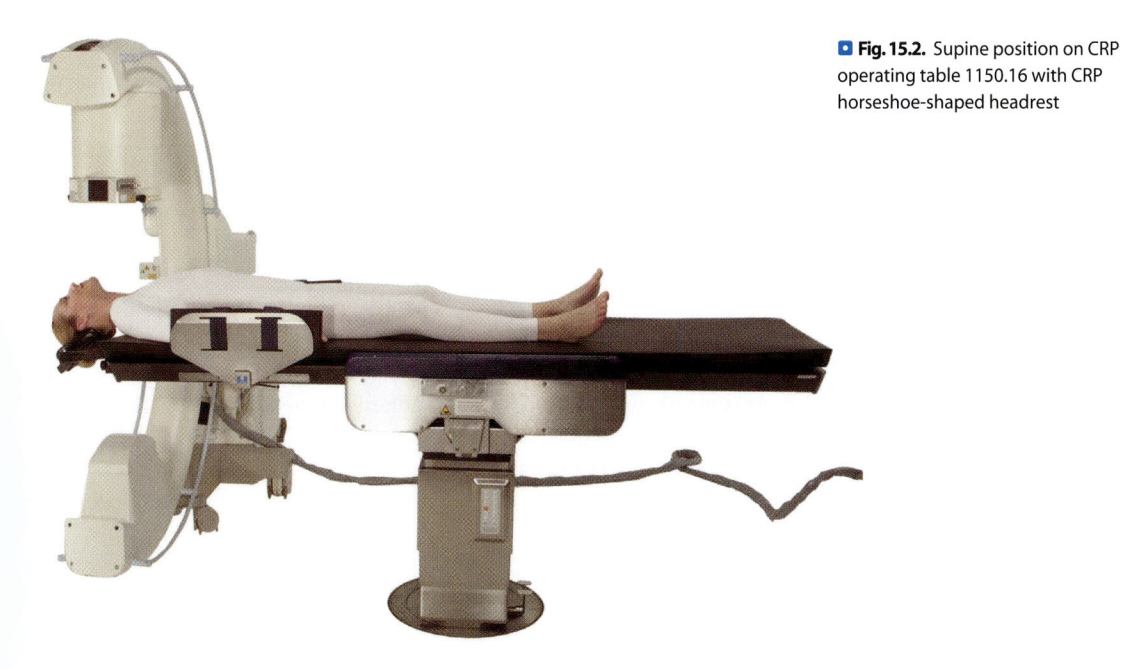

Fig. 15.2. Supine position on CRP operating table 1150.16 with CRP horseshoe-shaped headrest

15.1.2 Supine position/skull clamp

◘ Figs. 15.3, 15.4.

Indications

Ventral access to the upper and lower cervical vertebrae with the possibility of intraoperative, external reposition measures for:
- dens fractures, dens pseudarthrosis
- posttraumatic lesions, misalignment and fractures in the upper and lower cervical vertebrae
- tumours, spondylitis, spondylodiscitis

Preparations
- Arm positioning devices
- Padded arm protection
- Skull clamp
- Shaving in the area of the incision and preoperative skin cleansing

Positioning
- Standard operating table position 1, position 2 or universal operating table
- Anaesthetic preparation and induction in supine position with 2 adapted arm positioning devices
- Normal positioning of the operating table in the theatre
- When positioning the patient, take appropriate measures to prevent decubitus at areas which are subjected to pressure
- Fix and pre-position the skull clamp to the head part of the operating table
- Move the patient towards the head end until the shoulders are at the upper edge of the operating table, scapula still on the table
- Position and fix the head in the skull clamp
- Position both arms at the body with arm protection or secure the arms, possibly fixing with plasters
- Apply the neutral electrode and connect to the HF surgery device
- Arrange absorbent drapes or self-adhesive covers for preoperative skin disinfection
- Position the operating lights
- Patient warming system

Risks
- Iatrogenic injuries at the skull clamp
- Dislocation, reposition loss

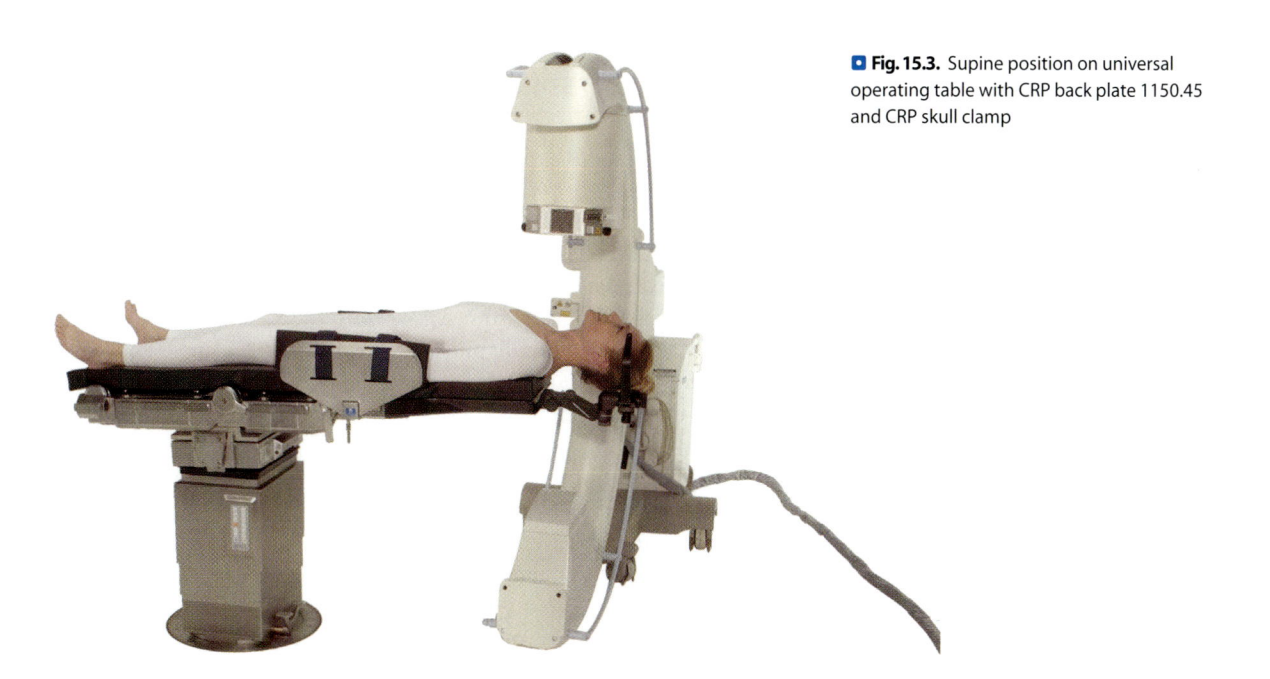

15.1 · Cervical spine

Fig. 15.3. Supine position on universal operating table with CRP back plate 1150.45 and CRP skull clamp

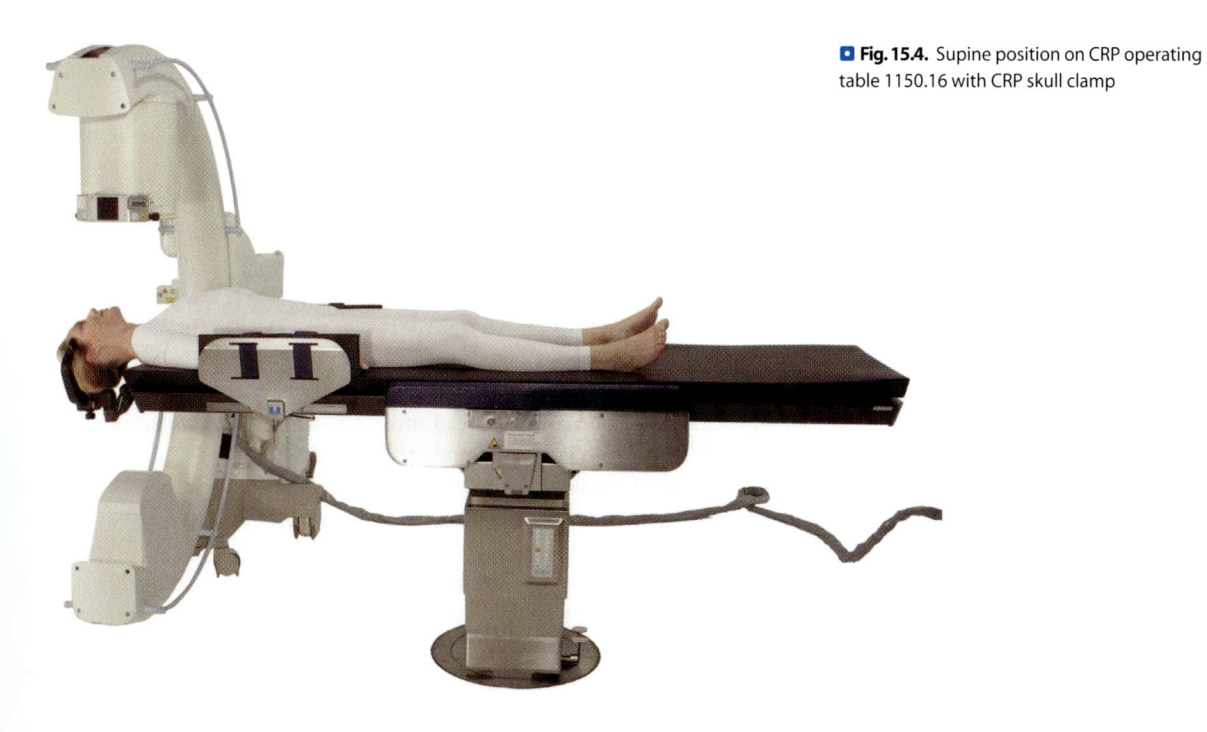

Fig. 15.4. Supine position on CRP operating table 1150.16 with CRP skull clamp

15.1.3 Supine position/spine holding unit MAQUET T554.0000

◘ Figs. 15.5, 15.6.

Indications

Ventral access to the upper and lower cervical vertebrae with the possibility of intraoperative, external reposition measures for:
- dens fractures, dens pseudarthrosis
- posttraumatic lesions, misalignment and fractures in the upper and lower cervical vertebrae
- tumours, spondylitis, spondylodiscitis

Preparations
- Arm positioning devices
- Padded arm protection
- Spine holding unit T544.0000
- Gel cushion
- Shaving in the area of the incision and preoperative skin cleansing

Positioning
- Standard operating table position 1, position 2 or universal operating table
- Anaesthetic preparation and induction in supine position with 2 adapted arm positioning devices
- Fit part 5 (special adapter with 4 short bars in ball bearings) to the ready positioned halo ring
- Normal positioning of the operating table in the theatre
- When positioning the patient, take appropriate measures to prevent decubitus at areas which are subjected to pressure
- Fit part 1 (adapter) to the side rails of the head plate
- Connect part 2 (telescopic bar) and part 3 (moving foot section) and fasten to part 1 (adapter)
- Fasten part 4 (screw tension device) to part 2 (telescopic bar)
- Move the patient towards the head end until the shoulders are at the upper edge of the operating table, scapula still on the table
- Fasten part 5 (special adapter) to part 4 (screw tension device)
- Position both arms at the body with arm protection or secure the arms, possibly fixing with plasters
- Possibly fit a radiolucent neck rest adjustable in height (hypomochlion, 6) to part 2 (telescopic bar) for intraoperative reposition and positioning
- Position the image converter
- Apply the neutral electrode and connect to the HF surgery device
- Arrange absorbent drapes or self-adhesive covers for preoperative skin disinfection
- Position the operating lights
- Patient warming system

Risks
- Injuries at the head and skull clamp from the halo ring
- Dislocation, reposition loss

15.1 · Cervical spine

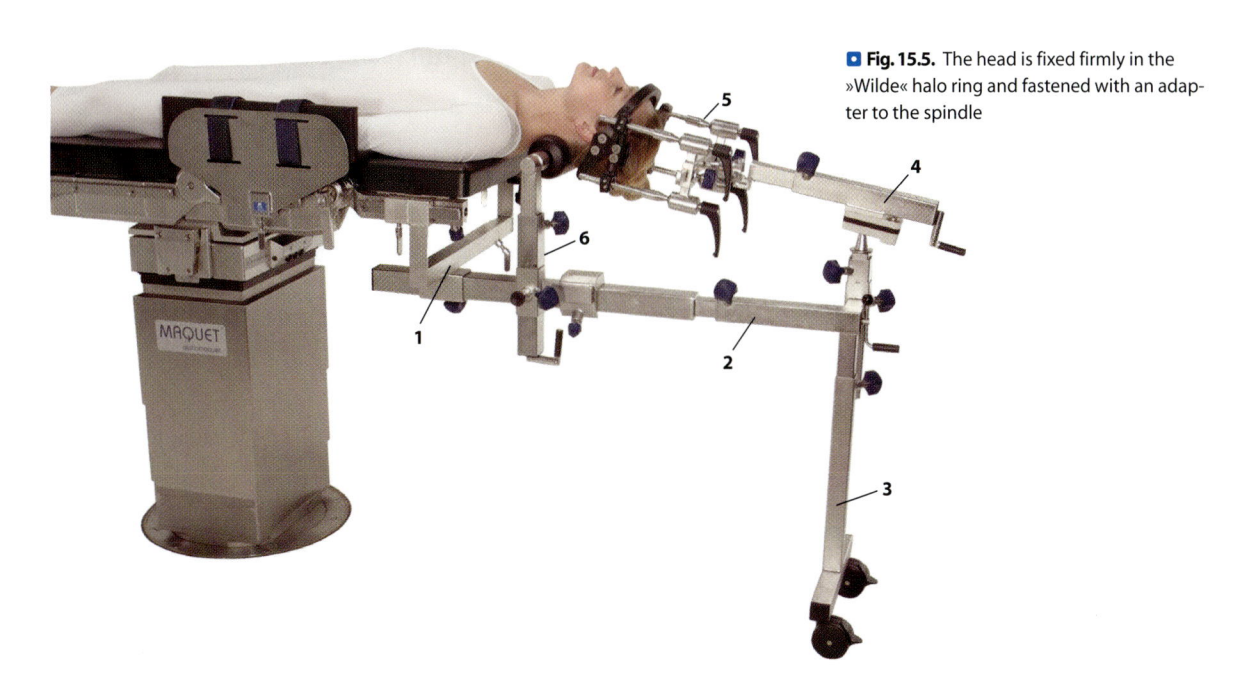

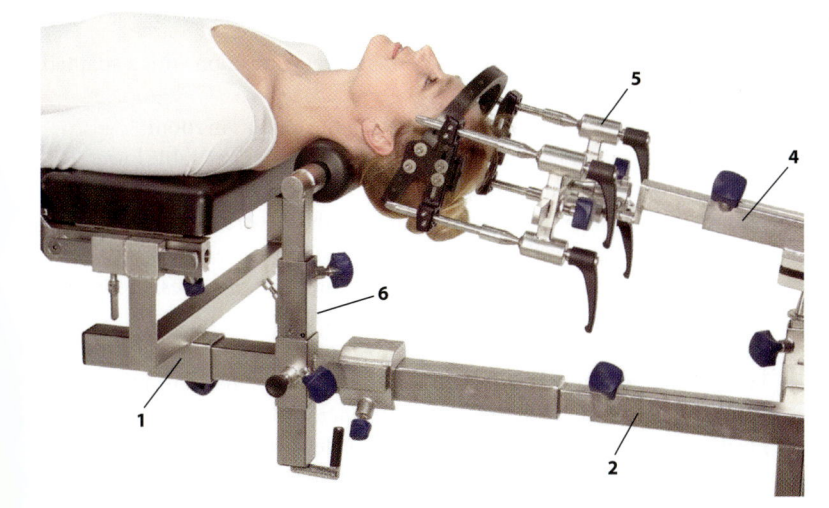

Fig. 15.5. The head is fixed firmly in the »Wilde« halo ring and fastened with an adapter to the spindle

Fig. 15.6. The hypomochlion is positioned under the vertebra being operated to support the cervical spine

15.1.4 Prone position/CRP horseshoe-shaped headrest

◘ Figs. 15.7, 15.8.

Indications

Rear access to the upper and lower cervical vertebrae without the possibility of intraoperative, external reposition measures for:
- pseudarthrosis in the upper cervical vertebrae
- posttraumatic lesions, fractures and misalignment at the occipitocervical junction and at the upper and lower cervical vertebrae
- tumours

Preparations
- Arm positioning devices
- Padded arm protection
- Thorax, pelvic and wedge cushions, padded roll
- Special bolster for prone position
- CRP horseshoe-shaped headrest
- Gel cushion
- Shaving in the area of the incision and preoperative skin cleansing

Positioning
- Standard operating table position 1, position 2 or universal operating table
- Anaesthetic preparation and induction in supine position with 2 adapted arm positioning devices
- Transfer to the prepared operating table in the induction room
- Position both tables next to each other, with the prepared table lowered
- Place the patient in the prone position on the padded cushion on the prepared operating table and take him into the theatre
- Normal positioning of the operating table in the theatre
- When positioning the patient, take appropriate measures to prevent decubitus at areas which are subjected to pressure
- Position the head on the special head positioning cushion
- Position the axillae freely with the thorax bolsters and ensure that the pelvic bolster finishes with the anterior superior iliac crest
- Position both arms on the arm positioning devices
- Apply the neutral electrode and connect to the HF surgery device
- Arrange self-adhesive drapes for preoperative skin disinfection
- Position the operating lights
- Patient warming system

Risks
- Iatrogenic injuries to the eyes and soft tissues (head fixing!)
- Dislocation, reposition loss

15.1 · Cervical spine

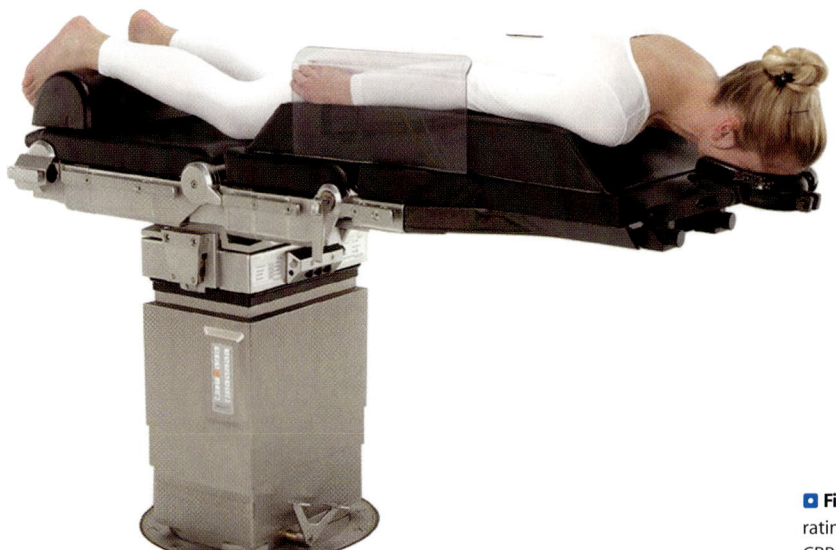

Fig. 15.7. Prone position on universal operating table with CRP back plate 1150.45 and CRP horseshoe-shaped headrest

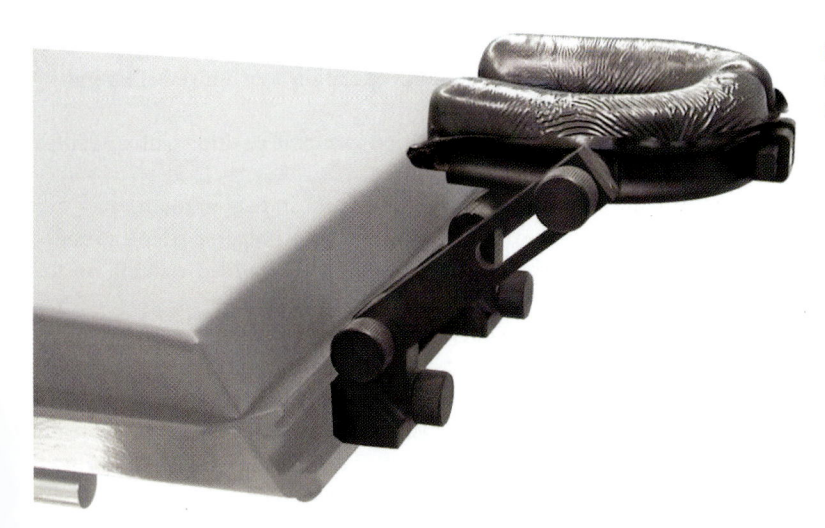

Fig. 15.8. CRP horseshoe-shaped headrest with gel padding for very comfortable positioning

15.1.5 Prone position/spine holding unit/skull clamp

◘ Figs. 15.9–15.12.

Indications
Rear access to the upper and lower cervical vertebrae with the possibility of intraoperative, external reposition measures for:
- pseudarthrosis in the upper cervical vertebrae
- posttraumatic lesions, fractures and misalignment at the occipitocervical junction and at the upper and lower cervical vertebrae
- tumours

Preparations
- Arm positioning devices
- Padded arm protection
- Thorax, pelvic and wedge cushions, padded roll
- Special bolster for prone position
- Vertebral column holding unit/skull clamp
- Gel cushion
- Shaving in the area of the incision and preoperative skin cleansing

Positioning
- Standard operating table position 1, position 2 or universal operating table
- Anaesthetic preparation and induction in supine position with 2 adapted arm positioning devices
- Transfer to the prepared operating table in the induction room
- Position both tables next to each other, with the prepared table lowered
- Place the patient in the prone position on the padded cushion on the prepared operating table and take him into the theatre
- Normal positioning of the operating table in the theatre
- When positioning the patient, take appropriate measures to prevent decubitus at areas which are subjected to pressure
- Fit part 5 (special adapter with 4 short bars in ball bearings) to the ready positioned halo ring
- Fit part 1 (adapter) to the side rails of the head plate
- Connect part 2 (telescopic bar) and part 3 (moving foot section) and fasten to part 1 (adapter)
- Fasten part 4 (screw tension device) to part 2 (telescopic bar)
- Fasten part 5 (special adapter) to part 4 (screw tension device)
- Position both arms at the body with arm protection or secure the arms, possibly fixing with plasters
- Position the axillae freely with the thorax bolsters and ensure that the pelvic bolster finishes with the anterior superior iliac crest
- Position the image intensifier
- Apply the neutral electrode and connect to the HF surgery device
- Arrange self-adhesive covers for preoperative skin disinfection
- Position the operating lights
- Patient warming system

Risks
- Iatrogenic injuries at the skull clamp
- Injuries to the head and at the skull clamp caused by the halo ring
- Dislocation, reposition loss

15.1 · Cervical spine

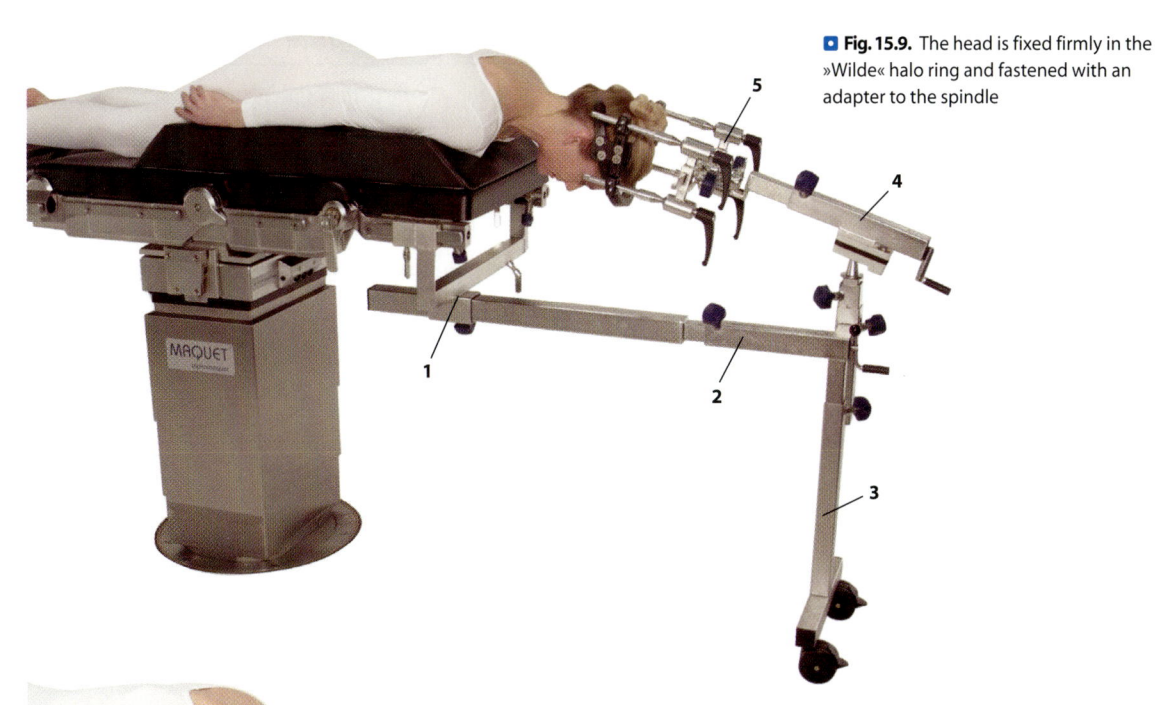

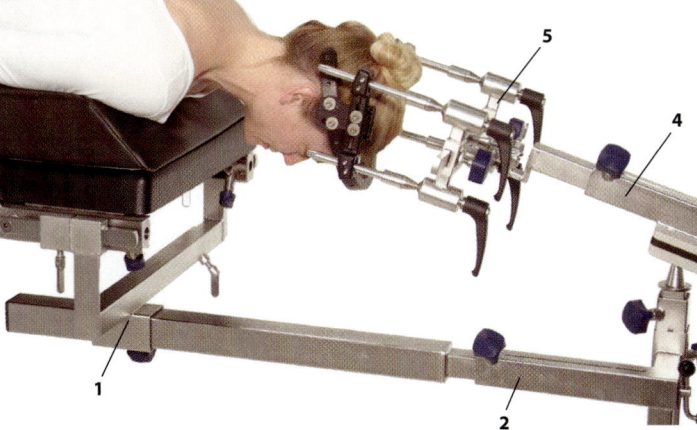

Fig. 15.9. The head is fixed firmly in the »Wilde« halo ring and fastened with an adapter to the spindle

Fig. 15.10. Stable fixing of the head with the halo ring

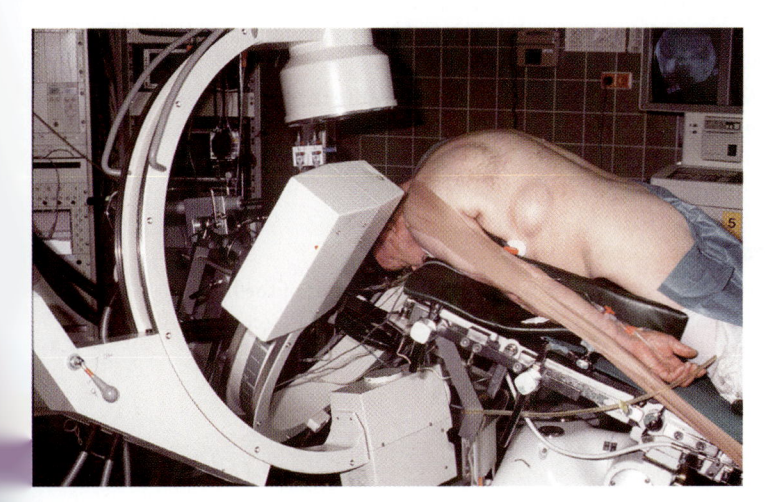

Fig. 15.11. Spine holding unit on Maquet 1120 with a Bekhterev patient in prone position

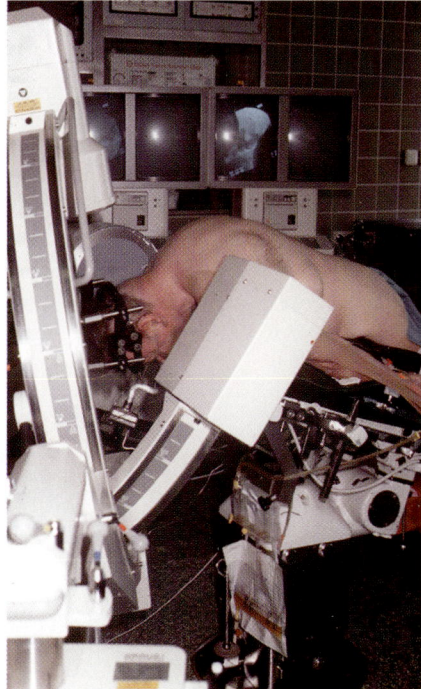

Fig. 15.12. One image intensifier for each scanning level

15.2 Thoracic spine, lumbar spine

15.2.1 Prone position

◘ Figs. 15.13–15.17.

Indications

Rear access to the thoracic and lumbar spine and costotransversectomy for operating:
- posttraumatic lesions, fractures and misalignment in the thoracic and lumbar spine
- tumours, spondylitis, spondylodiscitis
- scoliosis
- spondylolisthesis

Preparations
- Arm positioning devices
- Special head positioning cushion for prone position
- Thorax, pelvic and wedge cushions, padded roll
- Special bolster for prone position
- Shaving in the area of the incision and preoperative skin cleansing

Positioning
- Standard operating table position 1, position 2 or universal operating table
- Anaesthetic preparation and induction in supine position with 2 adapted arm positioning devices
- Transfer to the prepared operating table in the induction room
- Position both tables next to each other, with the prepared table lowered
- Place the patient in the prone position on the padded cushion on the prepared operating table and take him into the theatre
- Normal positioning of the operating table in the theatre
- When positioning the patient, take appropriate measures to prevent decubitus at areas which are subjected to pressure
- Position the head on the special head positioning cushion
- Position the axillae freely with the thorax bolsters and ensure that the pelvic bolster finishes with the anterior superior iliac crest
- Position both arms on the arm positioning devices
- Position the image intensifier
- Apply the neutral electrode and connect to the HF surgery device
- Arrange self-adhesive covers for preoperative skin disinfection
- Position the operating lights
- Patient warming system

Risks
- Iatrogenic injuries to the eyes and soft tissues of the head
- Intraoperative loss of the achieved positioning (secondary dislocation)

15.2 · Thoracic spine, lumbar spine

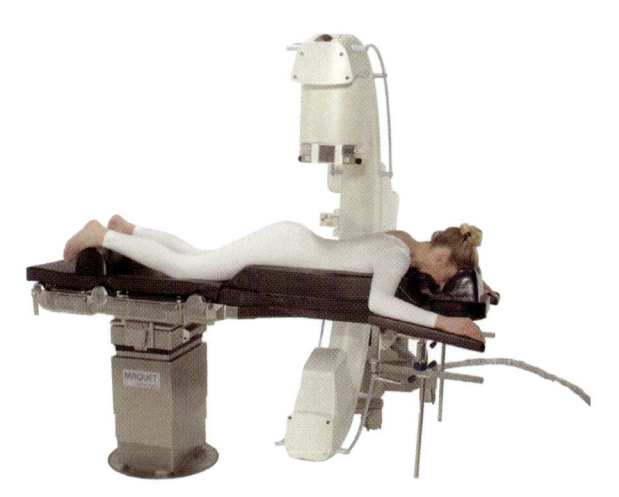

Fig. 15.13. Prone position on universal operating table with CRP back plate 1150.45 and CRP head plate

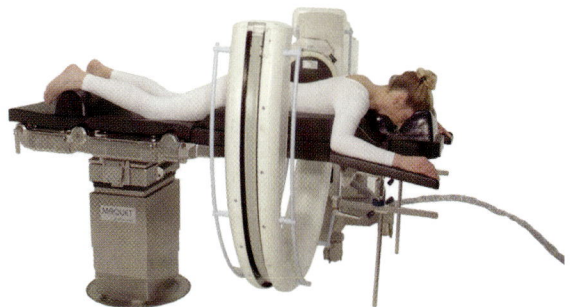

Fig. 15.14. By using the narrow CRP back plate 1150.45, the Iso-C3D can also be used in the prone position without any problems

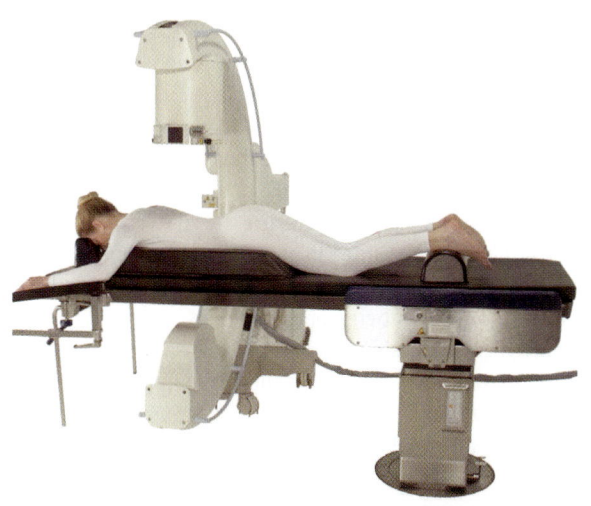

Fig. 15.15. Prone position on CRP operating table 1150.16 with CRP head plate for 360° use of image intensifier

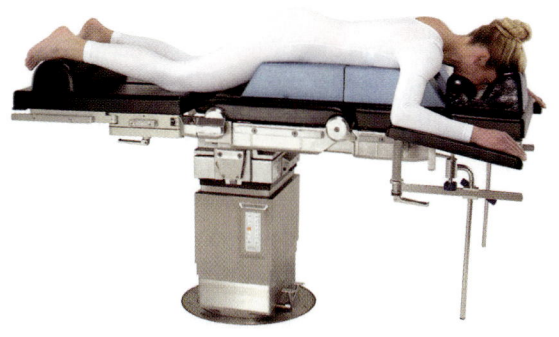

Fig. 15.16. Prone position on universal operating table 1150.30 with arm positioning in maximum 90° abduction

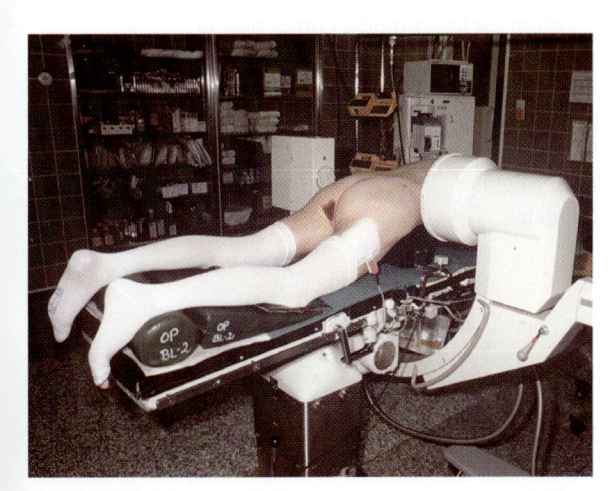

Fig. 15.17. The image intensifier remains in swivelled adjustment during the operation

15.2.2 Lateral position

◘ Figs. 15.18–15.22.

Indications

Thoracotomy, thoracolumbar access, lumbotomy for operating:
- posttraumatic lesions, fractures and misalignment in the thoracic and lumbar spine
- tumours, spondylitis, spondylodiscitis
- scoliosis
- spondylolisthesis

Preparations
- Arm positioning devices
- Gel ring, gel cushion, Goepel leg holder, lateral supports, radial adjusting clamps, padded cushions (normal and flat) and wedge cushions or tunnel cushions, body belts
- Shaving in the area of the incision and preoperative skin cleansing

Positioning
- Standard operating table position 1 or universal operating table
- Anaesthetic preparation and induction in supine position with 2 adapted arm positioning devices
- Normal positioning of the operating table in the theatre
- When positioning the patient, take appropriate measures to prevent decubitus at areas which are subjected to pressure
- Fit the radial adjusting clamp to the side rail of the head plate, position the Goepel leg holder
- Spread out the arm on the side not being operated
- Move the patient onto the healthy side
- Move the lower arm forwards so that the weight of the upper body does not lie directly on the shoulder
- Fit the radial adjusting clamps to the side rails of the leg plates/head plate and position the body support on the level of the sacrum, symphysis and scapula, with the tip of the scapula positioned freely
- 1st possibility: position the legs with the padded cushions (normal and flat) and possibly wedge cushions
- Fix the lower leg and positioning aids with the body belts
- 2nd possibility: position the legs with the tunnel cushion
- Position the image intensifier
- Apply the neutral electrode and connect to the HF surgery device
- Arrange absorbent drapes or self-adhesive covers for preoperative skin disinfection
- Position the operating lights
- Patient warming system

15.2 · Thoracic spine, lumbar spine

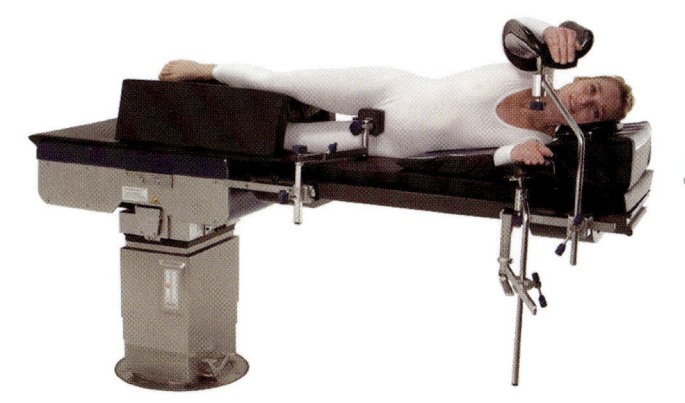

Fig. 15.18. Lateral position on CRP operating table 1150.16 with 2 CRP accessory adapters

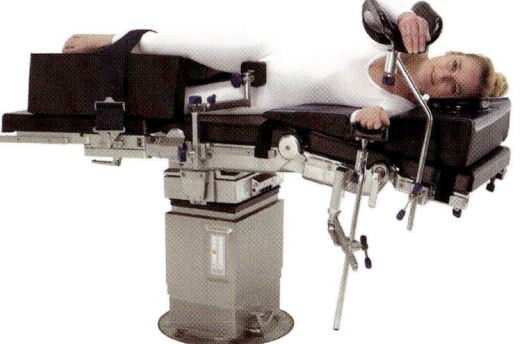

Fig. 15.19. Lateral position on universal operating table with side positioning cushions for anatomic positioning of the lower arm

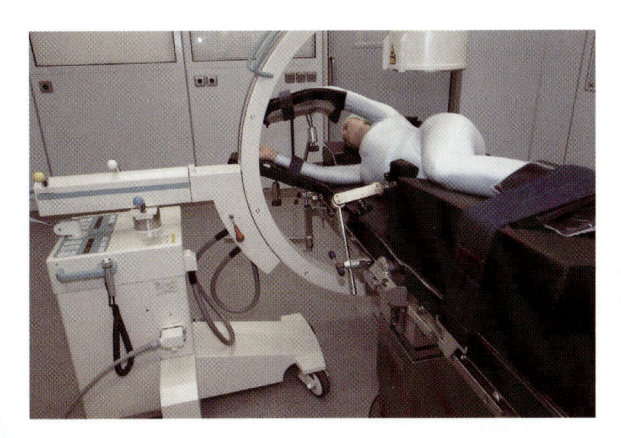

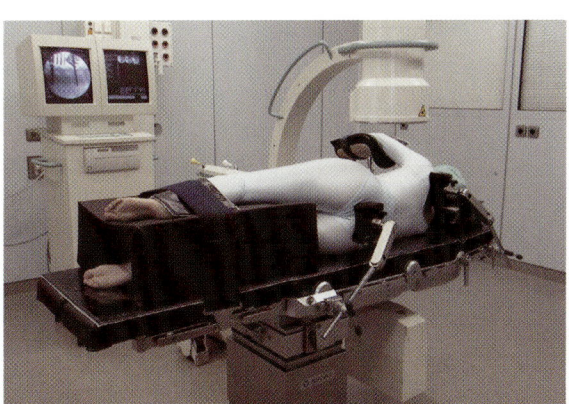

Fig. 15.20. Use of image intensifier from the side opposite the surgeon

Fig. 15.21. Back support at the scapula and sacrum

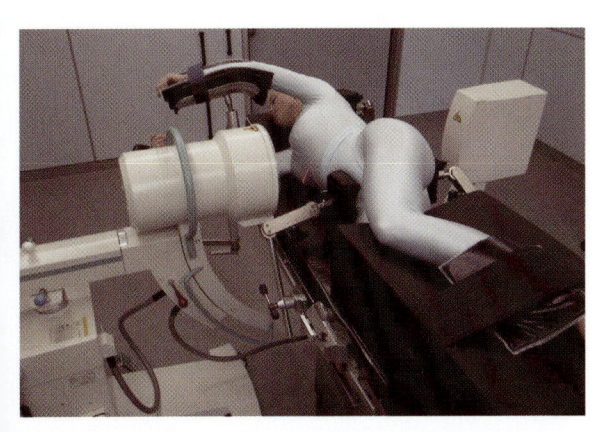

Fig. 15.22. The image intensifier remains in swivelled adjustment during the operation

15.2.3 Supine position

◨ Figs. 15.23–15.25.

Indications
Front access to the cervicothoracic junction and to the upper thoracic spine, thoracotomy, transperitoneal access, lumbotomy for operating:
- posttraumatic lesions, fractures and misalignment in the thoracic and lumbar spine and in the lumbosacral junction
- tumours, spondylitis, spondylodiscitis
- scoliosis
- spondylolisthesis

Preparations
- Arm positioning devices
- Shaving in the area of the incision and preoperative skin cleansing

Positioning
- Standard operating table position 1, universal operating table
- Anaesthetic preparation and induction in supine position with 2 adapted arm positioning devices
- Normal positioning of the operating table in the theatre
- When positioning the patient, take appropriate measures to prevent decubitus at areas which are subjected to pressure
- Position both arms in abduction position on the arm positioning devices
- Apply the neutral electrode and connect to the HF surgery device
- Arrange absorbent drapes or self-adhesive covers for preoperative skin disinfection
- Position the operating lights
- Patient warming system

15.2 · Thoracic spine, lumbar spine

Fig. 15.23. Supine position on CRP operating table 1150.16 with arm positioning in maximum 90° abduction for operations to the lumbar spine

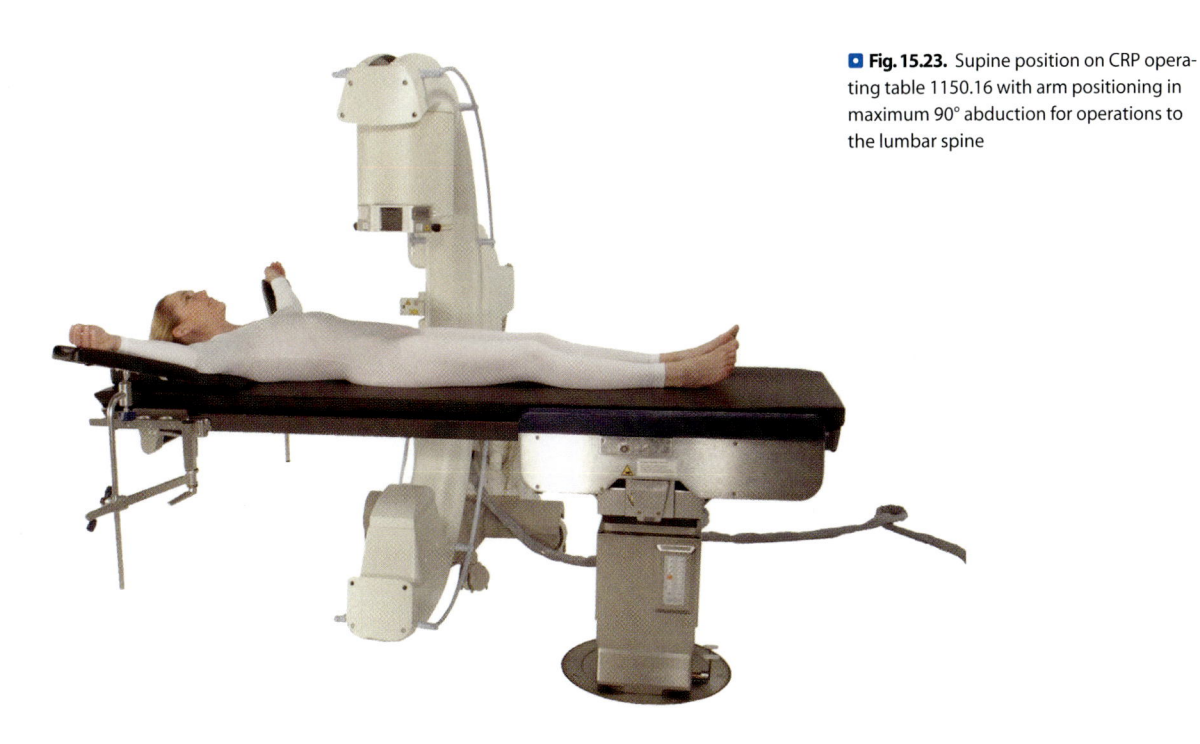

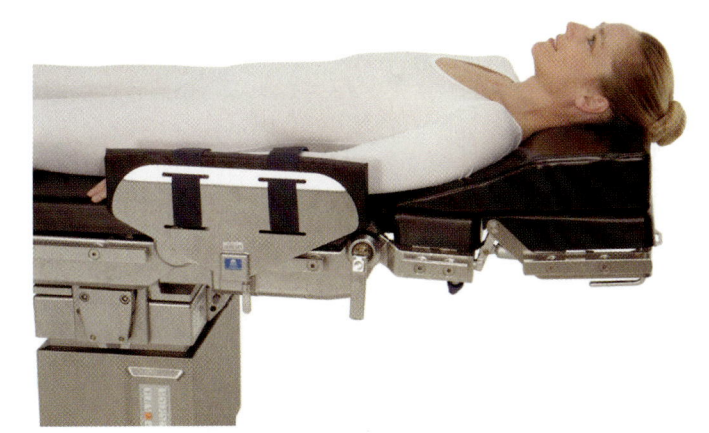

Fig. 15.24. Supine position on universal operating table with arms positioned at the body for operations to the thoracic spine

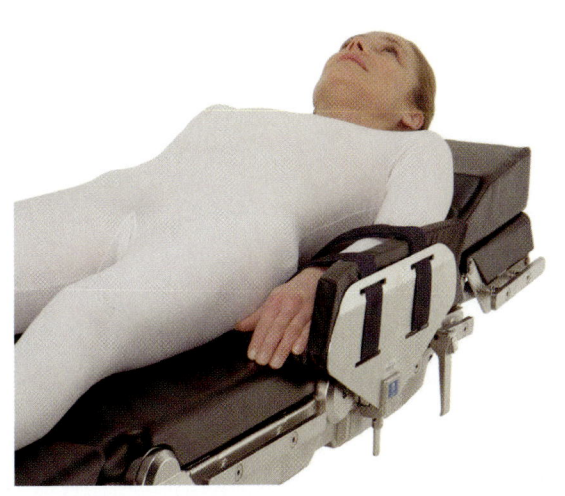

Fig. 15.25. Arm protection from the elbow to the hand with arms positioned at the body

16 Pelvis

16.1 Pelvic girdle – 204
16.1.1 Supine position – 204
16.1.2 Lateral position – 206
16.1.3 Prone position – 208

16.2 Acetabulum – 210
16.2.1 Supine position – 210
16.2.2 Lateral position – 212
16.2.3 Prone position – 214

16.1 Pelvic girdle

16.1.1 Supine position

◘ Figs. 16.1–16.6.

Indications

Access to the front pelvic girdle, ilium, iliosacral joint and hip joint (Pfannenstiel, modified Stoppa, ilioinguinal, anterolateral, Judet, Smith-Peterson) for operating:
- fractures, misalignment and posttraumatic lesions in the front pelvic girdle, ilium, iliosacral joint and at the symphysis
- tumours, osteomyelitis, ossification
- tamponade for pelvic bleeding
- placement of the pelvic cingulum

Preparations
- Arm positioning devices
- Possibly table extension
- Shaving in the area of the incision and preoperative skin cleansing

Positioning
- Standard operating table position 1, position 2 or universal operating table, possibly table extension
- Anaesthetic preparation and induction in supine position with 2 adapted arm positioning devices
- Normal positioning of the operating table in the theatre
- When positioning the patient, take appropriate measures to prevent decubitus at areas which are subjected to pressure
- Position both arms in the abduction position on the arm positioning devices
- Apply the neutral electrode and connect to the HF surgery device
- Arrange absorbent drapes or self-adhesive covers for preoperative skin disinfection
- Position the operating lights
- Patient warming system

16.1 · Pelvic girdle

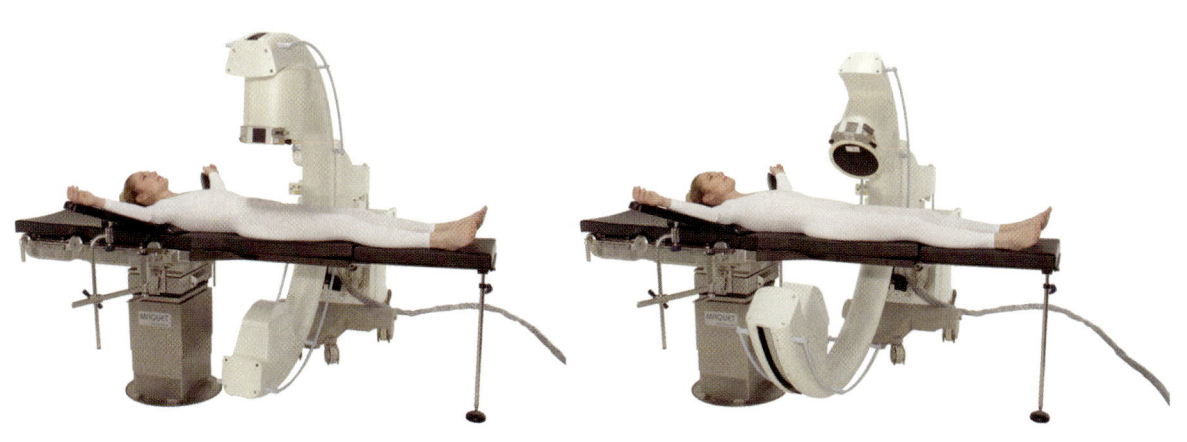

Fig. 16.1. Supine position on universal operating table with CRP back plate 1150.45 and supported extension plate

Fig. 16.2. By using the narrow CRP back plate 1150.45, the Iso-C3D can also be used in the supine position without any problems

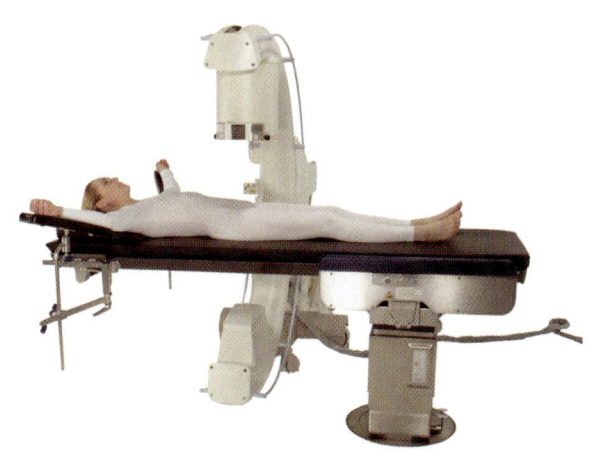

Fig. 16.3. Supine position on the CRP operating table 1150.16, using the image intensifier

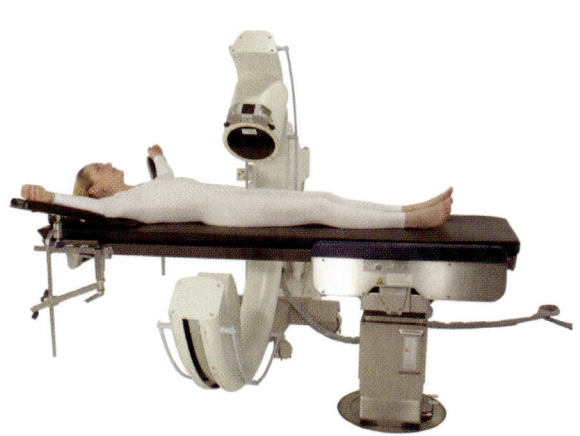

Fig. 16.4. Arms positioned with maximum 90° abduction and in supination position for 360° use of the image intensifier

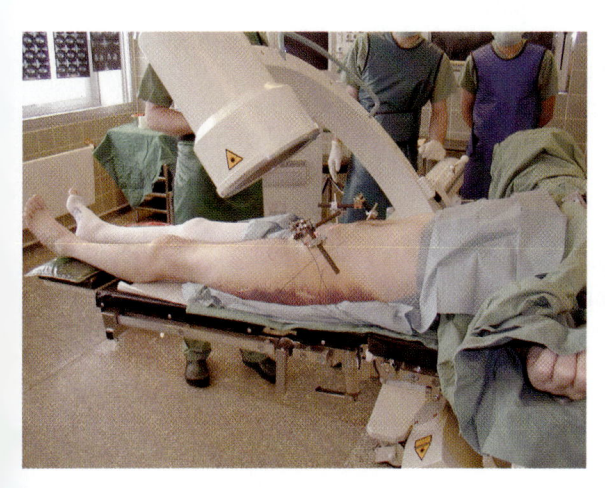

Fig. 16.5. System 1120 with leg plate extension

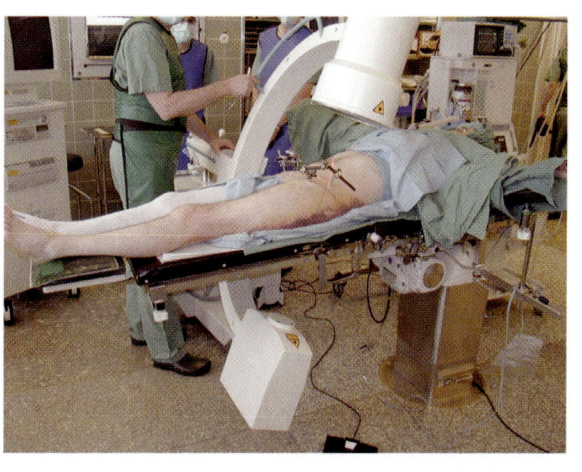

Fig. 16.6. Use of the image intensifier after placing a pelvis fixator

16.1.2 Lateral position

◘ Figs. 16.7–16.9.

Indications

Lateral, anterolateral and rear access to the ilium and iliosacral joint for operating:
- fractures, misalignment and posttraumatic lesions of the ilium, pelvic column and iliosacral joint
- tumours, osteomyelitis, ossification, gluteal compartment syndrome
- exposure of the sciatic nerve

Preparations
- Arm positioning devices
- Gel ring, gel cushion, Goepel leg holder, side supports, radial adjusting clamps, padded cushions (normal and flat) and wedge cushions, tunnel cushions, body belts, possibly table extension
- Shaving in the area of the incision and preoperative skin cleansing

Positioning
- Standard operating table position 1, position 2 or universal operating table, possibly table extension
- Anaesthetic preparation and induction in supine position with 2 adapted arm positioning devices
- Normal positioning of the operating table in the theatre
- When positioning the patient, take appropriate measures to prevent decubitus at areas which are subjected to pressure
- Fit the radial adjusting clamp to the rail of the head plate, position the Goepel leg holder
- Spread out the arm on the side not being operated
- Move the patient onto the healthy side
- Move the lower arm forwards so that the weight of the upper body does not lie directly on the shoulder
- Fit the radial adjusting clamps to the side rails of the leg plates/head plate and position the body supports on the level of the sacrum of the symphysis and the scapula
- **1st possibility:** position the legs with the padded cushions (normal and flat) and possibly wedge cushions
- Fix the lower leg and the positioning aids with the body belts
- **2nd possibility:** position the legs with the tunnel cushion
- Apply the neutral electrode and connect to the HF surgery device
- Arrange absorbent drapes or self-adhesive covers for preoperative skin disinfection
- Position the operating lights
- Patient warming system

16.1 · Pelvic girdle

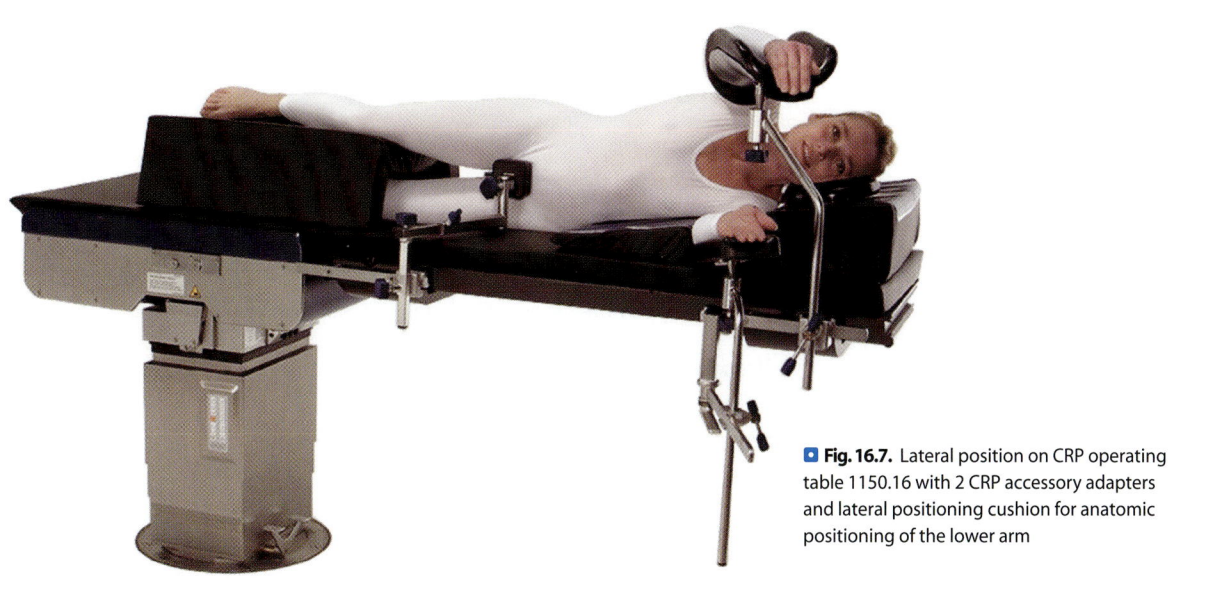

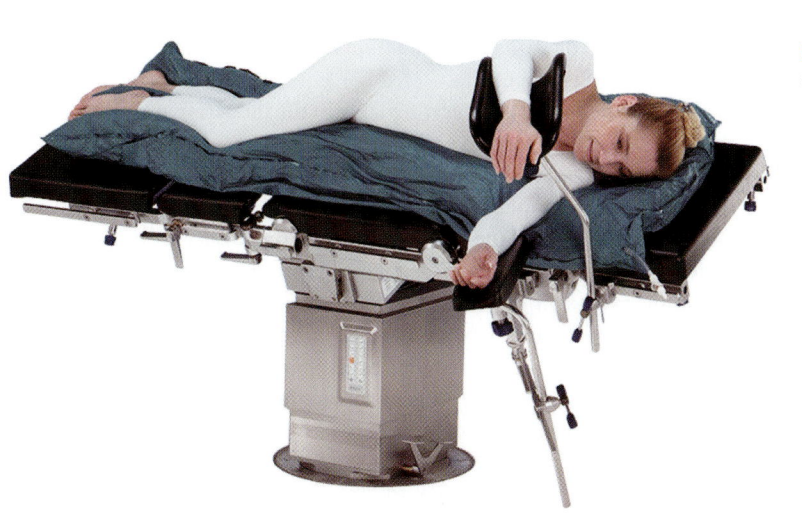

Fig. 16.7. Lateral position on CRP operating table 1150.16 with 2 CRP accessory adapters and lateral positioning cushion for anatomic positioning of the lower arm

Fig. 16.8. Lateral position on universal operating table with vacuum mat

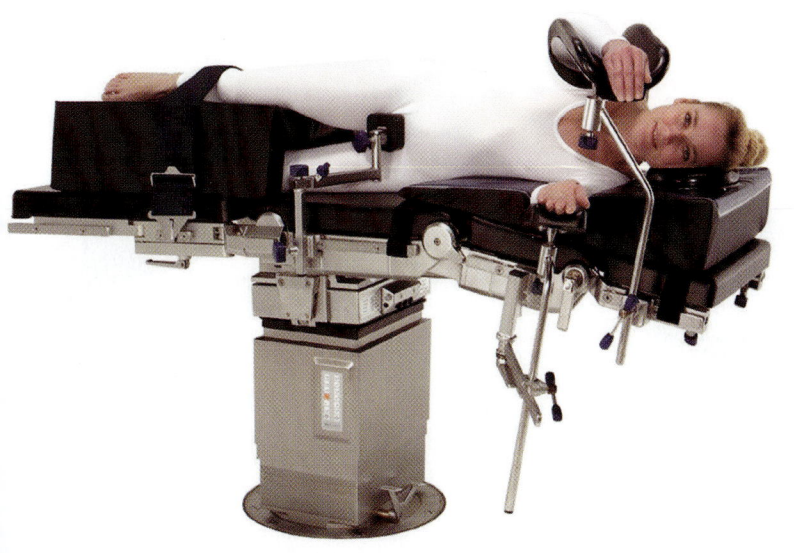

Fig. 16.9. Lateral position on universal operating table with lateral positioning cushion and operating table in flex position for neutral position of the spinal column

16.1.3 Prone position

Figs. 16.10–16.13.

Indications
Dorsal access to the sacrum, hip joint, iliosacral joint for:
- fractures, misalignment and posttraumatic lesions in the area of the sacrum, iliosacral joint and hip joint
- tumours, gluteal compartment syndrome
- exposure of the sacral nerve and the sciatic nerve

Preparations
- Arm positioning devices
- Special head positioning pillow for prone position
- Thorax, pelvic and wedge cushion, padded roll
- Possibly table extension
- Shaving in the area of the incision and preoperative skin cleansing

Positioning
- Standard operating table position 1, position 2 or universal operating table
- Anaesthetic preparation and induction in supine position with 2 adapted arm positioning devices
- Transfer to the prepared operating table in the induction room
- Position both tables next to each other, with the prepared table lowered
- Place the patient in prone position on the padded cushion of the prepared operating table and take him into the theatre
- Normal positioning of the operating table in the theatre
- When positioning the patient, take appropriate measures to prevent decubitus at areas which are subjected to pressure
- Position the head on the special head positioning cushion
- Position both arms on the arm positioning devices
- Apply the neutral electrode and connect to the HF surgery device
- Arrange self-adhesive covers for preoperative skin disinfection
- Position the operating lights
- Patient warming system

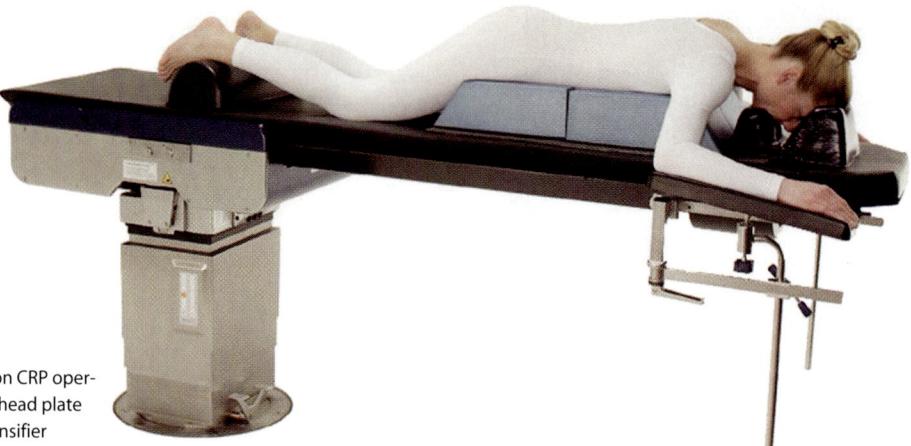

Fig. 16.10. Prone position on CRP operating table 1150.16 with CRP head plate for 360° use of the image intensifier

16.1 · Pelvic girdle

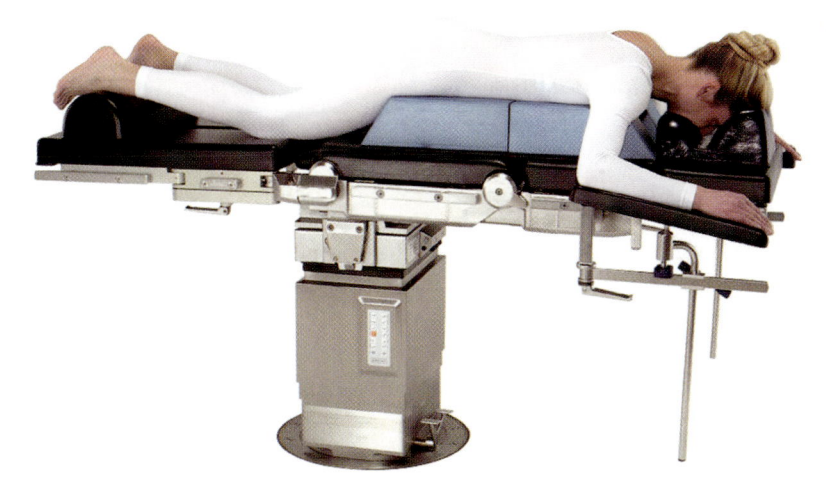

Fig. 16.11. Prone position on universal operating table 1150.30 with arms positioned in maximum 90° abduction

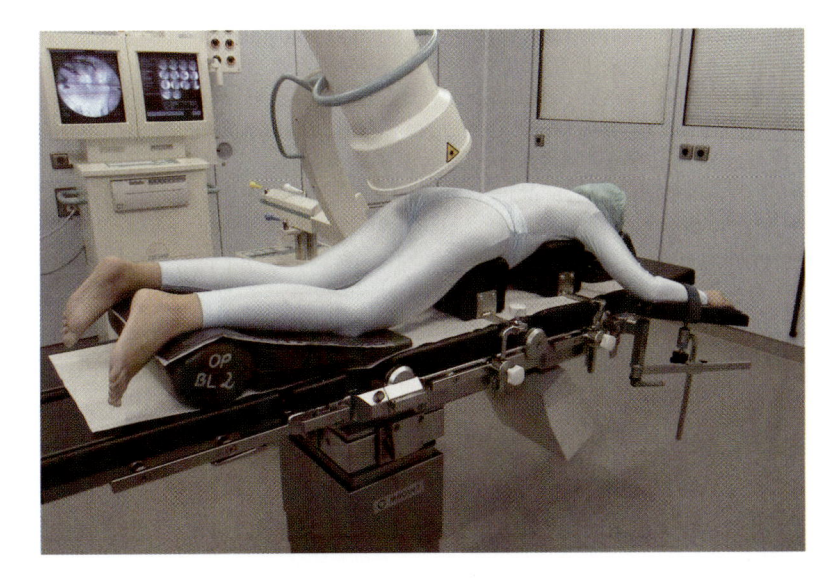

Fig. 16.12. Prone position on universal operating table 1150.30 with bolsters (MHH) and use of the image intensifier

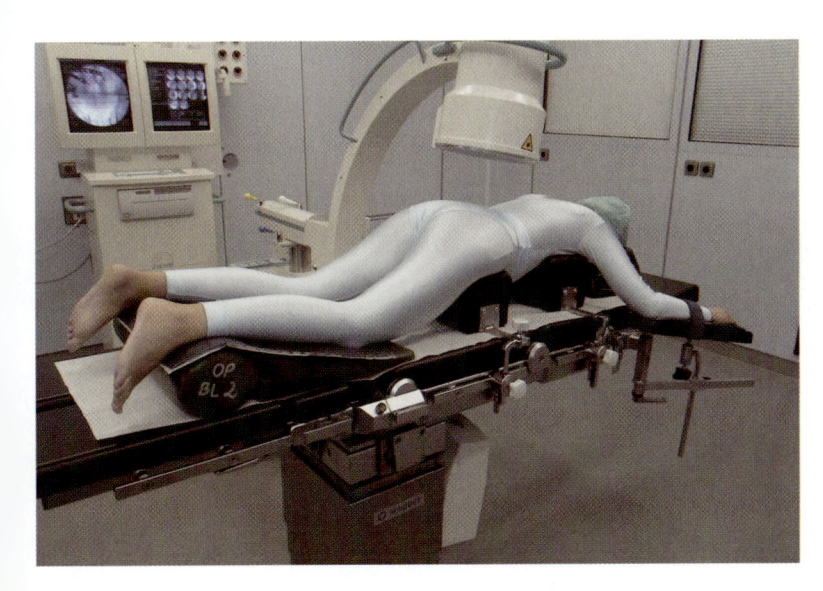

Fig. 16.13. Prone position on universal operating table 1150.30 with maximum longitudinal displacement toward the head for optimum use of the image intensifier

16.2 Acetabulum

16.2.1 Supine position

Figs. 16.14–16.17.

Indications

Operations for acetabulum fractures using the following access: ilioinguinal access, Smith-Peterson access, extended iliofemoral access, extended Pfannenstiel access, modified Stoppa access.

Preparations
- Arm positioning devices
- Shaving in the area of the incision and preoperative skin cleansing

Positioning
- Standard operating table position 1, position 2 or universal operating table
- Anaesthetic preparation and induction in supine position with 2 adapted arm positioning devices
- Normal positioning of the operating table in the theatre
- When positioning the patient, take appropriate measures to prevent decubitus at areas which are subjected to pressure
- Position both arms in abduction position on the arm positioning devices
- Apply the neutral electrode and connect to the HF surgery device
- Arrange absorbent drapes or self-adhesive covers for preoperative skin disinfection
- Position the operating lights
- Patient warming system

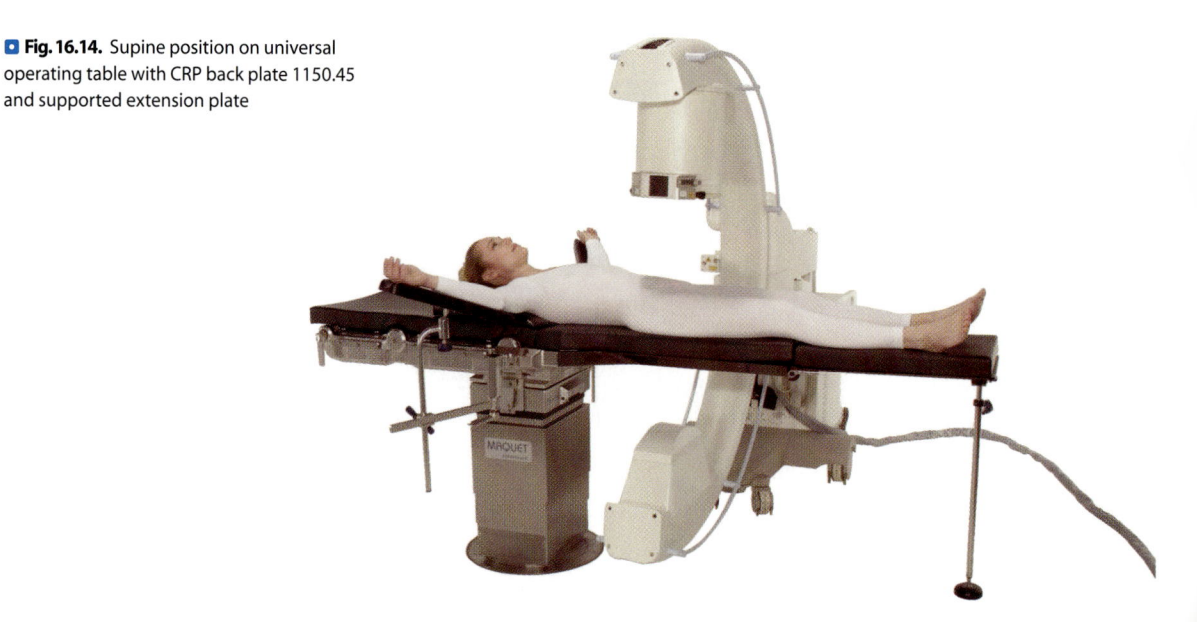

Fig. 16.14. Supine position on universal operating table with CRP back plate 1150.45 and supported extension plate

16.2 · Acetabulum

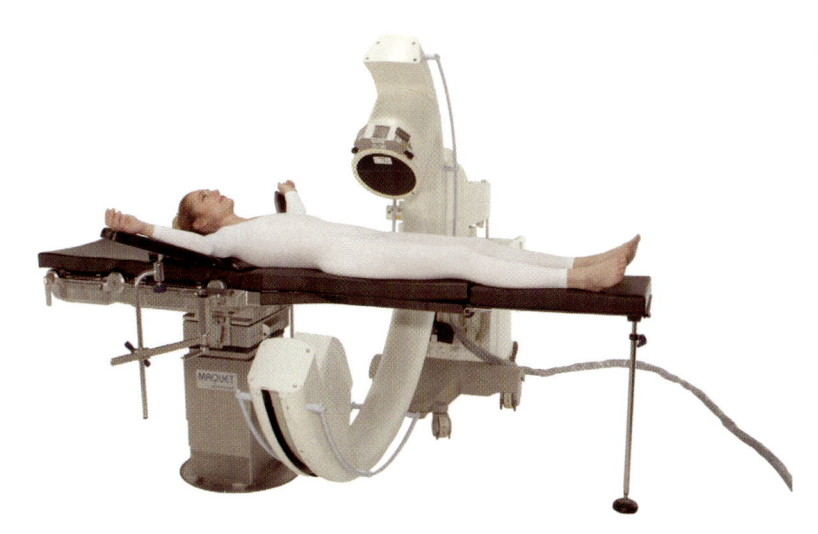

Fig. 16.15. By using the narrow CRP back plate 1150.45, the Iso-C3D can also be used in the supine position without any problems

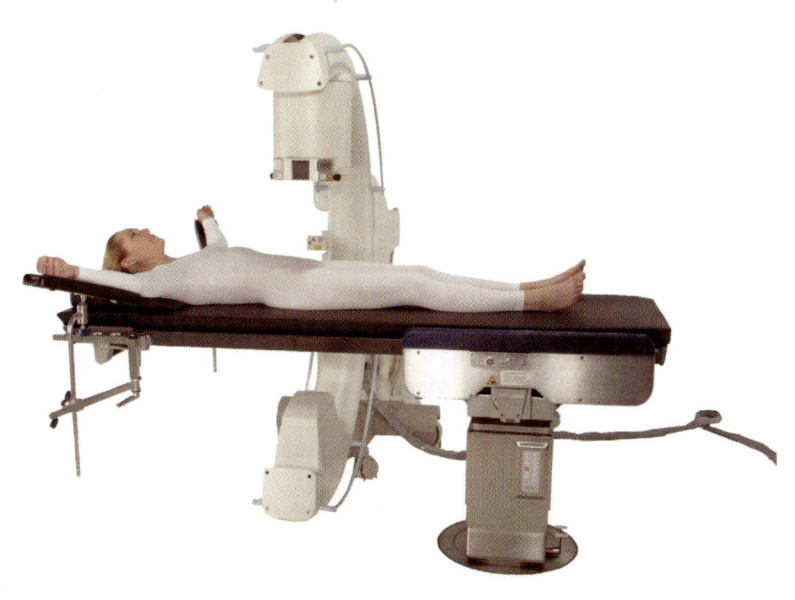

Fig. 16.16. Supine position on CRP operating table 1150.16 with use of the image intensifier

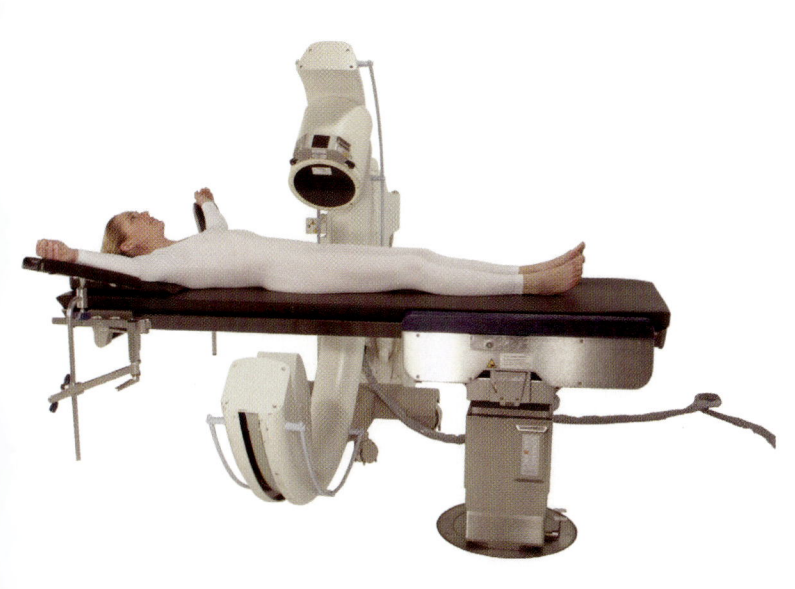

Fig. 16.17. Arms positioned in maximum 90° abduction and in supination position for 360° use of the image intensifier

16.2.2 Lateral position

◘ Figs. 16.18–16.20.

Indications

Operations for acetabulum fractures using the following access: Kocher-Langenbeck access, combined ventral/dorsal access, extended access.

Preparations
- Arm positioning devices
- Gel ring, gel cushion, Goepel leg holder, side supports, radial adjusting clamps, padded cushions (normal and flat) and wedge cushions, tunnel cushions, body belts,
- Shaving in the area of the incision and preoperative skin cleansing

Positioning
- Standard operating table position 1 or universal operating table
- Anaesthetic preparation and induction in supine position with 2 adapted arm positioning devices
- Normal positioning of the operating table in the theatre
- When positioning the patient, take appropriate measures to prevent decubitus at areas which are subjected to pressure
- Fit the radial adjusting clamp to the side rail of the head plate, position the Goepel leg holder
- Spread out the arm on the side not being operated
- Move the patient onto the healthy side
- Move the lower arm forwards so that the weight of the upper body does not lie directly on the shoulder
- Fit the radial adjusting clamps to the side rails of the leg plates/head plate and position the body supports on the level of the sacrum of the symphysis and the scapula
- **1st possibility:** position the legs with the padded cushions (normal and flat) and possibly wedge cushions
- Fix the lower leg and the positioning aids with the body belts
- **2nd possibility:** position the legs with the tunnel cushion
- Apply the neutral electrode and connect to the HF surgery device
- Arrange absorbent drapes or self-adhesive covers for preoperative skin disinfection
- Position the operating lights
- Patient warming system

16.2 · Acetabulum

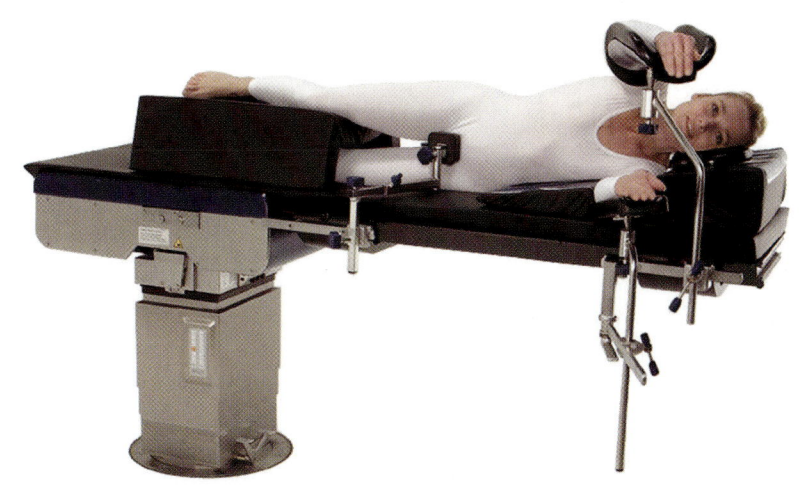

Fig. 16.18. Lateral position on CRP operating table 1150.16 with 2 CRP accessory adapters and lateral positioning cushion for anatomic positioning of the lower arm

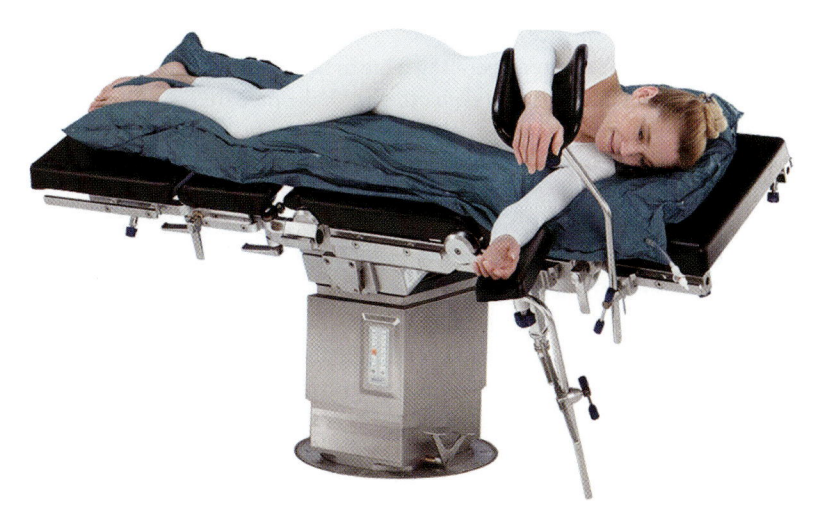

Fig. 16.19. Lateral position on universal operating table with vacuum mat

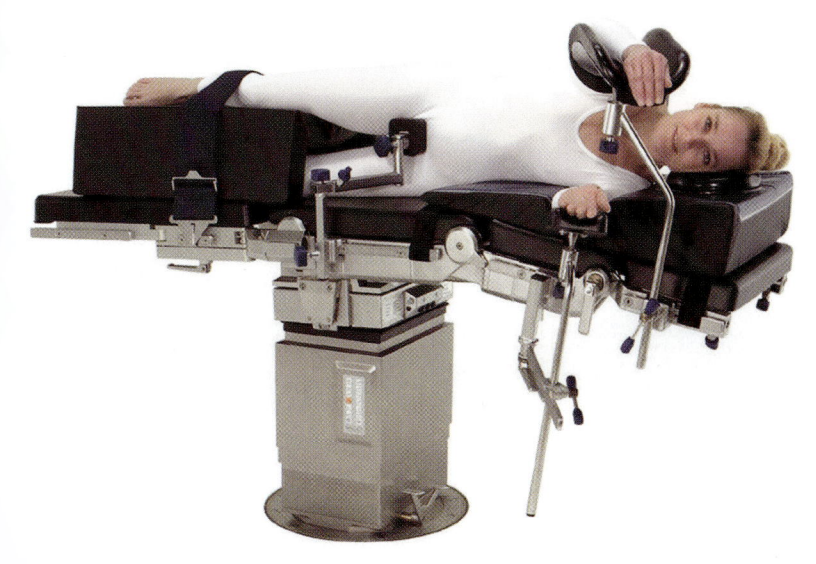

Fig. 16.20. Lateral position on universal operating table with lateral positioning cushion and operating table in flex position for neutral position of the spinal column

16.2.3 Prone position

Figs. 16.21–16.24.

Indications
Operations for acetabulum fractures using the Kocher-Langenbeck access.

Preparations
- Arm positioning devices
- Special head positioning cushion for prone position
- Thorax, pelvic and wedge cushion, padded roll
- Shaving in the area of the incision and preoperative skin cleansing

Positioning
- Standard operating table position 1, position 2 or universal operating table
- Anaesthetic preparation and induction in supine position with 2 adapted arm positioning devices
- Transfer to the prepared operating table in the induction room
- Position both tables next to each other, with the prepared table lowered
- Place the patient in prone position on the padded cushion of the prepared operating table and take him into the theatre
- Normal positioning of the operating table in the theatre
- When positioning the patient, take appropriate measures to prevent decubitus at areas which are subjected to pressure
- Position the head on the special head positioning cushion
- Position both arms on the arm positioning devices
- Apply the neutral electrode and connect to the HF surgery device
- Arrange self-adhesive covers for preoperative skin disinfection
- Position the operating lights
- Patient warming system

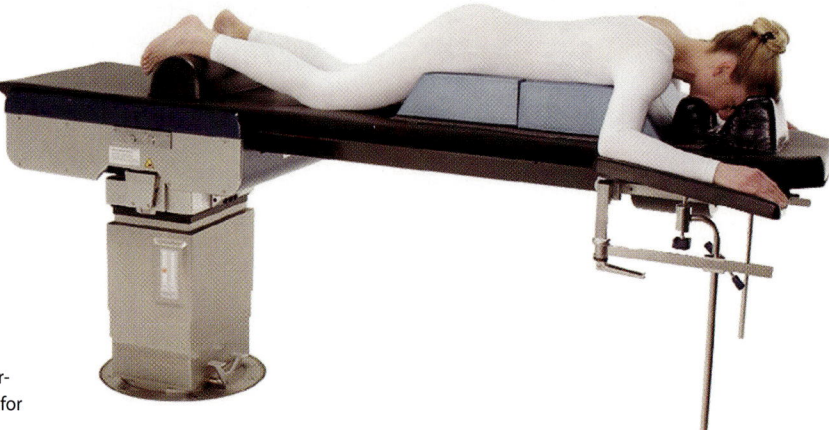

Fig. 16.21. Prone position on CRP operating table 1150.16 with CRP head plate for 360° use of the image intensifier

16.2 · Acetabulum

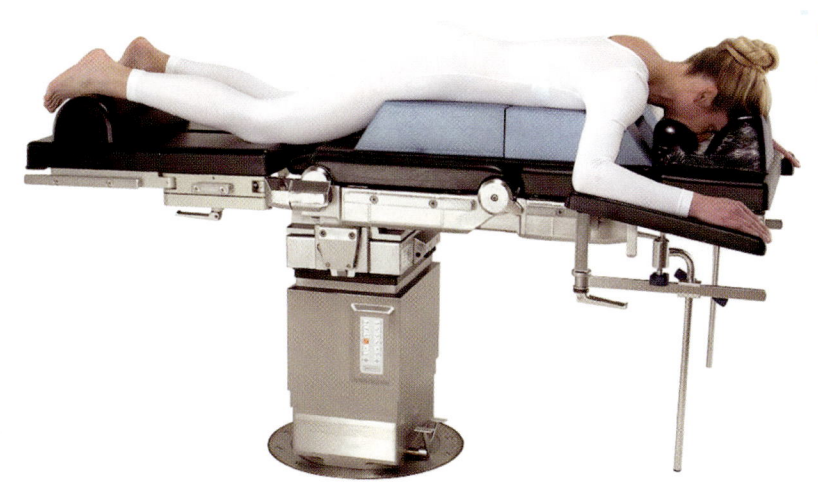

Fig. 16.22. Prone position on universal operating table 1150.30 with arms positioned in maximum 90° abduction

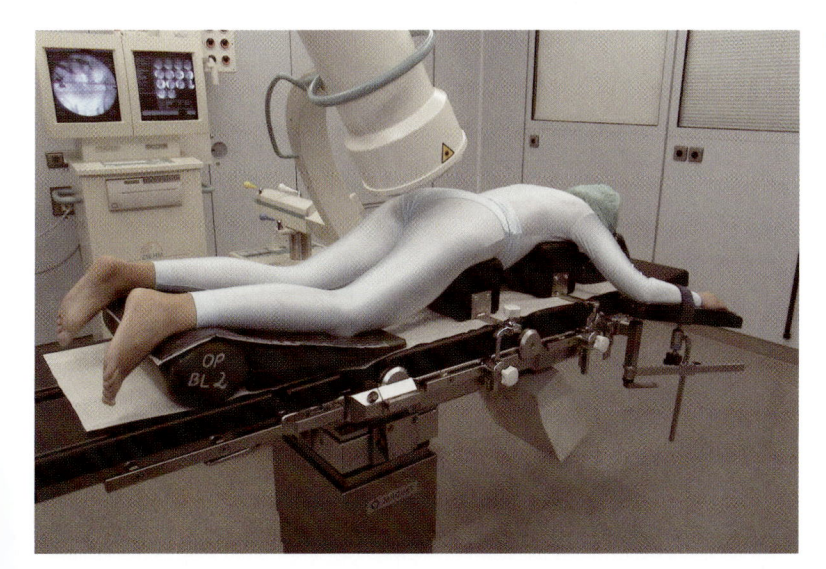

Fig. 16.23. Prone position on universal operating table 1150.30 with bolsters (MHH) and use of the image intensifier

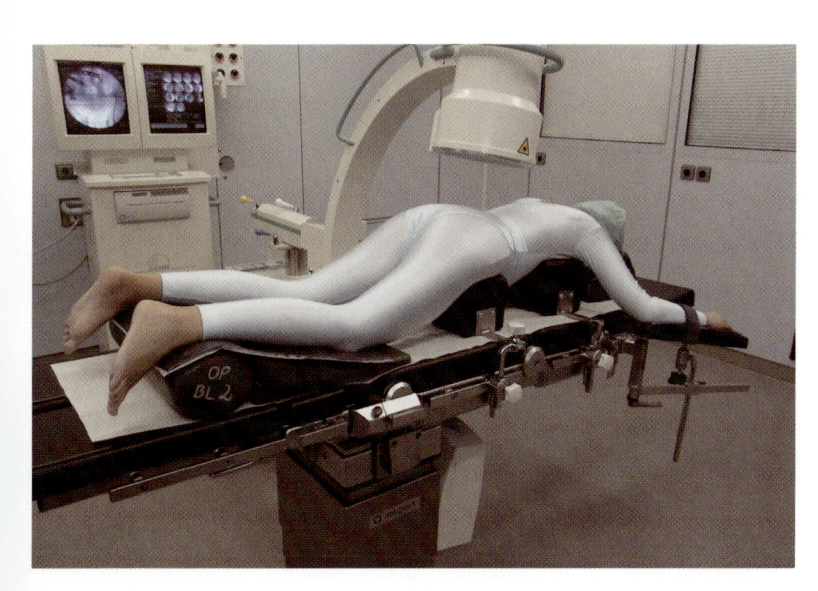

Fig. 16.24. Prone position on universal operating table 1150.30 with maximum longitudinal displacement towards the head for optimum use of the image intensifier

17 Upper extremities

17.1 Shoulder – 218
17.1.1 Supine position – 218
17.1.2 Beach-chair position – 220
17.1.3 Prone position – 222

17.2 Upper arm – 224
17.2.1 Supine position – 224
17.2.2 Prone position – 226

17.3 Elbow – 228
17.3.1 Supine position – 228
17.3.2 Prone position – 230

17.4 Forearm and hand – 232
17.4.1 Supine position – 232

17.1 Shoulder

17.1.1 Supine position

▪ Figs. 17.1, 17.2.

Indications

Ventral, axillary, transdeltoid access to the shoulder joint, access to the clavicle and to the acromioclavicular joint for fractures, pseudarthrosis, posttraumatic misalignment, luxation, instability, tumours, inflammation and rupture of the biceps tendon.

Preparations
- Arm positioning devices
- Remove Gilchrist bandage
- Gel ring
- Shaving in the area of the incision and preoperative skin cleansing

Positioning
- Standard operating table position 1, position 2 or universal operating table with X-ray protection, clavicle remains available for scanning
- Anaesthetic preparation and induction in supine position with 2 adapted arm positioning devices
- Crosswise positioning of the operating table in the theatre
- When positioning the patient, take appropriate measures to prevent decubitus at areas which are subjected to pressure
- Tilt the operating table in the Trendelenburg position, raise the back plate by 20–30°, lower the leg plates and the head section by hand
- Position the head on a gel ring, possibly slightly turned to the other side and reclined
- Position the infusion arm on an arm positioning device
- Pad the shoulder with a positioning aid, thus raising the operating site or joint being operated
- Cover the arm on the side being operated while leaving it free to move and position it at the body with arm protection or place it on the arm positioning device
- Apply the neutral electrode and connect to the HF surgery device
- Arrange self-adhesive covers for preoperative skin disinfection
- Position the operating lights
- Patient warming system

17.1 · Shoulder

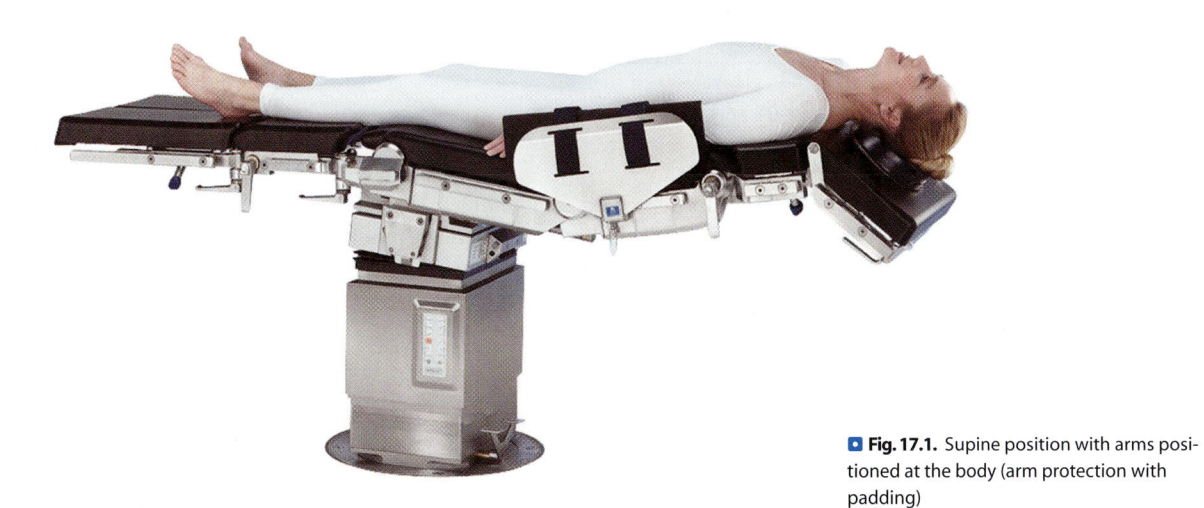

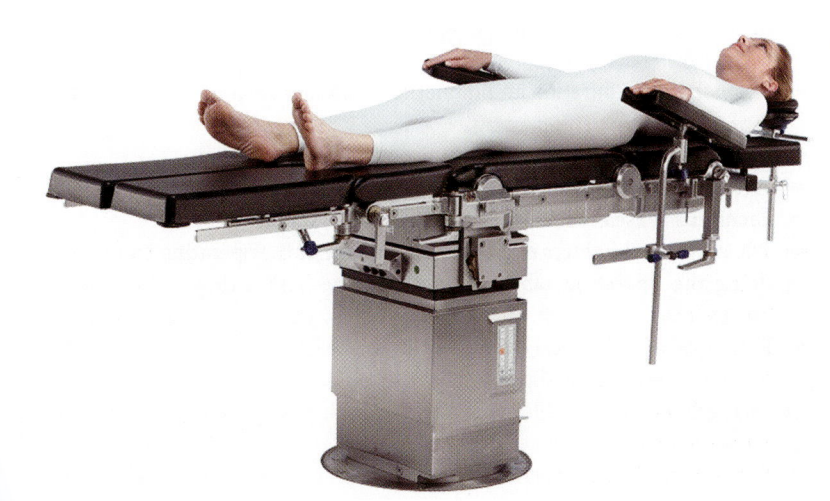

Fig. 17.1. Supine position with arms positioned at the body (arm protection with padding)

Fig. 17.2. Supine position on special shoulder plate with the advantage of scanning and the head on a one-piece horseshoe-shaped headrest

17.1.2 Beach-chair position

◘ Figs. 17.3–17.7.

Indications

Ventral, transdeltoid access to the shoulder joint, access to the clavicle and to the acromioclavicular joint for fractures, pseudarthrosis, posttraumatic misalignment, luxation, instability, tumours, inflammation, rupture of the biceps tendon, arthrosis, impingement syndrome and rotator cuff lesions.

Preparations

- Arm positioning devices
- Remove Gilchrist bandage
- Gel ring
- Shaving in the area of the incision and preoperative skin cleansing

Positioning

- Beach-chair (BC) operating table position 2 or universal operating table with special back plate
- Anaesthetic preparation and induction in supine position with 2 adapted arm positioning devices
- Crosswise positioning of the operating table in the theatre
- When positioning the patient, take appropriate measures to prevent decubitus at areas which are subjected to pressure
- The patient's shoulders end at the upper edge of the operating table
- Bring the operating table gradually to the half-sitting (beach-chair) position
- Raise the back plate and alternately lower the head of the complete operating table until the final position is reached
- Change the Bowden cable over and lower the legs to the horizontal position (system 1120)
- Position the head on a gel ring and fix with transparent plaster right across the forehead or use a head support for shoulder operation (U-shaped helmet)
- Position the infusion arm on an arm positioning device
- Cover the arm on the side being operated while leaving it free to move and position it at the body with arm protection or place it on the arm positioning device
- Apply the neutral electrode and connect to the HF surgery device
- Fit the thorax support to the side rail of the shoulder plate
- Arrange self-adhesive covers for preoperative skin disinfection
- Position the operating lights
- Patient warming system

Risks

- Iatrogenic injuries to the eyes and soft tissues (head fixing) when fixed with plaster or foil
- Secondary dislocation

17.1 · Shoulder

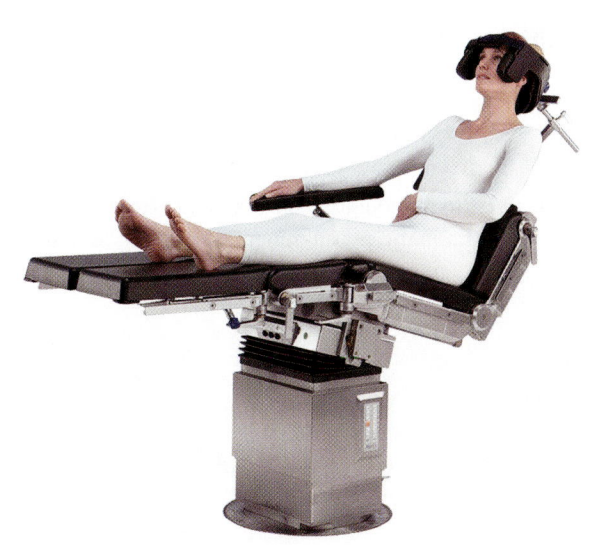

Fig. 17.3. Beach-chair positioning on special shoulder plate with helmet for safe positioning of the head

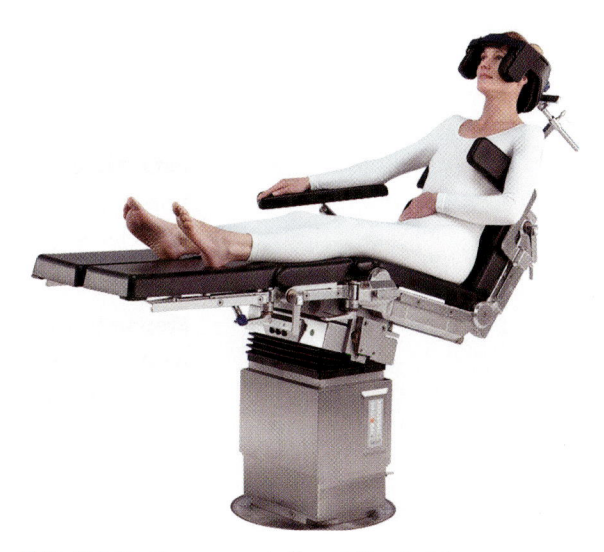

Fig. 17.4. The thorax support offers additional safety

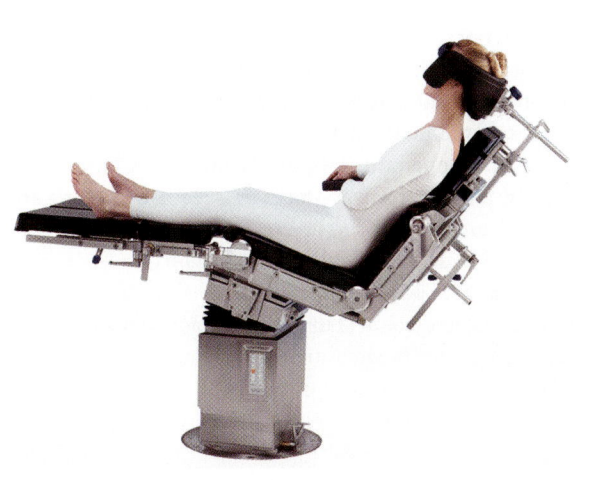

Fig. 17.5. The universal operating table with special shoulder plate is adapted to the body

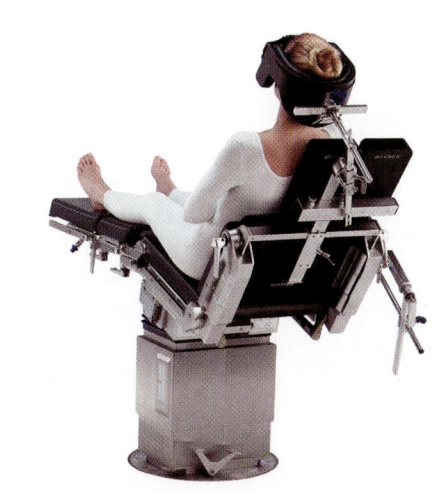

Fig. 17.6. A segment is removed to leave free access to the rear shoulder

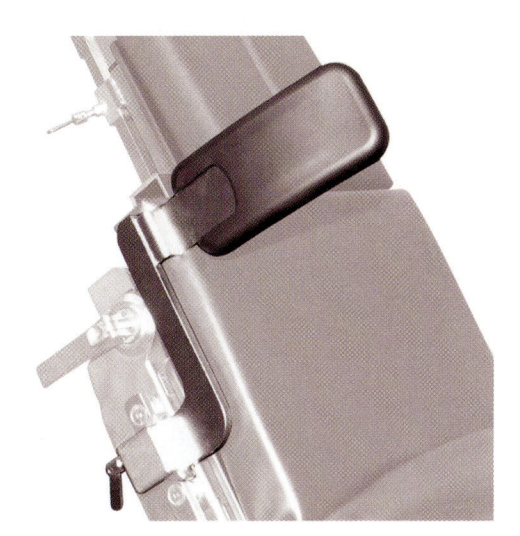

Fig. 17.7. Thorax support

17.1.3 Prone position

◘ Figs. 17.8, 17.9.

Indications

Dorsal and transacromial access to the shoulder joint and access to the scapula for luxation, fractures, posttraumatic misalignment, instability, tumours, rotator cuff lesions.

Preparations
- Arm positioning devices
- Special head positioning cushion for prone position
- Thorax, pelvic and wedge cushion, padded roll
- Shaving in the area of the incision and preoperative skin cleansing

Positioning
- Standard operating table position 1, position 2 or universal operating table
- Anaesthetic preparation and induction in supine position with 2 adapted arm positioning devices
- Transfer to the prepared operating table in the induction room
- Position both tables next to each other, with the prepared table lowered
- Place the patient in prone position on the padded cushion of the prepared operating table and take him into the theatre
- Crosswise positioning of the operating table in the theatre
- When positioning the patient, take appropriate measures to prevent decubitus at areas which are subjected to pressure
- Position the head on the special head positioning cushion
- Position both arms on the arm positioning devices
- Apply the neutral electrode and connect to the HF surgery device
- Arrange self-adhesive covers for preoperative skin disinfection
- Position the operating lights
- Patient warming system

17.1 · Shoulder

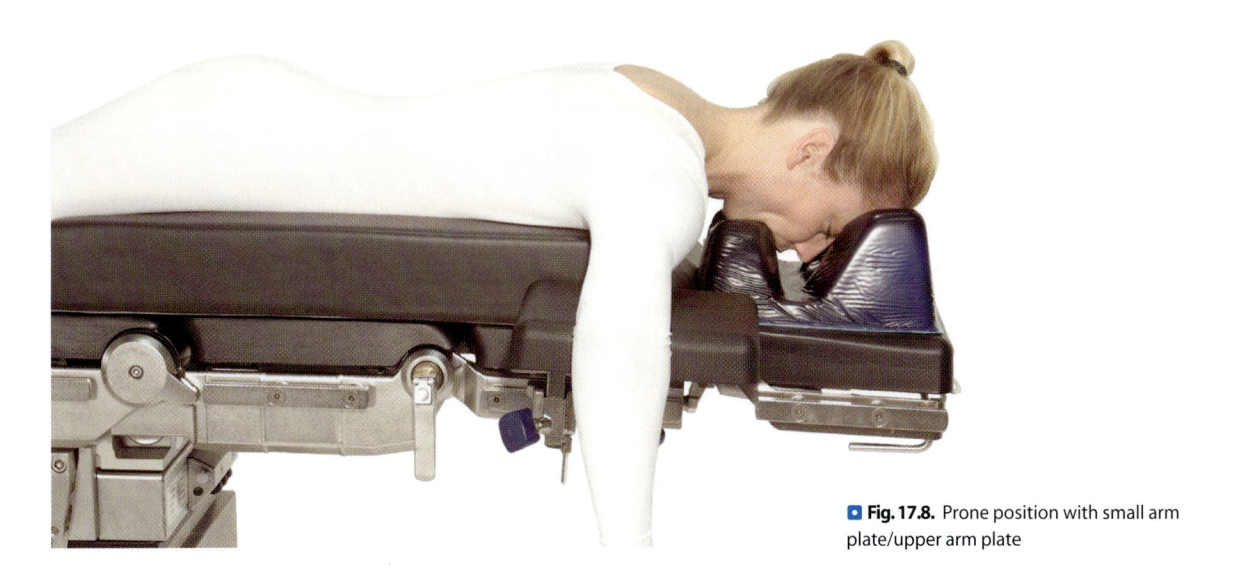

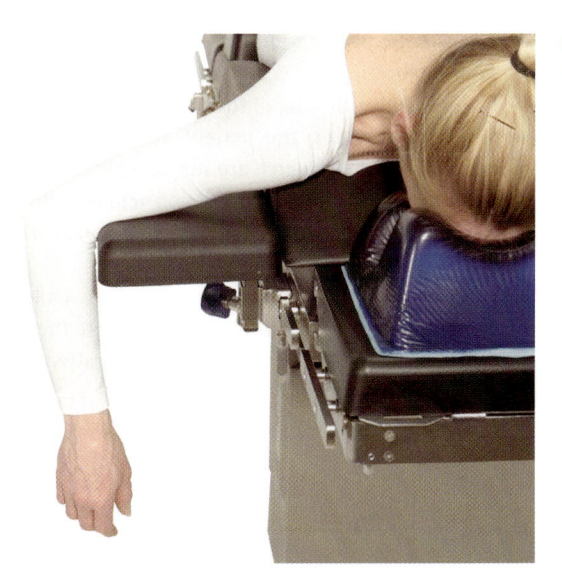

Fig. 17.8. Prone position with small arm plate/upper arm plate

Fig. 17.9. The distal joint is positioned lower than the proximal joint

17.2 Upper arm

17.2.1 Supine position

Figs. 17.10–17.13.

Indications

Extended ventral access to the shoulder joint and ventral, medial and lateral access to the humerus for fractures, pseudarthrosis, posttraumatic misalignment, tumours, inflammation, nerve lesions.

Preparations
- Arm positioning devices
- Remove Gilchrist bandage
- Shaving in the area of the incision and preoperative skin cleansing

Positioning
- Standard operating table position 1, position 2 or universal operating table with X-ray protection
- Anaesthetic preparation and induction in supine position with 2 adapted arm positioning devices
- Crosswise positioning of the operating table in the theatre
- When positioning the patient, take appropriate measures to prevent decubitus at areas which are subjected to pressure
- Standard supine position, infusion arm is spread out
- Remove the arm positioning device and fasten the large arm table to the side rail of the back plate
- Position the patient near to the edge of the table
- Apply the neutral electrode and connect to the HF surgery device
- Arrange self-adhesive covers for preoperative skin disinfection
- Position the operating lights
- Patient warming system

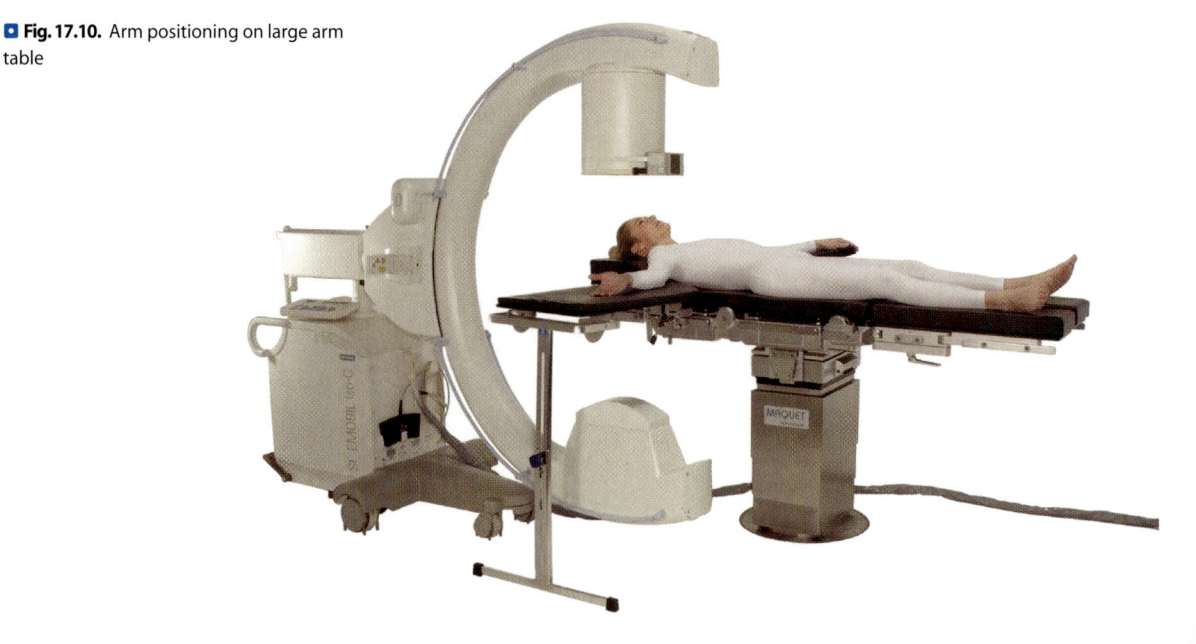

Fig. 17.10. Arm positioning on large arm table

17.2 · Upper arm

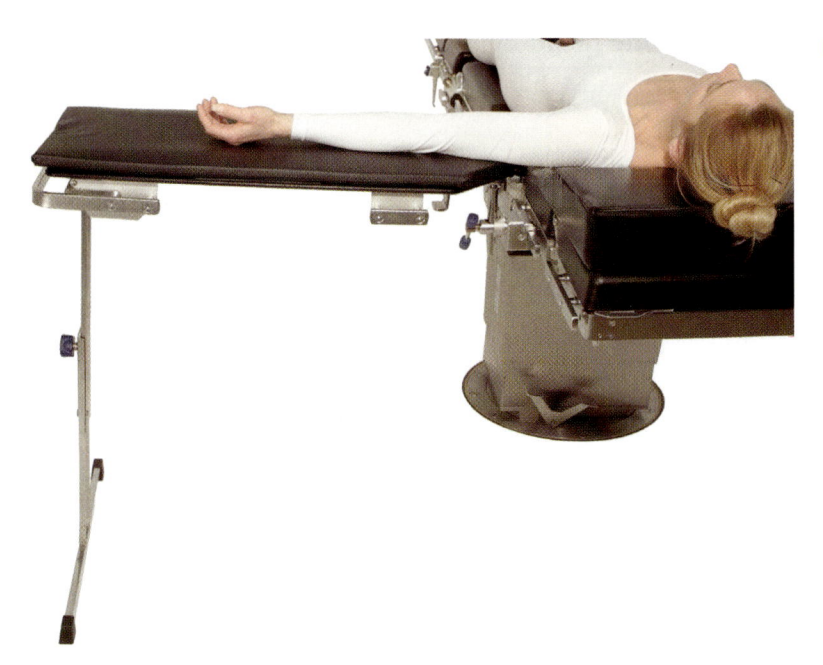

Fig. 17.11. 360° fluoroscopy possibility

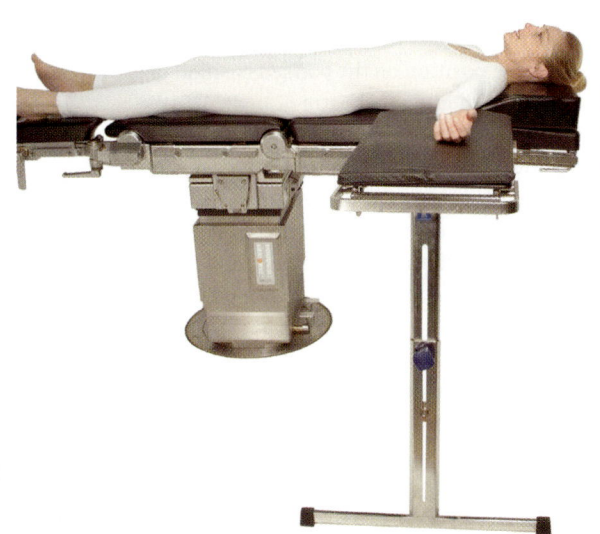

Fig. 17.12. Arms positioned with maximum 90° abduction in supination position

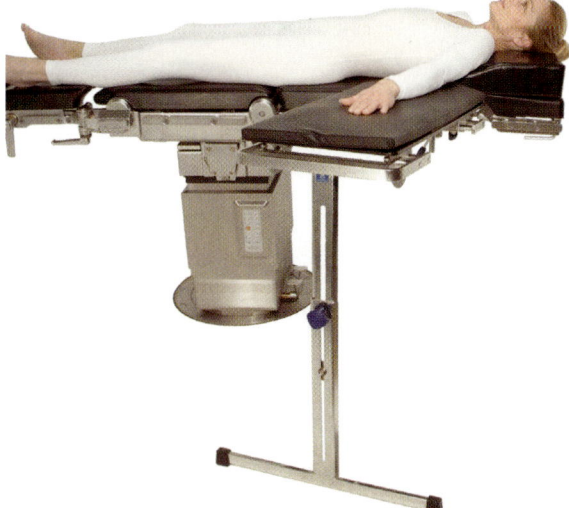

Fig. 17.13. Arms positioned with maximum approx. 50° abduction in pronation position

17.2.2 Prone position

◘ Figs. 17.14–17.16.

Indications

Dorsal access to the humerus for fractures, pseudarthrosis, posttraumatic misalignment, tumours, inflammation, nerve lesions.

Preparations
- Arm positioning devices
- Special head positioning cushion for prone position
- Thorax, pelvic and wedge cushion, padded roll
- Small arm rest, X-ray protection, C-arm (poss. G-arm) in the theatre
- Remove Gilchrist bandage
- Shaving in the area of the incision and preoperative skin cleansing

Positioning
- Standard operating table position 1, position 2 or universal operating table
- Anaesthetic preparation and induction in supine position with 2 adapted arm positioning devices
- Transfer to the prepared operating table in the induction room
- Position both tables next to each other, with the prepared table lowered
- Place the patient in prone position on the padded cushion of the prepared operating table and take him into the theatre
- Crosswise positioning of the operating table in the theatre
- When positioning the patient, take appropriate measures to prevent decubitus at areas which are subjected to pressure
- Position the head on the special head positioning cushion
- Position the infusion arm on the arm positioning device
- Position the patient near to the edge of the table, until the injured/fractured arm hangs at the elbow over the edge of the small arm rest with the lower arm in a vertical position
- Apply the neutral electrode and connect to the HF surgery device
- Arrange self-adhesive covers for preoperative skin disinfection
- Position the operating lights
- Patient warming system

17.2 · Upper arm

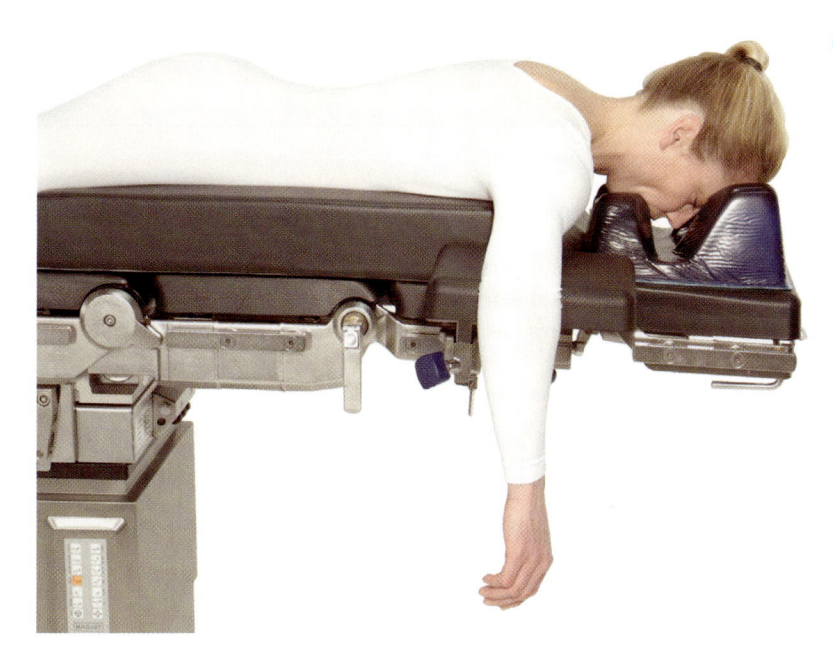

Fig. 17.14. Prone position with small arm plate/upper arm plate

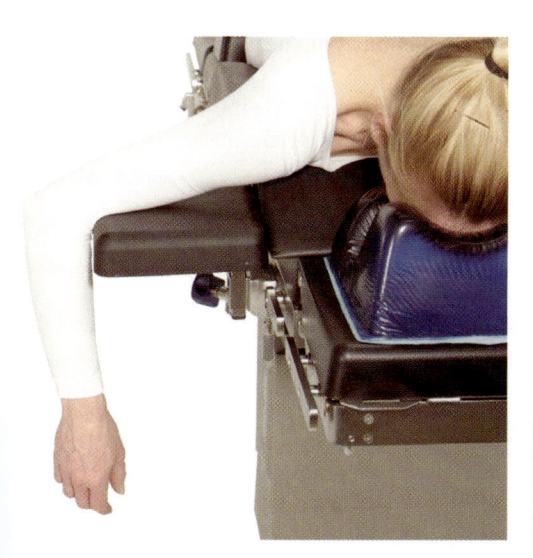

Fig. 17.15. The distal joint is positioned lower than the proximal joint

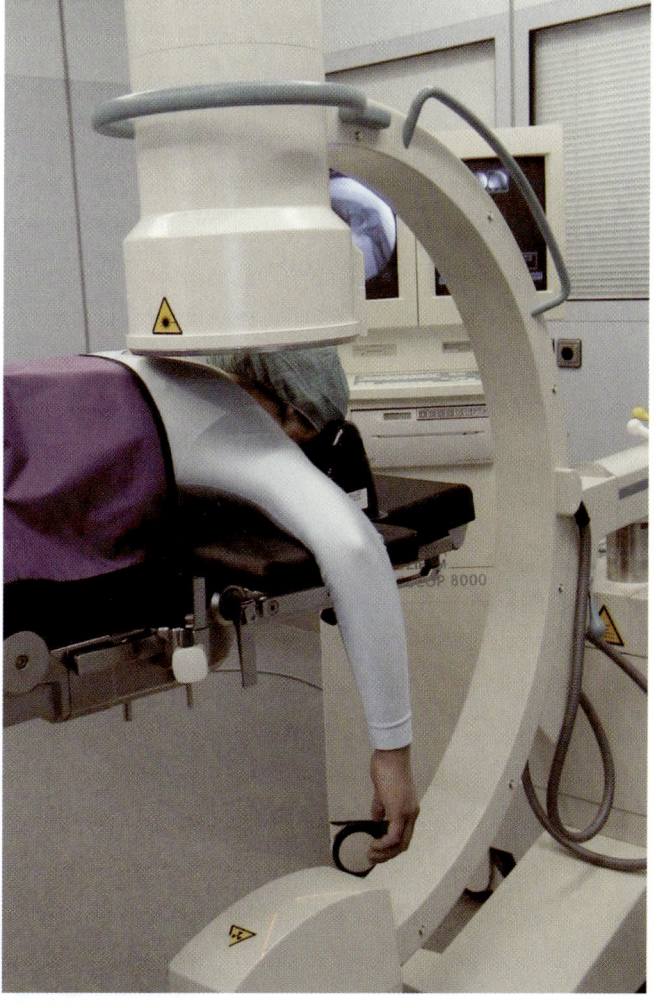

Fig. 17.16. Use of the image intensifier on the head side (here in anteroposterior position) offers optimum scope for swivelling round

17.3 Elbow

17.3.1 Supine position

◘ Figs. 17.17–17.20.

Indications
Lateral, medial, ventral and dorsal access to the elbow for fractures, posttraumatic misalignment, floating cartilage, inflammation, arthrosis, arthrofibrosis, soft tissue lesions, nerve lesions and contractures.

Preparations
- Arm positioning devices
- Remove Gilchrist bandage
- Large arm table
- Shaving in the area of the incision and preoperative skin cleansing
- Apply a tourniquet in position

Positioning
- Standard operating table position 1, position 2 or universal operating table with X-ray protection
- Anaesthetic preparation and induction in supine position with 2 adapted arm positioning devices
- Crosswise positioning of the operating table in the theatre
- When positioning the patient, take appropriate measures to prevent decubitus at areas which are subjected to pressure
- Standard supine position, infusion arm is in abduction
- 1st arm table: remove the arm positioning device and fasten the large arm table to the rail of the back plate
- Position the patient near to the edge of the table
- Apply the neutral electrode and connect to the HF surgery device
- Connect the compressed air device to the tourniquet
- Arrange self-adhesive covers for preoperative skin disinfection
- Position the operating lights
- Patient warming system

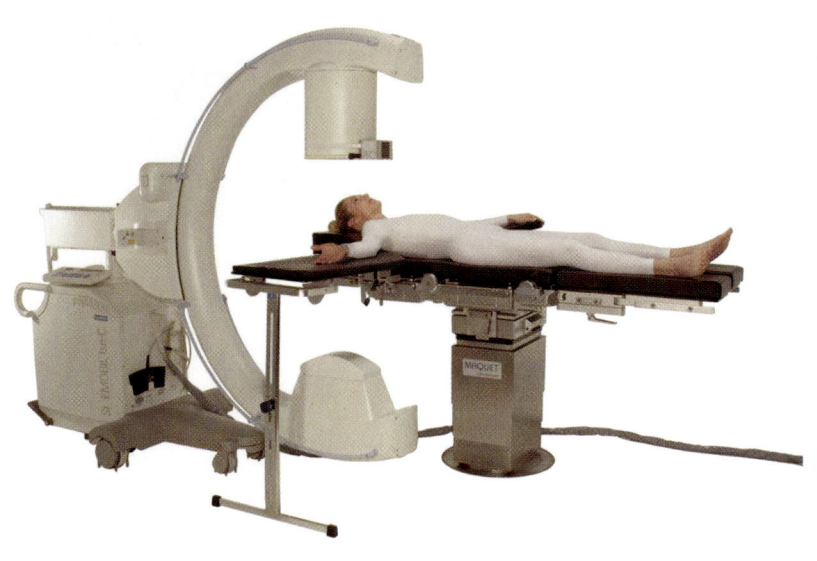

◘ **Fig. 17.17.** Arm positioning on large arm table

17.3 · Elbow

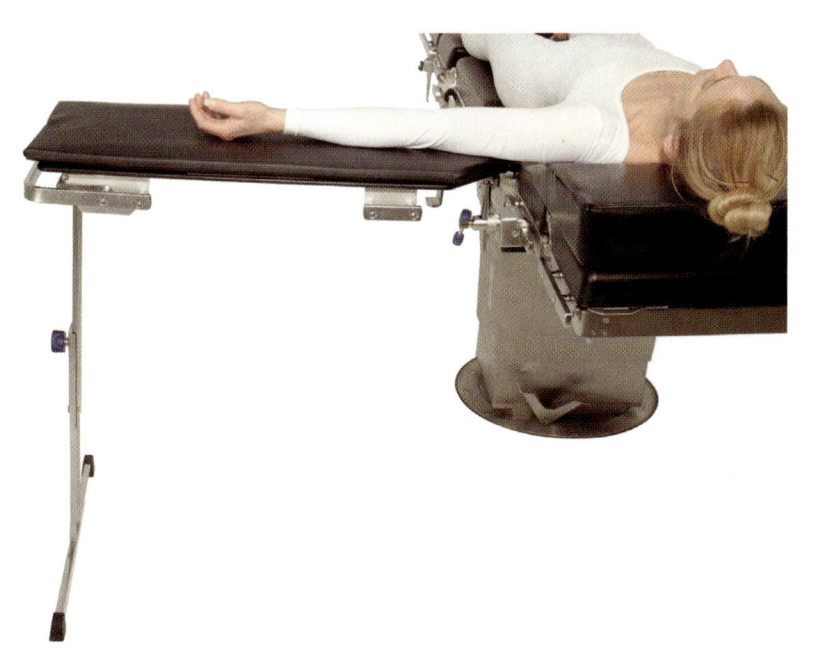

Fig. 17.18. 360° fluoroscopy possibility

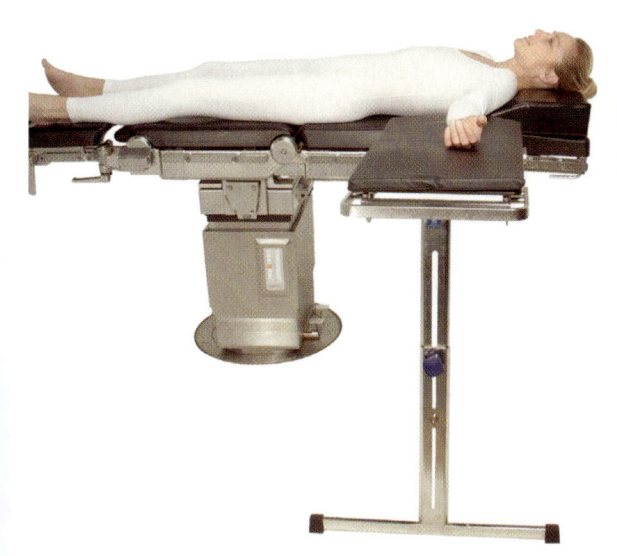

Fig. 17.19. Arms positioned with maximum 90° abduction in supination position

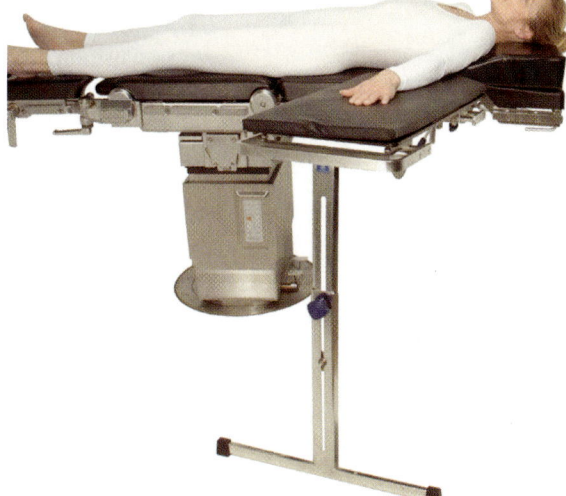

Fig. 17.20. Arms positioned with maximum approx. 50° abduction in pronation position

17.3.2 Prone position

◘ Figs. 17.21–17.23.

Indications
Dorsal access to the elbow for fractures, posttraumatic misalignment, floating cartilage, inflammation, arthrosis, arthrofibrosis, soft tissue lesions, nerve lesions and contractures.

Preparations
- Arm positioning devices
- Special head positioning cushion for prone position, thorax, pelvic and wedge cushion, padded roll
- Small arm rest, X-ray protection, C-arm (poss. G-arm) in the theatre
- Remove Gilchrist bandage
- Shaving in the area of the incision and preoperative skin cleansing
- Apply a tourniquet in position

Positioning
- Standard operating table position 1, position 2 or universal operating table
- Anaesthetic preparation and induction in supine position with 2 adapted arm positioning devices
- Transfer to the prepared operating table in the induction room
- Position both tables next to each other, with the prepared table lowered
- Place the patient in prone position on the padded cushion of the prepared operating table and take him into the theatre
- Crosswise positioning of the operating table in the theatre
- When positioning the patient, take appropriate measures to prevent decubitus at areas which are subjected to pressure
- Position the head on the special head positioning cushion
- Position the infusion arm on the arm positioning device
- Position the patient near to the edge of the table, until the injured/fractured arm hangs at the elbow over the edge of the small arm rest with the lower arm in a vertical position
- Apply the neutral electrode and connect to the HF surgery device
- Connect the compressed air device to the tourniquet
- Arrange self-adhesive covers for preoperative skin disinfection
- Position the operating lights
- Patient warming system

17.3 · Elbow

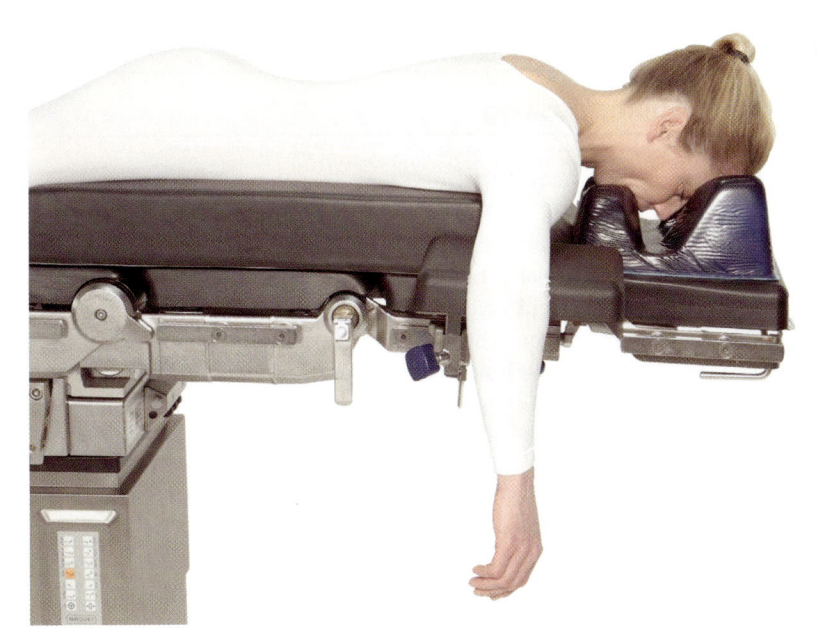

Fig. 17.21. Prone position with small arm plate/upper arm plate

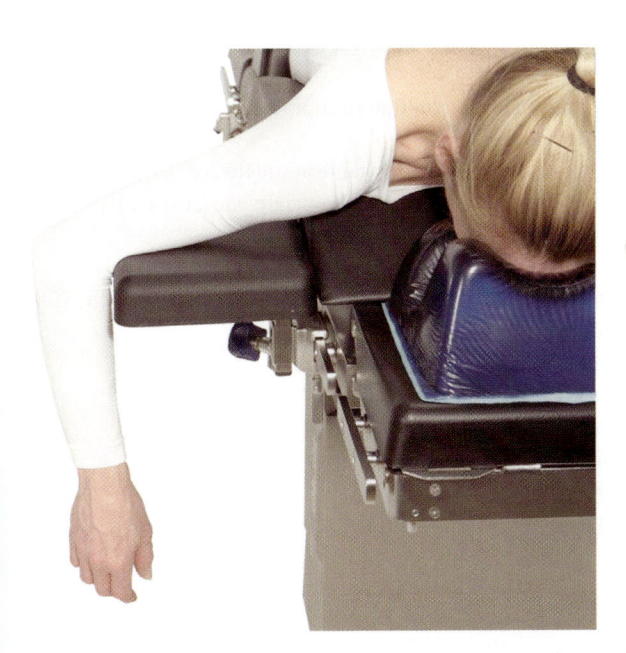

Fig. 17.22. The distal joint is positioned lower than the proximal joint

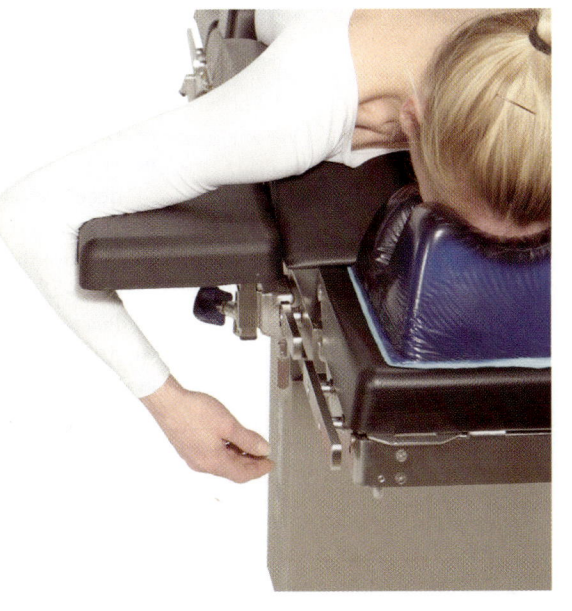

Fig. 17.23. The small arm plate/upper arm plate should have a narrow surface so that the arm can be bent

17.4 Forearm and hand

17.4.1 Supine position

Figs. 17.24–17.29.

Indications

Ventral, dorsal and dorsolateral access to the forearm, dorsal and palm access to the wrist and to the hand, access to the thumb and first finger for fractures, posttraumatic misalignment, pseudarthrosis, luxation, inflammation, arthrosis, soft tissue lesions, nerve lesions, contractures, tumours, operations to tendons, synovial sheaths and carpal tunnel.

Preparations
- Arm positioning devices
- Remove splints from extremity
- Large arm table
- Shaving in the area of the incision and preoperative skin cleansing
- Apply a tourniquet in position

Positioning
- Standard operating table position 1, position 2 or universal operating table with X-ray protection
- Anaesthetic preparation and induction in supine position with 2 adapted arm positioning devices
- Crosswise positioning of the operating table in the theatre
- When positioning the patient, take appropriate measures to prevent decubitus at areas which are subjected to pressure
- Standard supine position, infusion arm is spread out
- Remove the arm positioning device and fit the large arm table to the side rail of the back plate
- Position the patient near to the edge of the table
- Apply the neutral electrode and connect to the HF surgery device
- Connect the compressed air device to the tourniquet
- Arrange self-adhesive covers for preoperative skin disinfection
- Position the operating lights
- Patient warming system

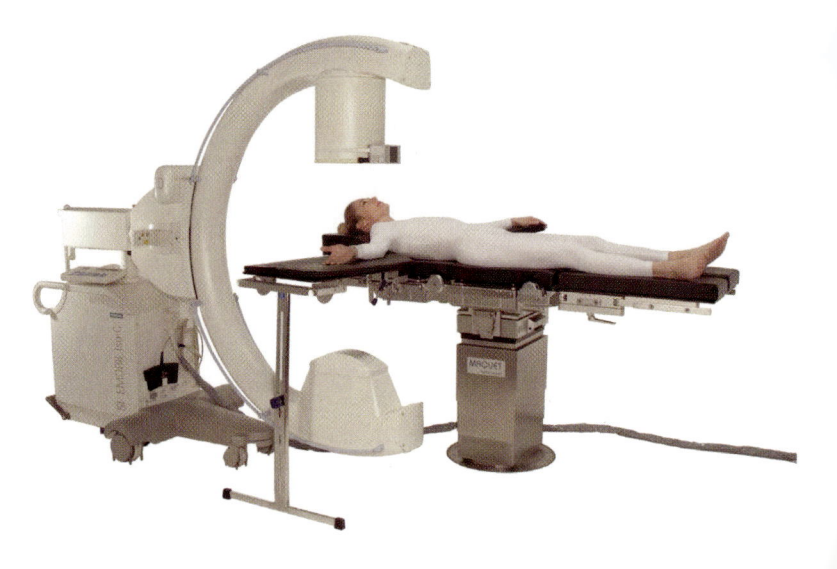

Fig. 17.24. Arm positioning on large arm table

17.4 · Lower arm and hand

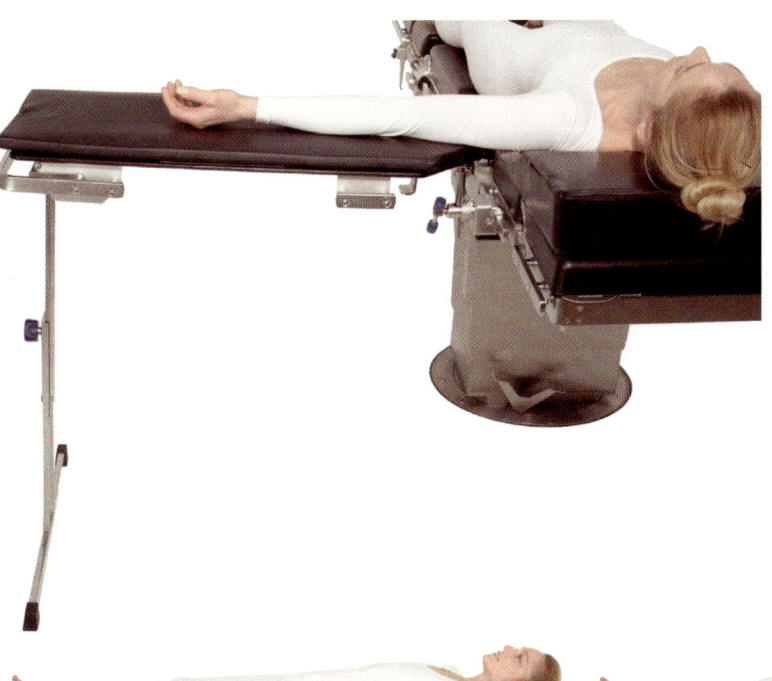

Fig. 17.25. 360° fluoroscopy possibility

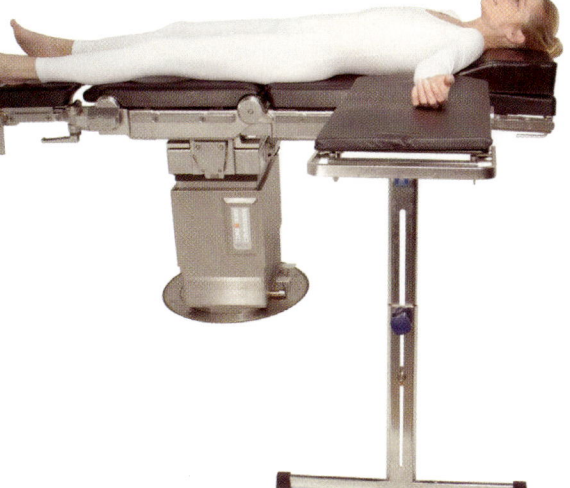

Fig. 17.26. Arms positioned with maximum 90° abduction in supination position

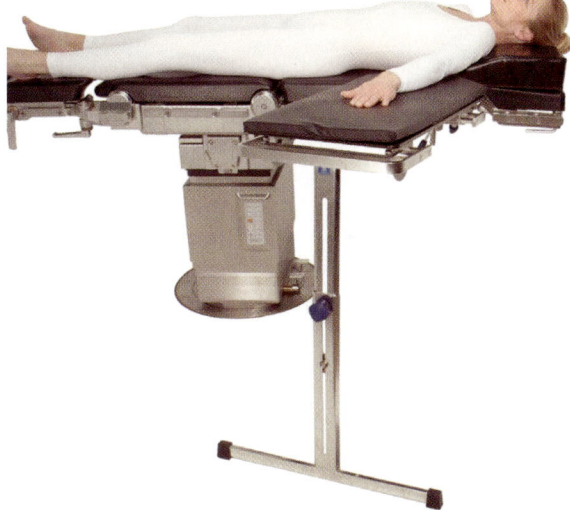

Fig. 17.27. Arms positioned with maximum approx. 50° abduction in pronation position

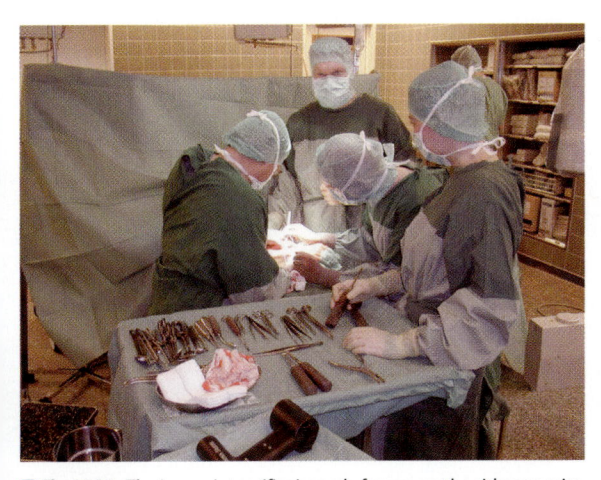

Fig. 17.28. The image intensifier is ready for use on the side opposite the surgeon

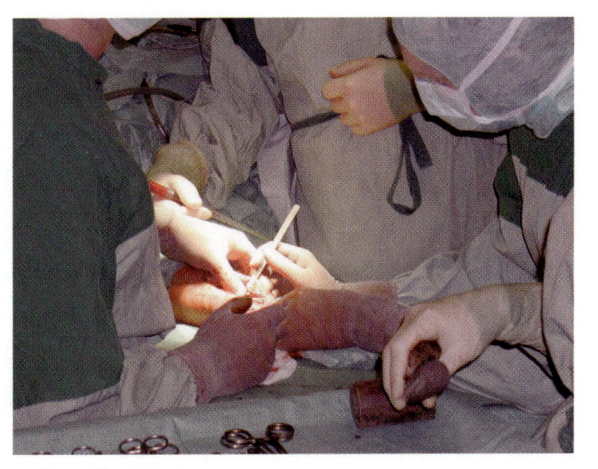

Fig. 17.29. Operation scene

18 Lower extremities

18.1 Hips – 236
18.1.1 Supine position – 236
18.1.2 Lateral position – 238

18.2 Thigh – 240
18.2.1 Supine position – 240
18.2.2 Modified supine position – 242
18.2.3 Lateral position – 244

18.3 Knee – 246
18.3.1 Supine position – 246
18.3.2 Prone position – 248

18.4 Lower leg – 250
18.4.1 Supine position – 250

18.5 Foot – 252
18.5.1 Supine position – 252
18.5.2 Lateral position – 254
18.5.3 Prone position – 256

18.1 Hips

18.1.1 Supine position

◘ Figs. 18.1–18.5.

Indications

Ventral, anterolateral and lateral access to the hip joint for coxarthrosis, fracture of the neck of the femur, loosening of a hip replacement, necrosis of the head of the hip and tumours.

Preparations
- Arm positioning devices
- Shaving in the area of the incision and preoperative skin cleansing

Positioning
- Standard operating table position 1, position 2 or universal operating table
- Anaesthetic preparation and induction in supine position with 2 adapted arm positioning devices
- Normal positioning of the operating table in the theatre
- When positioning the patient, take appropriate measures to prevent decubitus at areas which are subjected to pressure
- Position both arms on the arm positioning device in abduction position
- Apply the neutral electrode and connect to the HF surgery device
- Arrange absorbent drapes or self-adhesive covers for preoperative skin disinfection
- Position the operating lights
- Patient warming system

Risks
- Secondary dislocation

18.1 · Hips

Fig. 18.1. Supine position on universal operating table with CRP back plate 1150.45 and supported extension plate

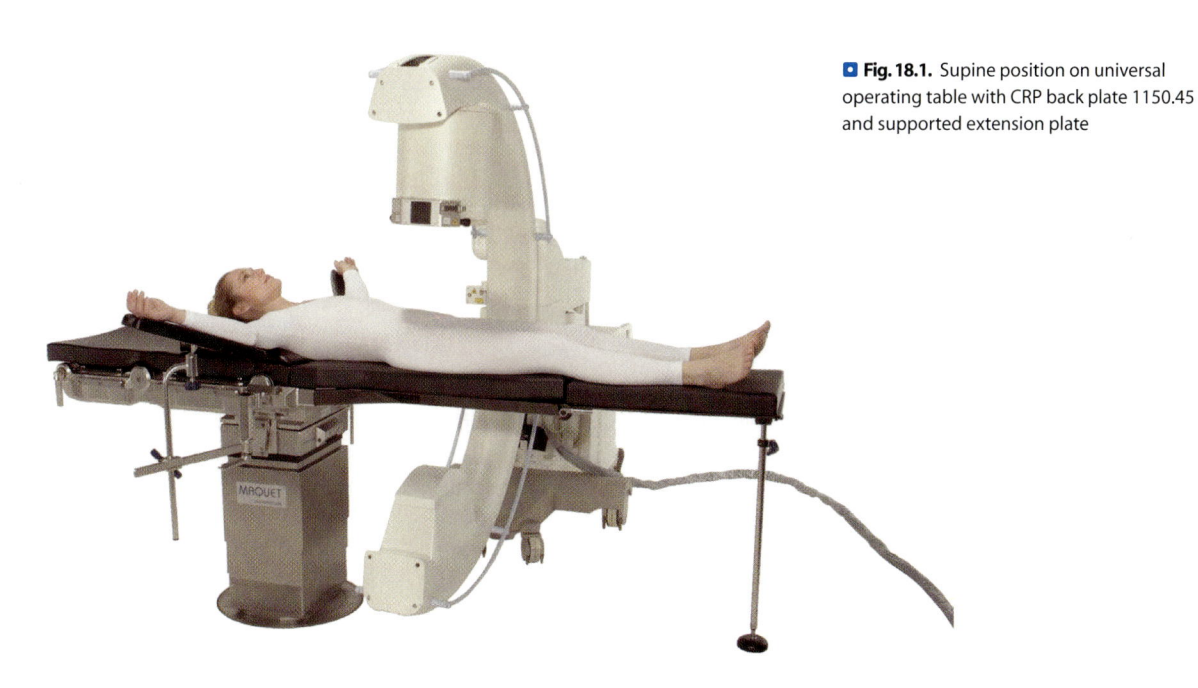

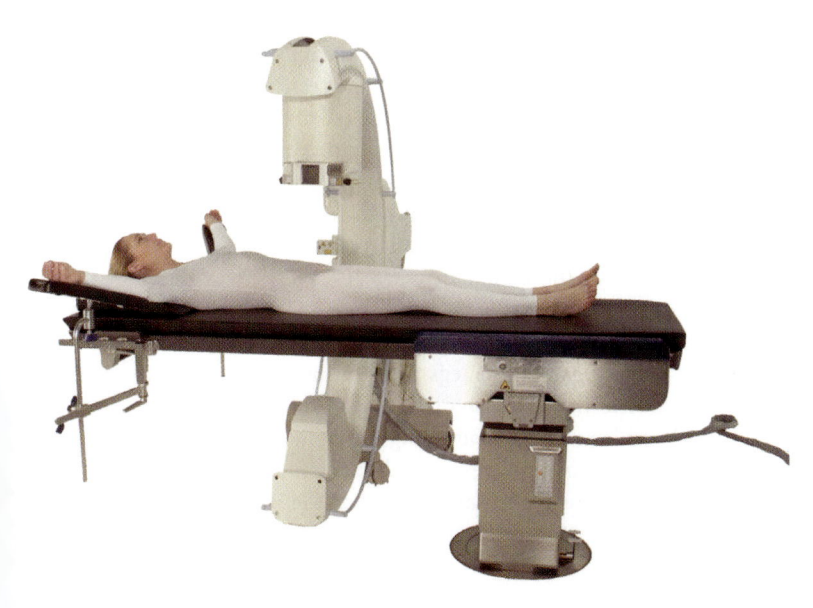

Fig. 18.2. Supine position on CRP operating table 1150.16 for 360° use of the image intensifier

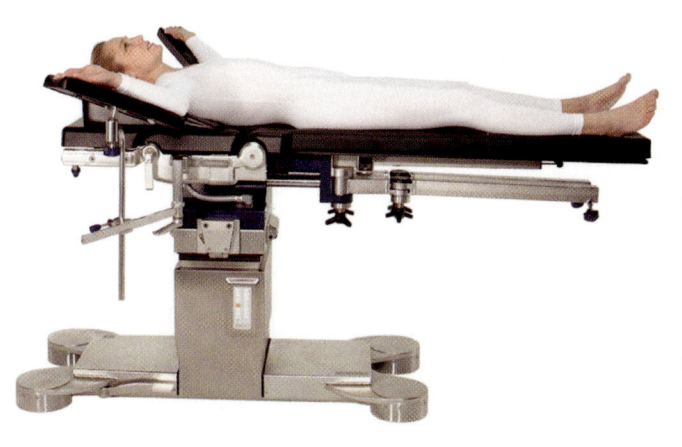

Fig. 18.3. Supine position on operating extension table (1150.20) with special leg plates for optimum fluoroscopy of the hips

Fig. 18.4. Masking the extremity for preoperative skin disinfection and additional moisture protection also during the operation (▶ see Fig. 18.15 on p. 243)

Fig. 18.5. Good covering techniques allow for movement of the extremity (▶ see Fig. 18.17 on p. 243)

18.1.2 Lateral position

◧ Figs. 18.6–18.8.

Indications
Anterolateral and lateral access to the hip joint for coxarthrosis, fracture of the neck of the femur, coxitis, loosening of a hip replacement, resection arthroplasty and tumours.

Preparations
- Arm positioning devices
- Shaving in the area of the incision and preoperative skin cleansing
- Gel ring, gel cushion, Goepel leg holder, side supports, radial adjusting clamps, padded cushions (normal and flat) and wedge cushions or tunnel cushions, body belts

Positioning
- Standard operating table position 1, position 2 or universal operating table
- Anaesthetic preparation and induction in supine position with 2 adapted arm positioning devices
- Normal positioning of the operating table in the theatre
- When positioning the patient, take appropriate measures to prevent decubitus at areas which are subjected to pressure
- Fit the radial adjusting clamp to the side rail of the head plate, position the Goepel leg holder and place a gel padded mat on the operating table
- Spread out the arm on the side not being operated
- Move the patient over onto the healthy side
- Move the lower arm forwards so that the weight of the upper body does not lie directly on the shoulder
- Fit the body supports to the rails and brace on the level of the sacrum and symphysis
- **1st possibility:** position the legs with the padded cushions (normal and flat) and possibly wedge cushions
- Fix the lower leg and the positioning aids with the body belts
- **2nd possibility:** position the legs with the tunnel cushion
- Apply the neutral electrode and connect to the HF surgery device
- Arrange absorbent drapes or self-adhesive covers for preoperative skin disinfection
- Position the operating lights
- Patient warming system

Risks
- Secondary dislocation

18.1 · Hips

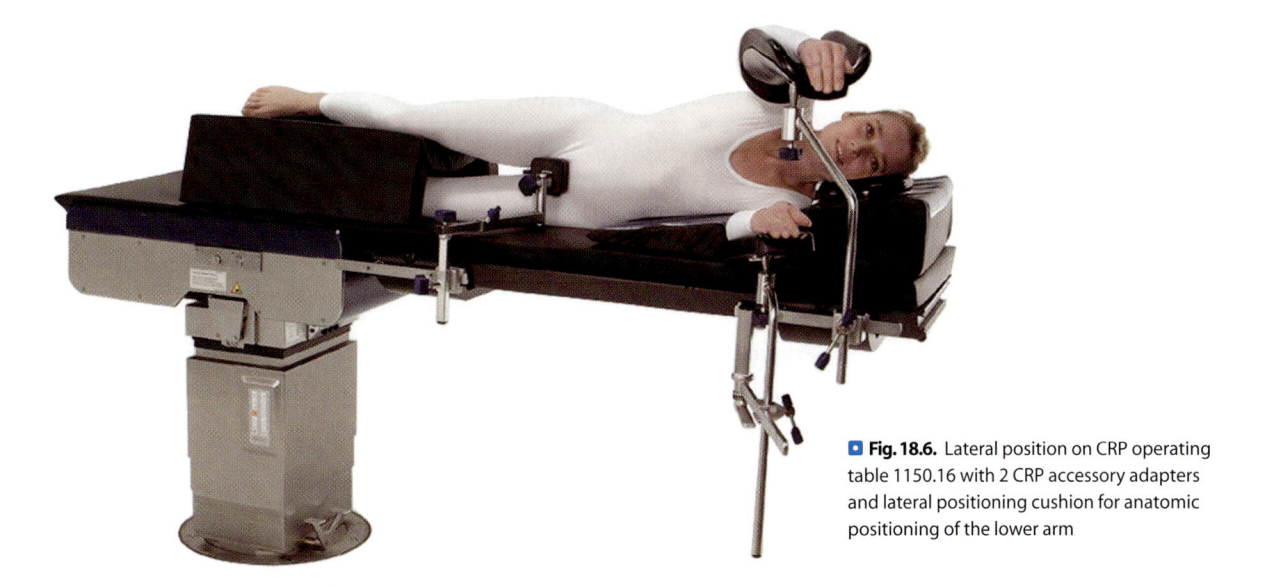

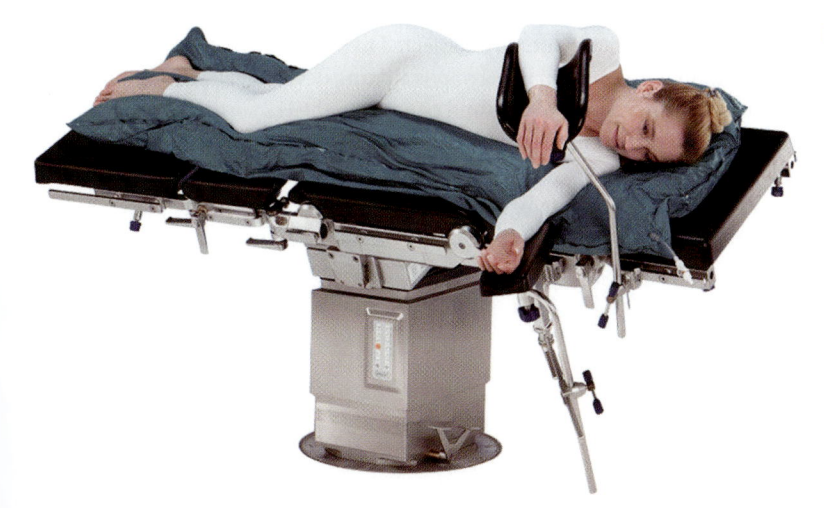

Fig. 18.6. Lateral position on CRP operating table 1150.16 with 2 CRP accessory adapters and lateral positioning cushion for anatomic positioning of the lower arm

Fig. 18.7. Lateral position on universal operating table with vacuum mat

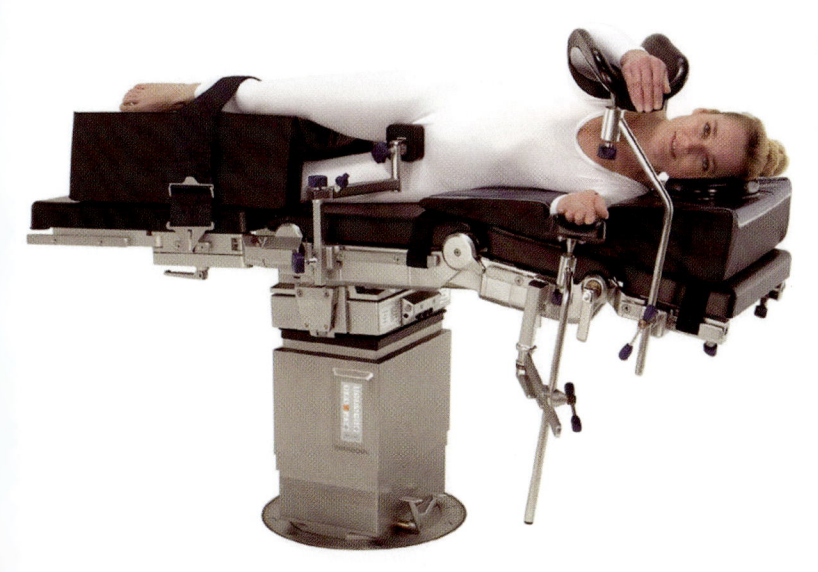

Fig. 18.8. Lateral position on universal operating table with lateral positioning cushion and operating table in flex position for neutral position of the spinal cord

18.2 Thigh

18.2.1 Supine position

◘ Figs. 18.9–18.13.

Indications

Ventral, lateral and medial access to the femur for fractures, posttraumatic misalignment, osteitis and tumours.

Preparations
- Arm positioning devices
- Shaving in the area of the incision and preoperative skin cleansing

Positioning
- Standard operating table position 1, position 2 or universal operating table
- Anaesthetic preparation and induction in supine position with 2 adapted arm positioning devices
- Normal positioning of the operating table in the theatre
- When positioning the patient, take appropriate measures to prevent decubitus at areas which are subjected to pressure
- Position both arms on the arm positioning device in abduction position
- Apply the neutral electrode and connect to the HF surgery device
- Arrange absorbent drapes or self-adhesive covers for preoperative skin disinfection
- Position the operating lights
- Patient warming system

Risks
- Secondary dislocation

18.2 · Thigh

Fig. 18.9. Supine position on universal operating table with CRP back plate 1150.45 and supported extension plate

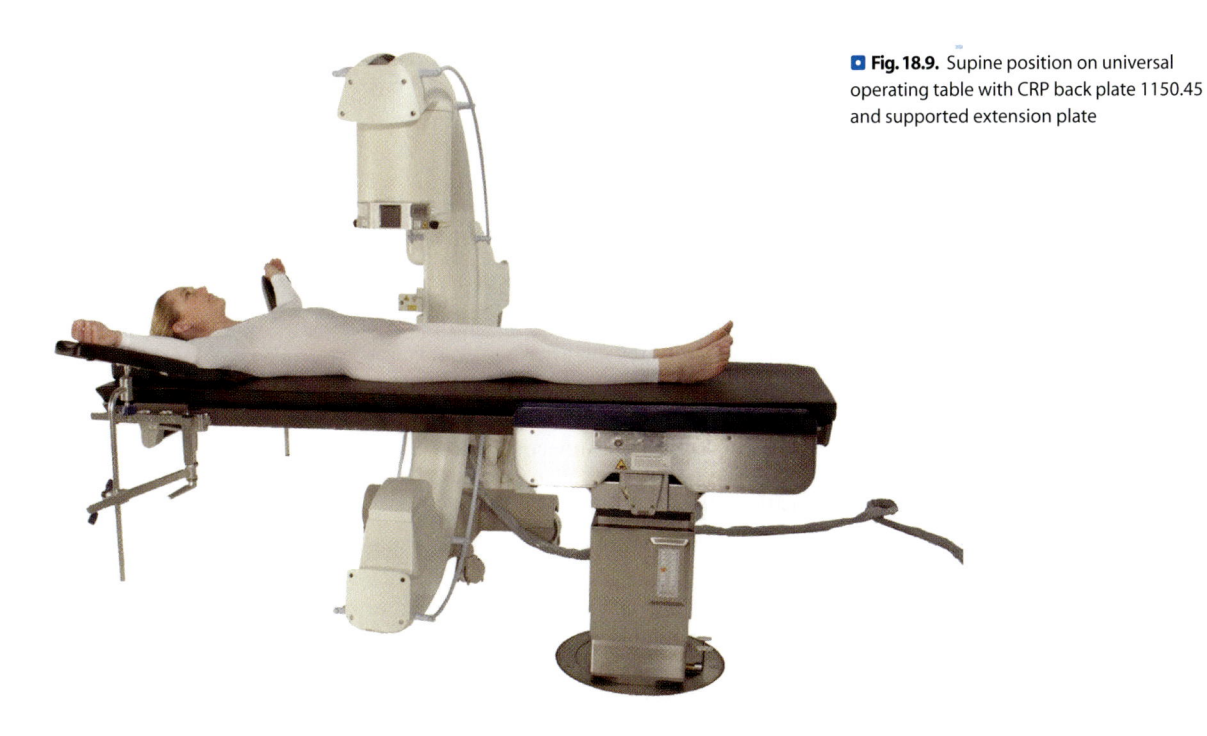

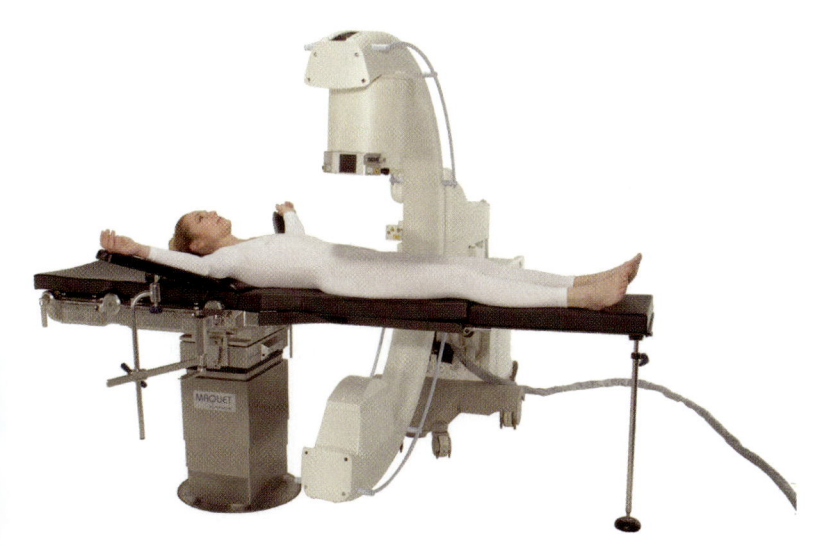

Fig. 18.10. Supine position on CRP operating table 1150.16 for 360° use of the image intensifier

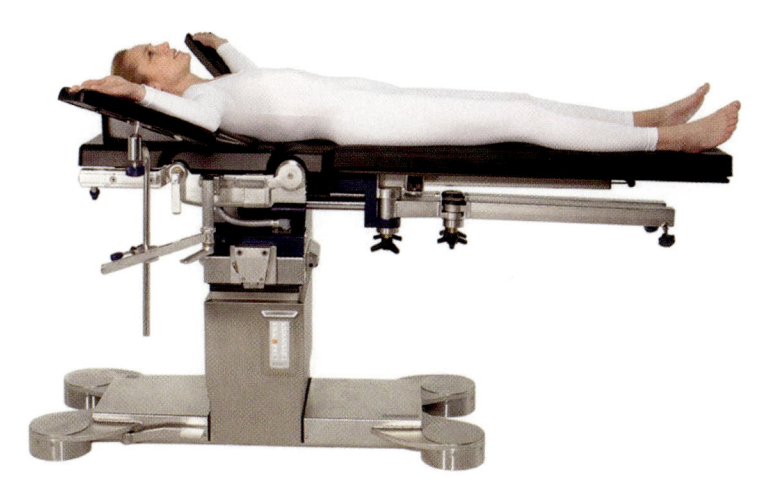

Fig. 18.11. Supine position on operating extension table (1150.20) with special leg plates for optimum fluoroscopy

Fig. 18.12. Masking the extremity for preoperative skin disinfection and additional moisture protection also during the operation (▶ see Fig. 18.15 on p. 243)

Fig. 18.13. Good covering techniques allow for movement of the extremity (▶ see Fig. 18.17 on p. 243)

18.2.2 Modified supine position

◘ Figs. 18.14–18.17.

Indications

Closed and open osteosynthesis procedures to the femur requiring intraoperative fluoroscopy with a lateral ray path.

Preparations
- Arm positioning devices
- Shaving in the area of the incision and preoperative skin cleansing
- Anaesthesia screen, Goepel leg holders, radial adjusting clamps, gel cushion, side rail connection piece

Positioning
- Standard operating table position 1, position 2 or universal operating table
- Anaesthetic preparation and induction in supine position with 2 adapted arm positioning devices
- Normal positioning of the operating table in the theatre
- When positioning the patient, take appropriate measures to prevent decubitus at areas which are subjected to pressure
- Fit the radial adjusting clamp to the side rail of the head plate on the side not being operated and fix the anaesthesia screen
- Position the arm on the healthy side on the arm positioning device in the abduction position and fix the other arm with Velcro straps to the anaesthesia screen over the thorax
- Fit the side rail connection piece to the short side rail of the seat plate on the side not being operated (operating table 1120)
- Fit the radial adjusting clamp and Goepel leg holder
- Position the healthy leg on the Goepel leg holder
- Apply the neutral electrode and connect to the HF surgery device
- Arrange absorbent drapes or self-adhesive covers for preoperative skin disinfection
- Position the operating lights
- Patient warming system

Risks
- Secondary dislocation
- Nerve injuries (pudendal nerve)

18.2 · Thigh

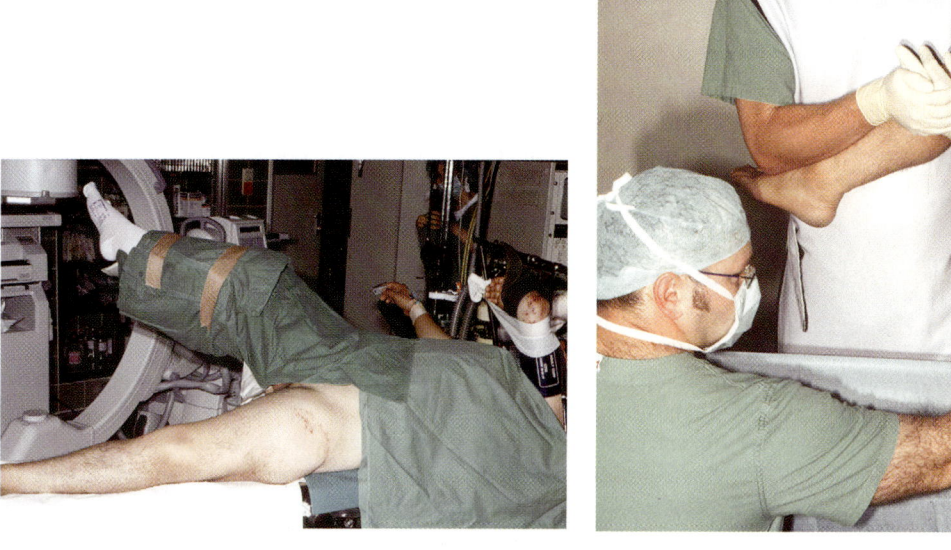

Fig. 18.14. Supine position with leg in abduction on Goepel leg holder and left arm positioned at the anaesthesia screen (use of the image intensifier swivelled through)

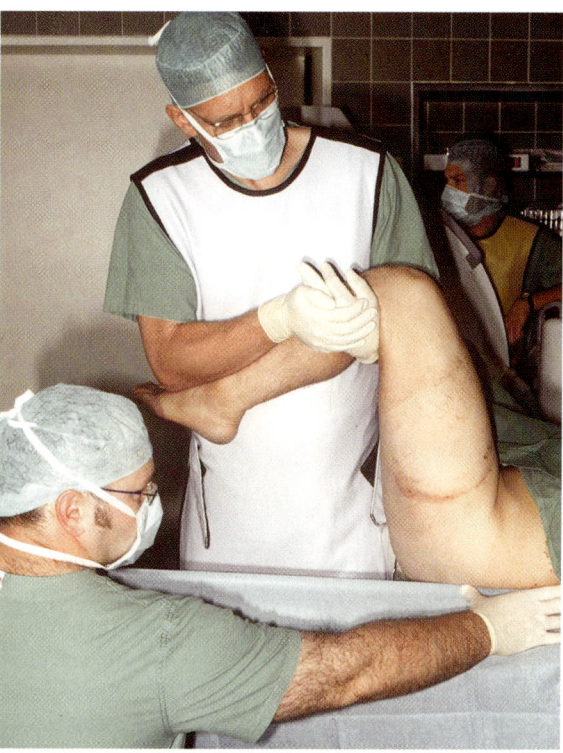

Fig. 18.15. Masking the extremity for preoperative skin disinfection and additional moisture protection also during the operation

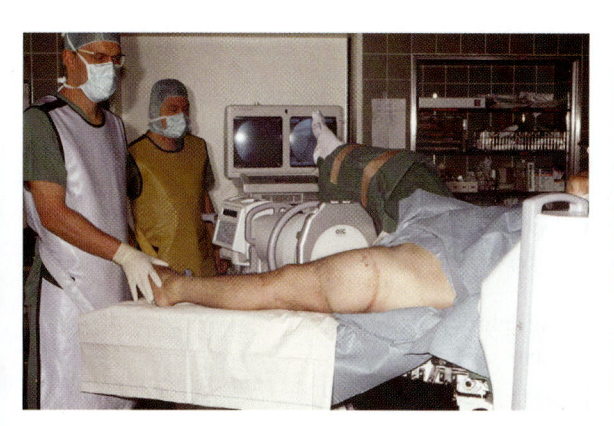

Fig. 18.16. Positioning the fractured leg on a leg plate with use of the image intensifier

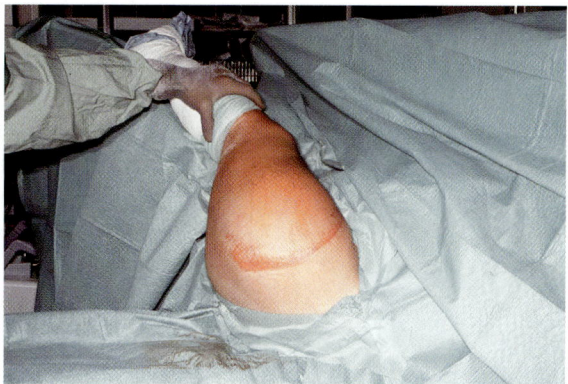

Fig. 18.17. Good covering techniques allow for movement of the extremity

18.2.3 Lateral position

◨ Figs. 18.18–18.20.

Indications

Lateral access to the femur for fractures, posttraumatic misalignment, osteitis and tumours.

Preparations
- Arm positioning devices
- Shaving in the area of the incision and preoperative skin cleansing
- Gel ring, gel cushion, Goepel leg holder, side supports, radial adjusting clamps, padded cushions (normal and flat) and wedge cushions or tunnel cushions, body belts

Positioning
- Standard operating table position 1, position 2 or universal operating table
- Anaesthetic preparation and induction in supine position with 2 adapted arm positioning devices
- Normal positioning of the operating table in the theatre
- When positioning the patient, take appropriate measures to prevent decubitus at areas which are subjected to pressure
- Fit the radial adjusting clamp to the rail of the head plate, position the Goepel leg holder
- Spread out the arm on the side not being operated
- Move the patient onto the healthy side
- Move the lower arm forwards so that the weight of the upper body does not lie directly on the shoulder
- Fit the body supports to the side rails and brace on the level of the sacrum and symphysis
- **1st possibility:** position the legs with the padded cushions (normal and flat) and possibly wedge cushions
- Fix the lower leg and the positioning aids with the body belts
- **2nd possibility:** position the legs with the tunnel cushion
- Apply the neutral electrode and connect to the HF surgery device
- Arrange absorbent drapes or self-adhesive covers for preoperative skin disinfection
- Position the operating lights
- Patient warming system

Risks
- Injury to the peroneal nerve

18.2 · Thigh

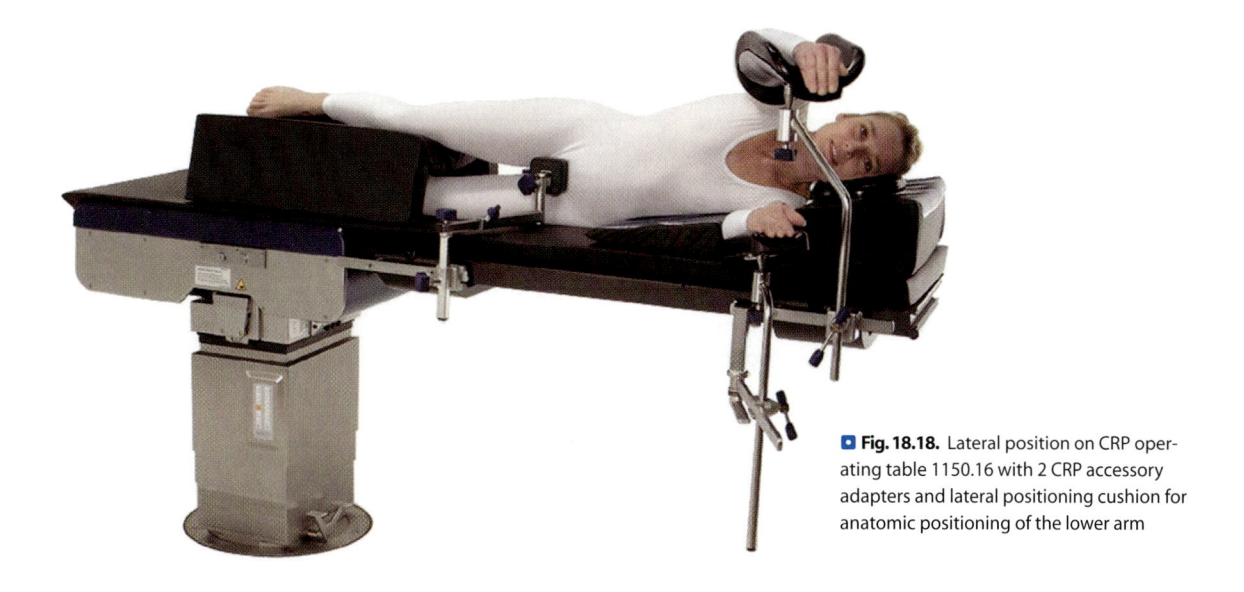

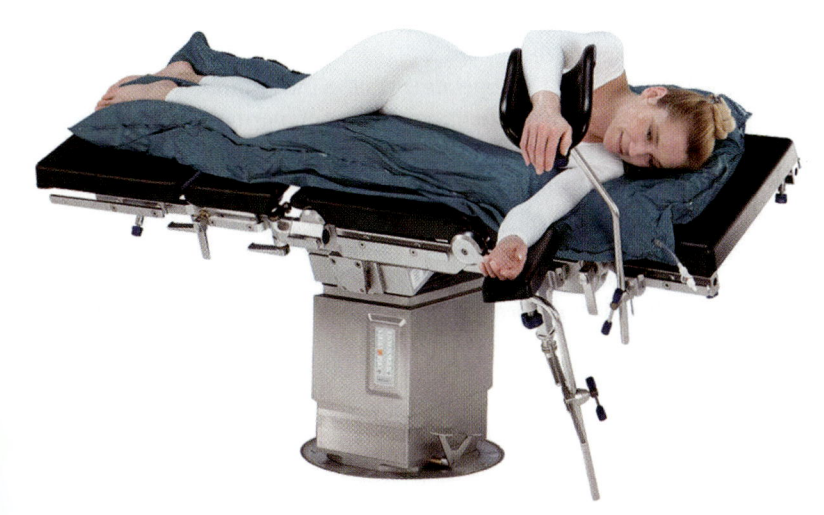

Fig. 18.18. Lateral position on CRP operating table 1150.16 with 2 CRP accessory adapters and lateral positioning cushion for anatomic positioning of the lower arm

Fig. 18.19. Lateral position on universal operating table with vacuum mat

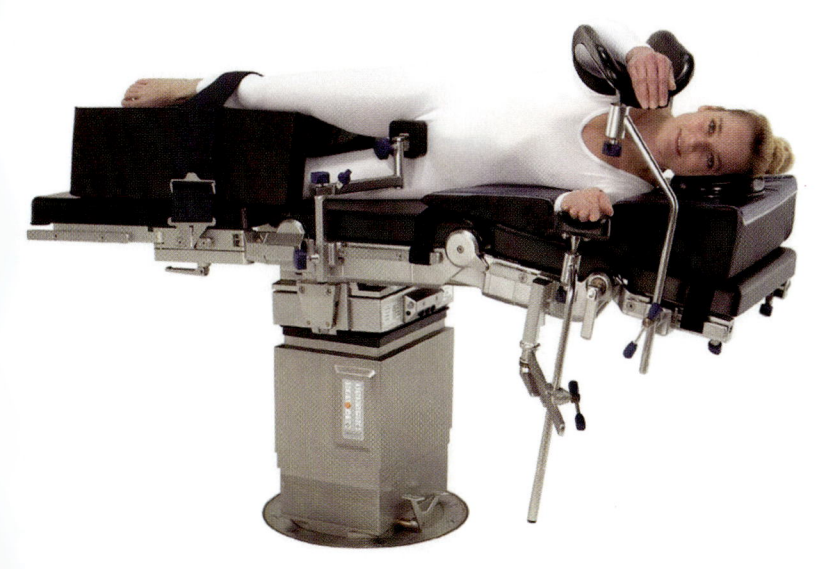

Fig. 18.20. Lateral position on universal operating table with lateral positioning cushion and operating table in flex position for neutral position of the spinal cord

18.3 Knee

18.3.1 Supine position

◘ Figs. 18.21–18.25.

Indications

Lateral, medial, posteromedial, para- and transpatellar access to the knee joint for gonarthrosis, fractures, posttraumatic misalignment, infection, loosening of knee replacements, synovitis, tumours, ligament injuries and arthrofibrosis.

Preparations
- Arm positioning devices
- Shaving in the area of the incision and preoperative skin cleansing
- Apply a tourniquet in position

Positioning
- Standard operating table position 1, position 2 or universal operating table
- Anaesthetic preparation and induction in supine position with 2 adapted arm positioning devices
- Normal positioning of the operating table in the theatre
- When positioning the patient, take appropriate measures to prevent decubitus at areas which are subjected to pressure
- Position both arms on the arm positioning devices in the abduction position
- Apply the neutral electrode and connect to the HF surgery device
- Connect the compressed air supply to the tourniquet
- Arrange absorbent drapes or self-adhesive covers for preoperative skin disinfection
- Position the operating lights
- Patient warming system

18.3 · Knee

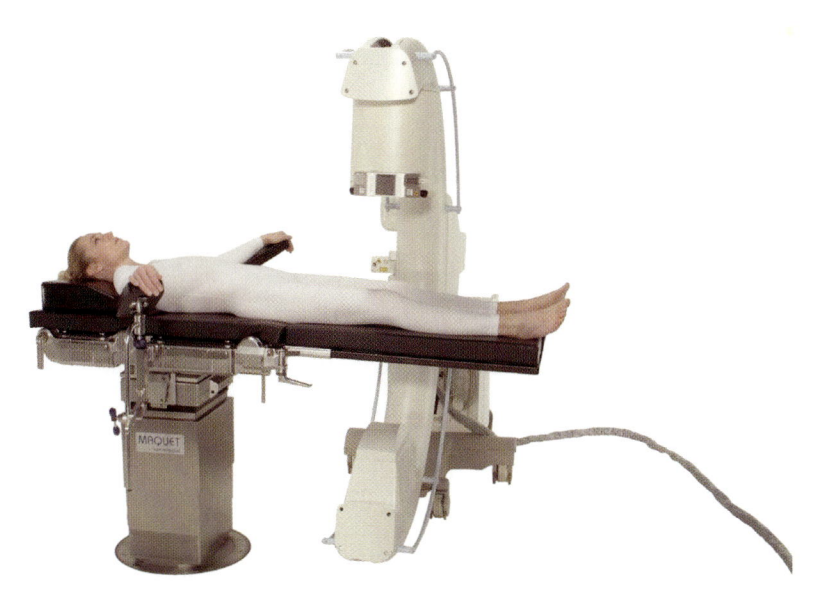

Fig. 18.21. Legs positioned on divided leg plates with individual adjustment

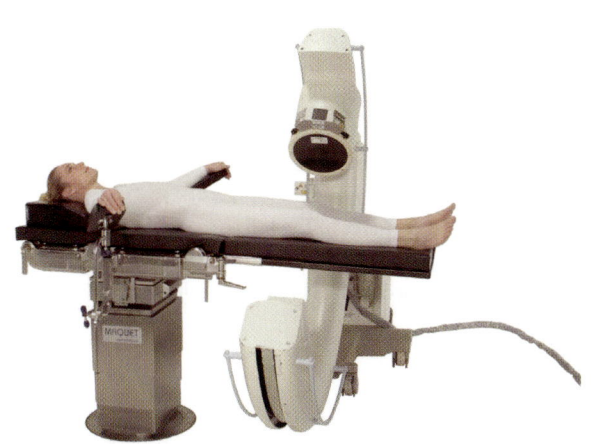

Fig. 18.22. Scanning possible through 360°

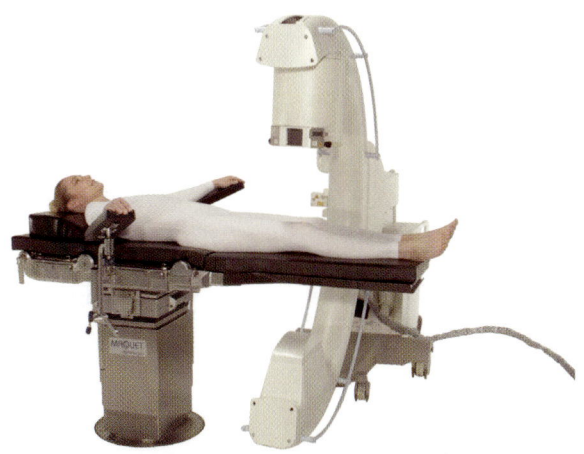

Fig. 18.23. Legs positioned on single-section CRP module 1150.45

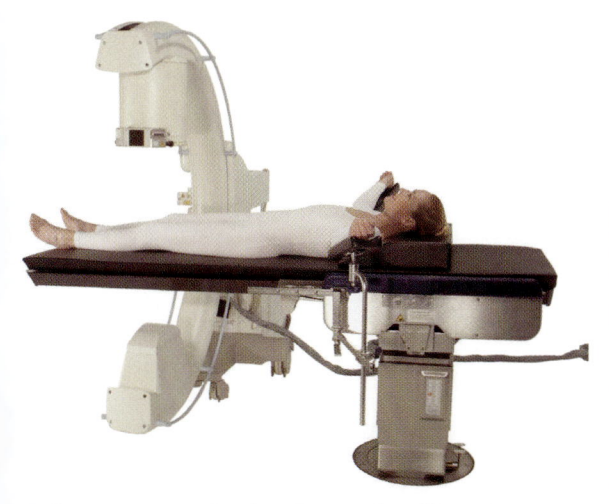

Fig. 18.24. Legs positioned on CRP operating table 1150.16

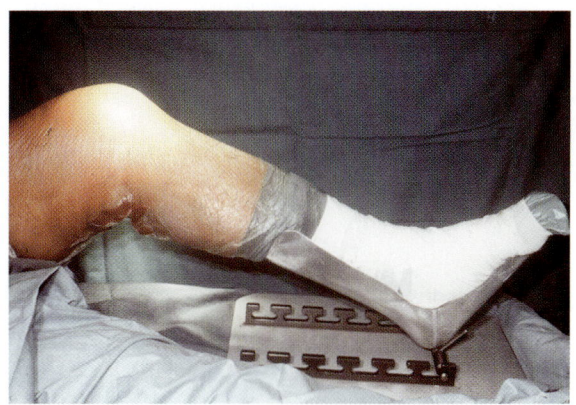

Fig. 18.25. Foot holder for total replacement of the knee joint

18.3.2 Prone position

◨ Figs. 18.26, 18.27.

Indications
Rear access to the knee joint for ligament injuries, tumours, vessel and nerve lesions.

Preparations
- Arm positioning devices
- Shaving in the area of the incision and preoperative skin cleansing
- Apply a tourniquet in position

Positioning
- Standard operating table position 1, position 2 or universal operating table
- Anaesthetic preparation and induction in supine position with 2 adapted arm positioning devices
- Transfer to the prepared operating table in the induction room
- Position both tables next to each other, with the prepared table lowered
- Place the patient in prone position on the padded cushion of the prepared operating table and take him into the theatre
- Normal positioning of the operating table in the theatre
- When positioning the patient, take appropriate measures to prevent decubitus at areas which are subjected to pressure
- Position the head on the special head positioning cushion
- Position both arms on the arm positioning devices
- Apply the neutral electrode and connect to the HF surgery device
- Connect the compressed air supply to the tourniquet
- Arrange self-adhesive covers for preoperative skin disinfection
- Position the operating lights
- Patient warming system

18.3 · Knee

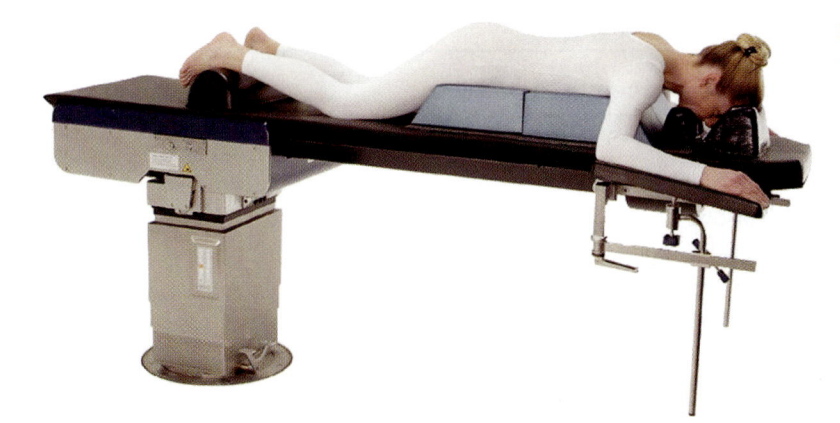

Fig. 18.26. Prone position on CRP operating table 1150.16 with CRP head plate for 360°C use of the image intensifier at the knee

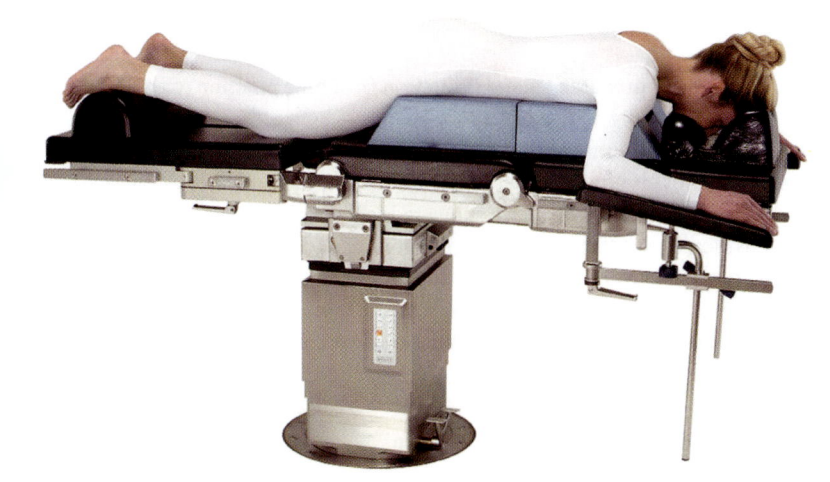

Fig. 18.27. Prone position on universal operating table 1150.30 with arms positioned in maximum 90° abduction

18.4 Lower leg

18.4.1 Supine position

◘ Figs. 18.28–18.33.

Indications

Access to the shaft of the tibia, lateral access to the fibula, lateral and medial access to the head of the tibia for fractures, misalignment, pseudarthrosis, osteitis, tumour and fibula removal.

Preparations
- Arm positioning devices
- Shaving in the area of the incision and preoperative skin cleansing
- Apply a tourniquet in position

Positioning
- Standard operating table position 1, position 2 or universal operating table
- Anaesthetic preparation and induction in supine position with 2 adapted arm positioning devices
- Normal positioning of the operating table in the theatre
- When positioning the patient, take appropriate measures to prevent decubitus at areas which are subjected to pressure
- Position both arms on the arm positioning devices in abduction position
- Apply the neutral electrode and connect to the HF surgery device
- Connect the compressed air supply to the tourniquet
- Arrange absorbent drapes or self-adhesive covers for preoperative skin disinfection
- Position the operating lights
- Patient warming system

18.4 · Lower leg

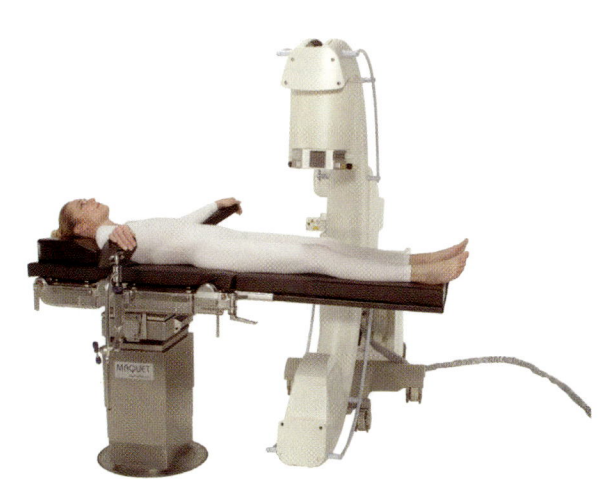

Fig. 18.28. Legs positioned on divided CRP leg plates with individual adjustment

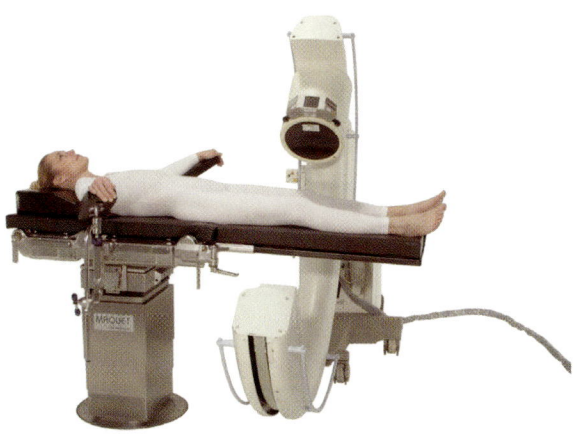

Fig. 18.29. Fluoroscopy possible through 360°

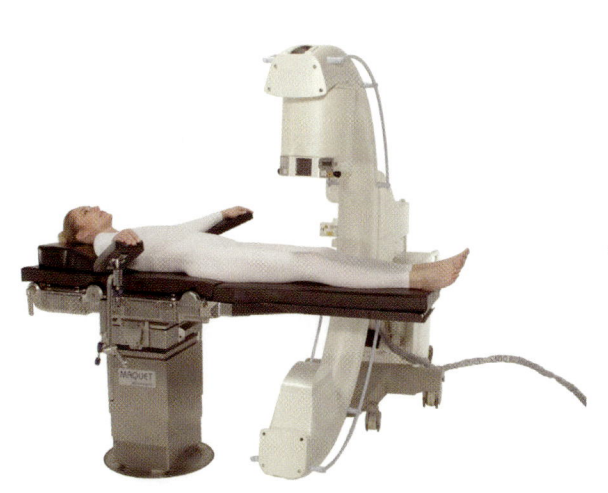

Fig. 18.30. Legs positioned on single-section CRP module 1150.45

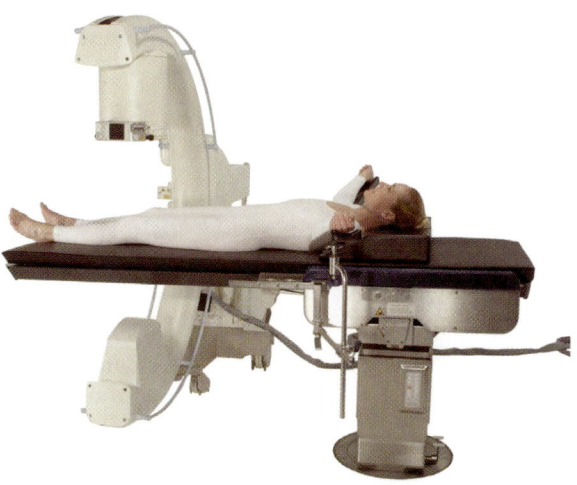

Fig. 18.31. Legs positioned on CRP operating table 1150.16

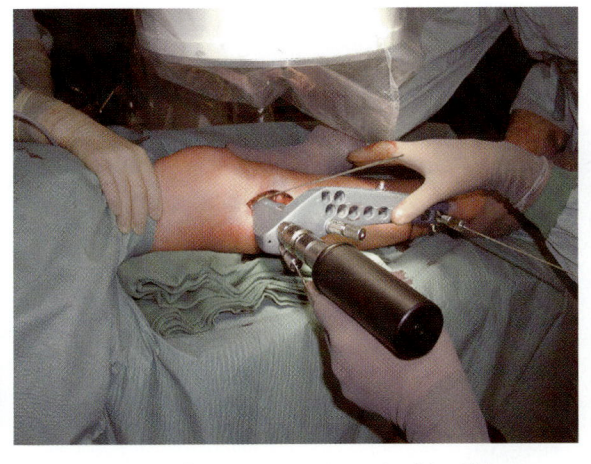

Fig. 18.32. Minimally invasive operation to the tibia with image intensifier in anteroposterior position

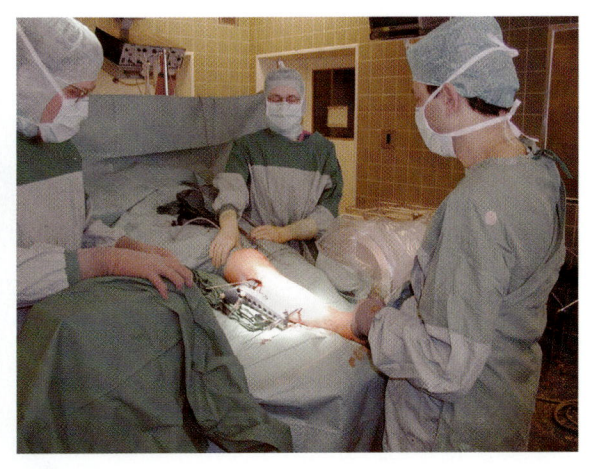

Fig. 18.33. Lateral fluoroscopy of the tibia with left leg lowered

18.5 Foot

18.5.1 Supine position

◘ Figs. 18.34–18.39.

Indications

Ventral, anterolateral, medial and posteromedial access to the ankle joint, access to the inner malleolus and outer malleolus, lateral and medial access to the talocalcaneonavicular, front, medial and plantar access to the middle foot and to the toes for fractures, posttraumatic, congenital and acquired misalignment, arthrosis, synovitis, osteochondral lesions, soft tissue lesions and tumours.

Preparations
- Arm positioning devices
- Wedge cushion, body support
- Shaving in the area of the incision and preoperative skin cleansing
- Apply a tourniquet in position

Positioning
- Standard operating table position 1, position 2 or universal operating table
- Anaesthetic preparation and induction in supine position with 2 adapted arm positioning devices
- Normal positioning of the operating table in the theatre
- When positioning the patient, take appropriate measures to prevent decubitus at areas which are subjected to pressure
- Position both arms on the arm positioning device in abduction position
- Apply the neutral electrode and connect to the HF surgery device
- Connect the compressed air supply to the tourniquet
- Arrange absorbent drapes or self-adhesive covers for preoperative skin disinfection
- Position the operating lights
- Patient warming system

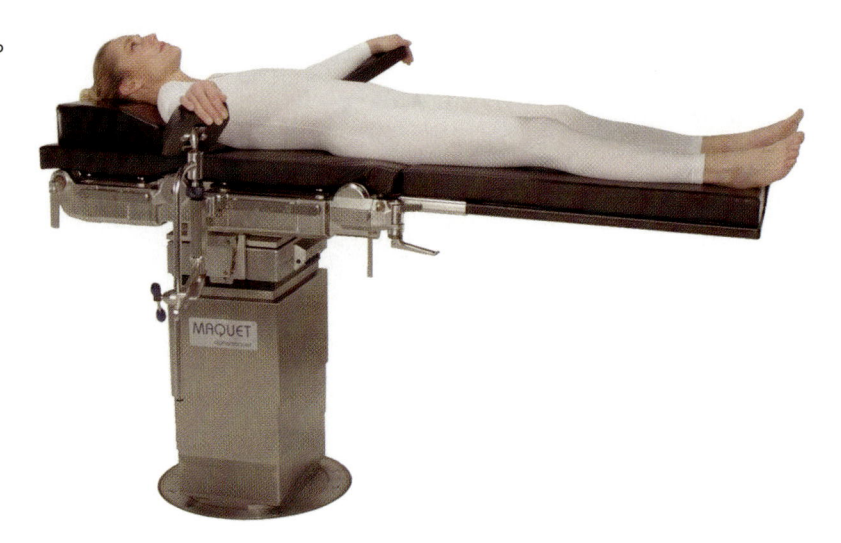

◘ **Fig. 18.34.** Legs positioned on divided CRP leg plates with individual adjustment

18.5 · Foot

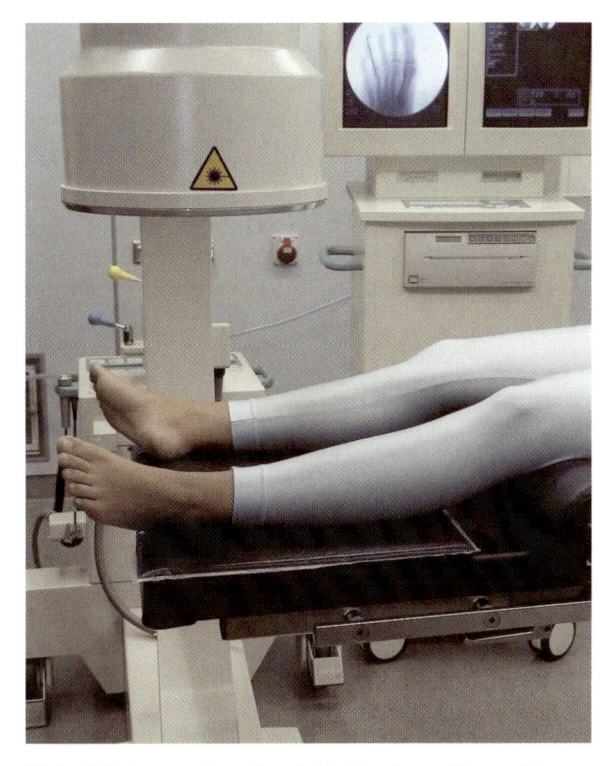

Fig. 18.35. Legs positioned on divided leg plates with use of the image intensifier

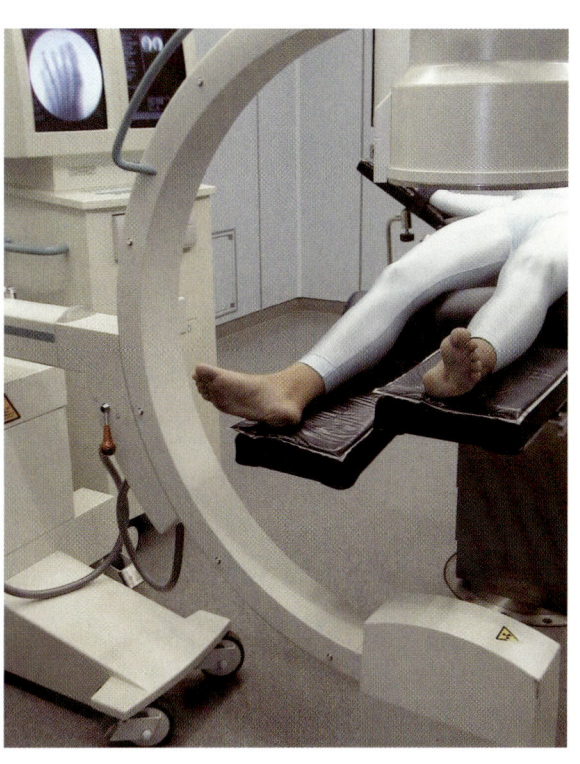

Fig. 18.36. Divided leg plates with individual adjustment

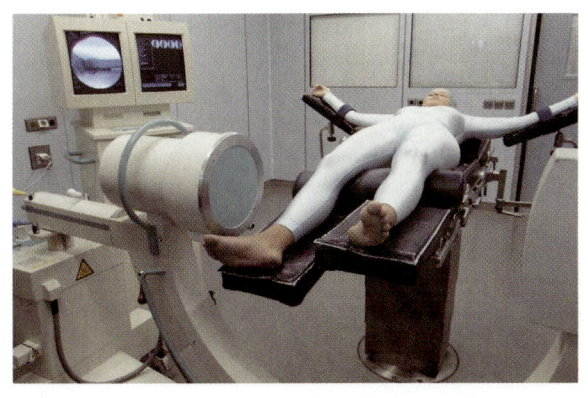

Fig. 18.37. Optimum scanning possibility with lateral ray path due to lowered leg plate

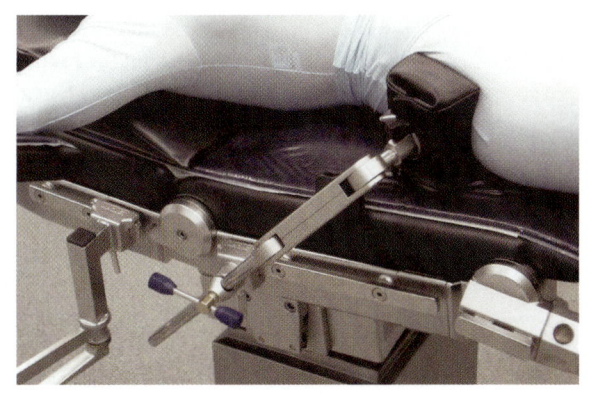

Fig. 18.38. Body support with wedge cushion padding under the pelvis on the other side

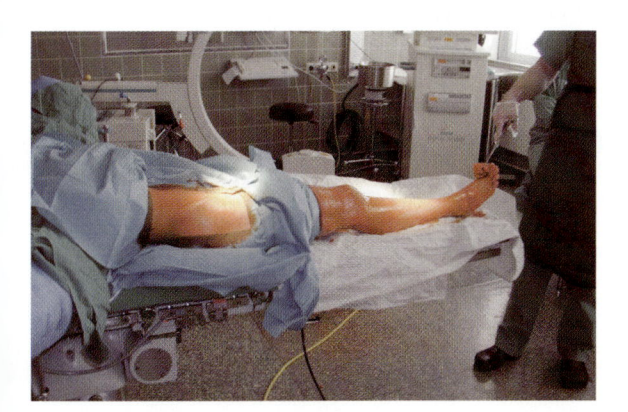

Fig. 18.39. Preoperative skin disinfection and additional moisture protection during the operation

18.5.2 Lateral position

◘ Figs. 18.40–18.43.

Indications

Access to the fibula and Achilles tendon, lateral access to the calcaneus and talocalcaneonavicular, medial and posteromedial access to the calcaneus and talocalcaneonavicular for fractures, posttraumatic, congenital and acquired misalignment, arthrosis, synovitis, osteochondral lesions, tumours and soft tissue lesions.

Preparations

- Arm positioning devices
- Gel ring, gel cushion, Goepel leg holder, lateral supports, radial adjusting clamps, padded cushions (normal and flat) and wedge cushions or tunnel cushions, body belts
- Shaving in the area of the incision and preoperative skin cleansing
- Apply a tourniquet in position

Positioning

- Standard operating table position 1, position 2 or universal operating table
- Anaesthetic preparation and induction in supine position with 2 adapted arm positioning devices
- Normal positioning of the operating table in the theatre
- When positioning the patient, take appropriate measures to prevent decubitus at areas which are subjected to pressure
- Fit the radial adjusting clamp to the side rail of the head plate, position the Goepel leg holder and place a gel mat on the operating table
- Spread out the arm on the side not being operated
- Move the patient onto the healthy side
- Move the lower arm forwards so that the weight of the upper body does not lie directly on the shoulder
- Fit the radial adjusting clamps to the side rails of the back plate and position the body supports on the level of the coccyx and symphysis
- **1st possibility:** position the legs with the padded cushions (normal and flat) and possibly wedge cushions
- Fix the lower leg and the positioning aids with the body belts
- **2nd possibility:** position the legs with the tunnel cushion
- Apply the neutral electrode and connect to the HF surgery device
- Connect the compressed air supply to the tourniquet
- Arrange absorbent drapes or self-adhesive covers for preoperative skin disinfection
- Position the operating lights
- Patient warming system

18.5 · Foot

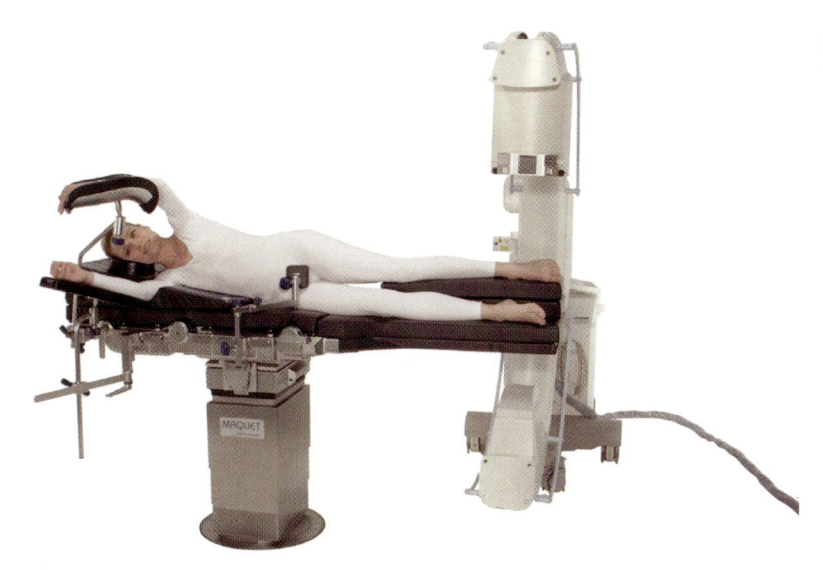

Fig. 18.40. Legs positioned on single-section CRP module 1150.45 with padded cushion

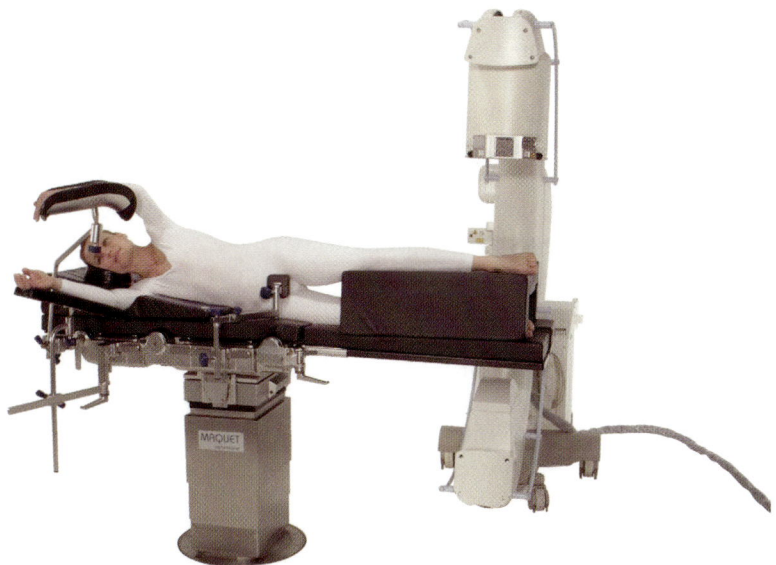

Fig. 18.41. Legs positioned on divided CRP leg plates with tunnel cushion

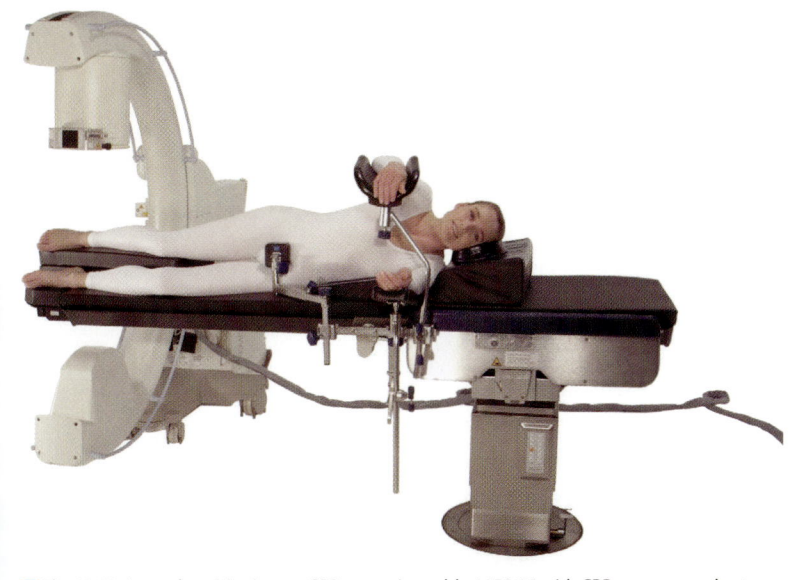

Fig. 18.42. Lateral positioning on CRP operating table 1150.16 with CRP accessory adapter and lateral positioning cushion for anatomic positioning of the lower arm

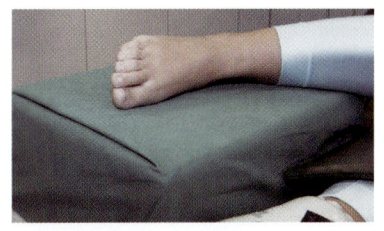

Fig. 18.43. Stable positioning of the foot and optimum access for the surgeon with use of the image intensifier from the opposite side in both levels

18.5.3 Prone position

■ Figs. 18.44, 18.45.

Indications

Posterolateral access to the talocalcaneonavicular and concealed osteosynthesis in the calcaneal part of the foot.

Preparations
- Arm positioning devices
- Shaving in the area of the incision and preoperative skin cleansing
- Apply a tourniquet in position

Positioning
- Standard operating table position 1, position 2 or universal operating table
- Anaesthetic preparation and induction in supine position with 2 adapted arm positioning devices
- Transfer to the prepared operating table in the induction room
- Position both tables next to each other, with the prepared table lowered
- Place the patient in prone position on the padded cushion of the prepared operating table and take him into the theatre
- Normal positioning of the operating table in the theatre
- When positioning the patient, take appropriate measures to prevent decubitus at areas which are subjected to pressure
- Position the head on the special head positioning cushion
- Position both arms on the arm positioning devices
- Apply the neutral electrode and connect to the HF surgery device
- Connect the compressed air supply to the tourniquet
- Arrange self-adhesive covers for preoperative skin disinfection
- Position the operating lights
- Patient warming system

18.5 · Foot

Fig. 18.44. Prone position on universal operating table 1150.30 with arms positioned in maximum 90° abduction

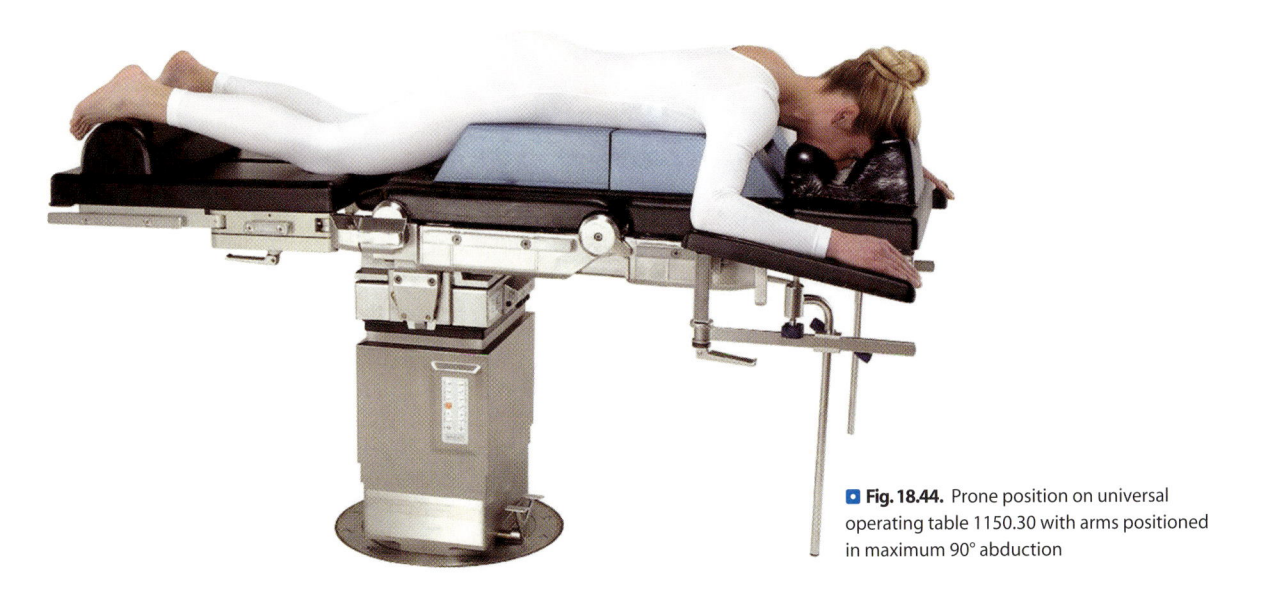

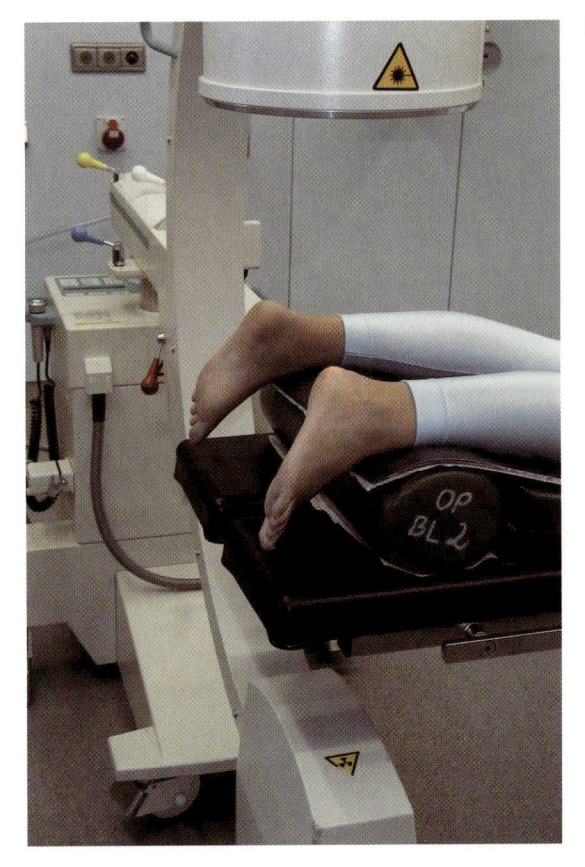

Fig. 18.45. Use of the image intensifier in anteroposterior position. C-arm with coloured handles for better communication between surgeon and operator

19 Positioning on the extension table

19.1 Extension table proximal femur – 260
19.1.1 Supine position – 260

19.2 Extension table thigh – 262
19.2.1 Supine position – 262

19.3 Extension table lower leg – 264
19.3.1 Supine position – 264

19.1 Extension table proximal femur

19.1.1 Supine position

◘ Figs. 19.1–19.5.

Indications

Osteosynthesis of the proximal femur entailing reposition with the possibility of extension and fluoroscopy in two levels, and displacement osteotomy of the proximal femur.

Preparations
- Arm positioning devices
- Extension table accessories
- Shaving in the area of the incision and preoperative skin cleansing
- G-arm, alternatively 1 or 2 C-arms

Positioning
- Universal operating table for traumatology and orthopaedic procedures (extension table)
- Anaesthetic preparation and induction in supine position with 2 adapted arm positioning devices
- If necessary, diagonal positioning of the operating table in the theatre
- When positioning the patient, take appropriate measures to prevent decubitus at areas which are subjected to pressure
- Longitudinal adjustment of the operating table towards the feet (1150.20)
- Swivel the extension bars in a V-shape towards the feet
- Insert the countertraction post on the side being treated
- Insert the long telescopic bar in the extension bar on the side not being operated
- Insert the short telescopic bar in the extension bar on the side being operated
- Fit the foot plate adapter
- Fit the screw tension device
- Fit the rotating and tilting clamp to the screw tension device
- Place a double wedge cushion on the operating table
- Fit the arm positioning device to the side rails of the lower back plate on the side not being operated
- Fit the anaesthesia screen with a radial adjusting clamp to the side rail of the upper back plate on the left-hand side
- Fit the anaesthesia screen extensions and possibly suspend 2 arm straps
- Position the foot plates before transferring the patient
- Transfer the patient from the induction table to the prepared operating table in supine position
- Fit the positioned foot plates to the screw tension device and foot plate adapter, constantly pulling the legs at the rotating and tilting clamp
- Position the arms
- Reposition the fracture using the image intensifier and position the legs
- Check all screwed and clamped connections
- Apply the neutral electrode and connect to the HF surgery device
- Arrange self-adhesive covers for preoperative skin disinfection
- Position the operating lights
- Patient warming system

Risks
- Secondary dislocation
- Nerve injuries (n. pudendus)

19.1 · Extension table proximal femur

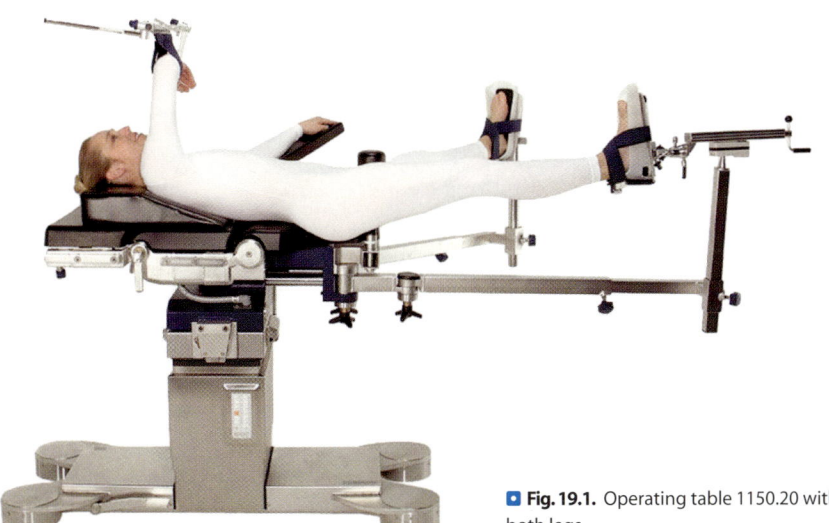

Fig. 19.1. Operating table 1150.20 with foot plates fitted for both legs

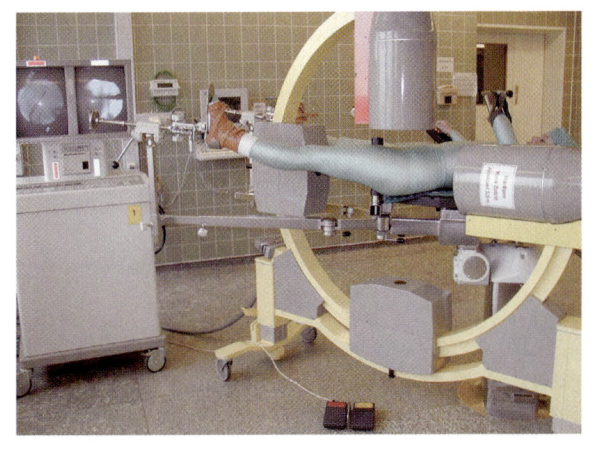

Fig. 19.2. Operating table 1140.20 with foot plates fitted for both legs and use of the G-arm

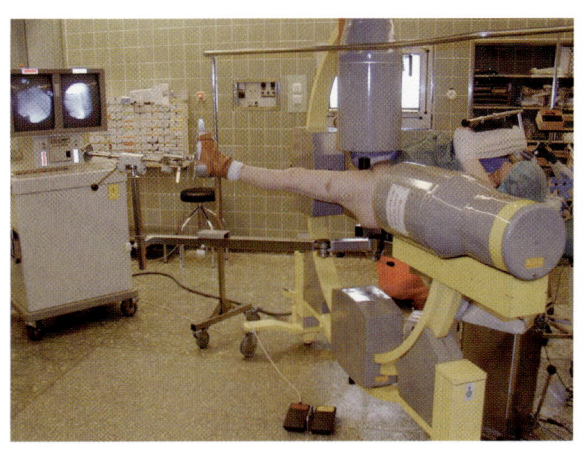

Fig. 19.3. Operating table 1140.20 with foot plates fitted for both legs and use of the G-arm for DHS operation (*DHS,* dynamic hip screw)

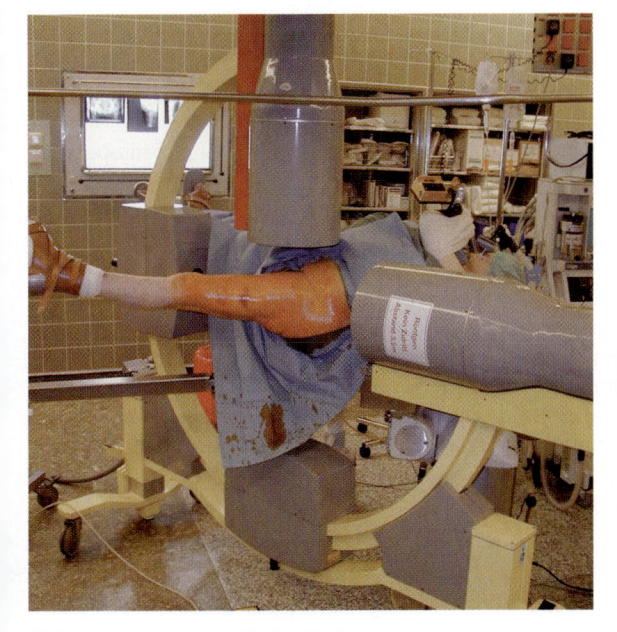

Fig. 19.4. Preoperative skin disinfection

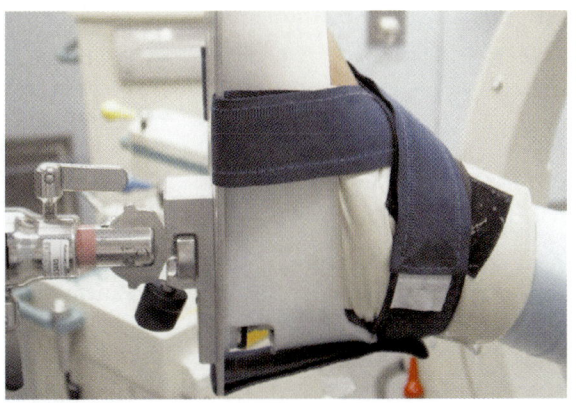

Fig. 19.5. Foot plate fitted to the rotating and tilting clamp with padded, fixed foot

19.2 Extension table thigh

19.2.1 Supine position

◘ Figs. 19.6–19.8.

Indications
Medullary nailing, intramedullary reaming.

Preparations
- Two arm positioning devices
- Extension table accessories
- Shaving in the area of the incision and preoperative skin cleansing

Positioning
- Universal operating table for traumatology and orthopaedic procedures (extension table)
- Anaesthetic preparation and induction in supine position with 2 adapted arm positioning devices
- If necessary, diagonal positioning of the operating table in the theatre
- When positioning the patient, take appropriate measures to prevent decubitus at areas which are subjected to pressure
- Longitudinal adjustment of the operating table towards the feet (1150.20)
- Swivel the extension bars in a V-shape towards the feet on the side being operated
- Insert the countertraction post on the side being treated
- Insert the short telescopic bar in the extension bar on the side being operated
- Fit the screw tension device
- Fit the rotating and tilting clamp to the screw tension device
- Place a double wedge cushion on the operating table
- Fit the arm positioning device to the rails of the lower back plate on the side not being operated
- Fit the side rail extension to the side rail of the seat plate
- Fit the Goepel leg holder to the side rail extension with a radial adjusting clamp
- Fit the anaesthesia screen with a radial adjusting clamp to the side rail of the upper back plate on the left-hand side
- Fit the anaesthesia screen extensions and possibly suspend 2 arm straps
- Fit the Kirschner wire bow before transferring the patient
- Transfer the patient from the induction table to the prepared operating table in supine position
- Fit the positioned Kirschner wire bow to the traction stirrup clamp with rotation, constantly pulling the leg
- Position the left leg in the Goepel leg holder
  Position the arms
- Reposition the fracture using the image intensifier
- To stabilise the patient, possibly support the thorax from the side
- Check all screwed and clamped connections
- Apply the neutral electrode and connect to the HF surgery device
- Arrange self-adhesive covers for preoperative skin disinfection
- Position the operating lights
- Patient warming system

Risks
- Iatrogenic damage caused by inserting the Steinmann nail
- Pressure injuries
- Compartment syndrome from overdistraction

19.2 · Extension table thigh

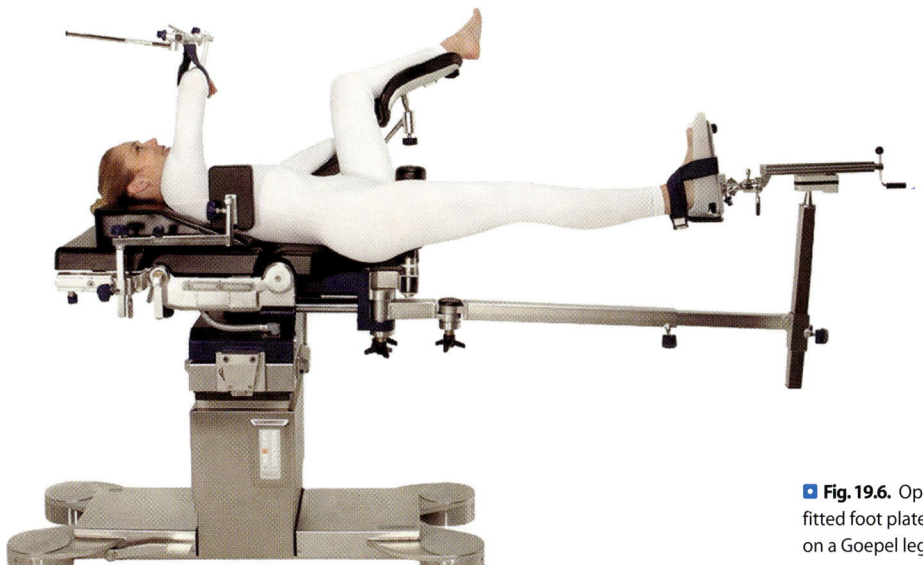

Fig. 19.6. Operating table 1150.20 with fitted foot plate, healthy leg is in abduction on a Goepel leg holder

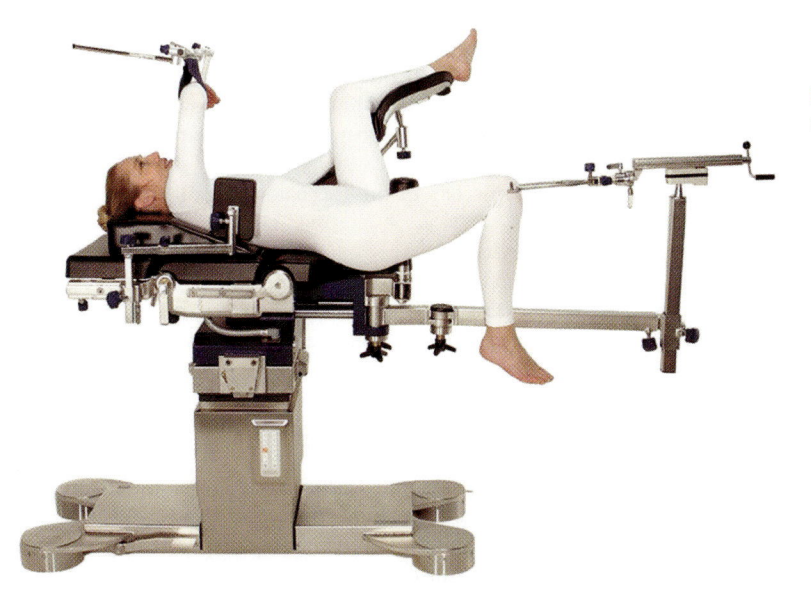

Fig. 19.7. Operating table 1150.20 with fitted Kirschner wire bow and thorax support

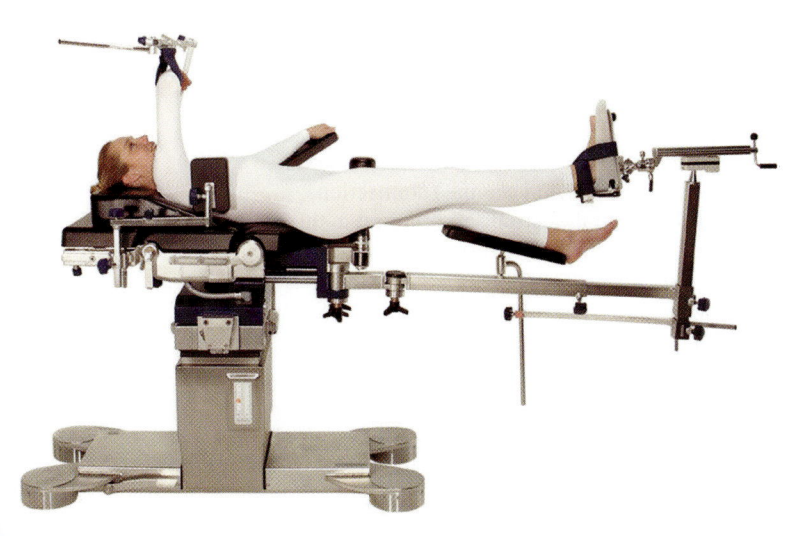

Fig. 19.8. Operating table 1150.20 with fitted foot plate, healthy leg is positioned downwards on a special support

19.3 Extension table lower leg

19.3.1 Supine position

◘ Figs. 19.9–19.11.

Indications
Medullary nailing, intramedullary reaming.

Preparations
- Two arm positioning devices
- Shaving in the area of the incision and preoperative skin cleansing

Positioning
- Universal operating table for traumatology and orthopaedic procedures (extension table)
- Anaesthetic preparation and induction in supine position with 2 adapted arm positioning devices
- If necessary, diagonal positioning of the operating table in the theatre
- When positioning the patient, take appropriate measures to prevent decubitus at areas which are subjected to pressure
- Longitudinal adjustment of the operating table towards the feet (1150.20)
- Fit the tibia device to the seat plate on the side being operated
- Unlock the unit at the lower radial joint and lower towards the feet to improve scanning the knee in anteroposterior ray path after positioning
- Lock the safety lever again
- Insert the short telescopic bar in the extension bar on the side being operated
- Fit the screw tension device
- Fit the rotation tilt clamp to the screw tension device
- Place a double wedge cushion on the operating table
- Fit the arm positioning device to the side rails of the lower back plate on the side not being operated
- Fit the side rails extension to the side rail of the seat plate
- Fit the Goepel leg holder to the side rail extension with a radial adjusting clamp
- Fit the anaesthesia screen with a radial adjusting clamp to the side rail of the upper back plate on the side not being operated
- Fit the anaesthesia screen extensions and possibly suspend 2 arm straps
- Fit the tension hoop before transferring the patient
- Transfer the patient from the induction table to the prepared operating table in supine position
- Fit the positioned Kirschner wire bow to the traction stirrup clamp with rotation, constantly pulling the leg
- Position the healthy leg in the Goepel leg holder
- Position the arms
- Reposition the fracture using the image intensifier
- Check all screwed and clamped connections
- Apply the neutral electrode and connect to the HF surgery device
- Arrange self-adhesive covers for preoperative skin disinfection
- Position the operating lights
- Patient warming system

Risks
- Iatrogenic damage caused by inserting the Steinmann nail
- Pressure injuries
- Compartment syndrome from overdistraction

19.3 · Extension table lower leg

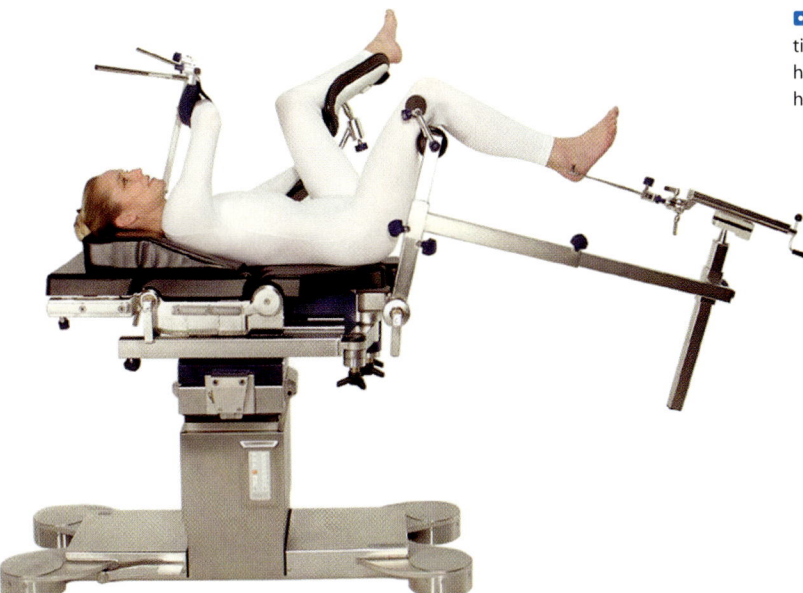

Fig. 19.9. Operating table 1150.20 with tibia device and fitted Kirschner wire bow, healthy leg is spread out on a Goepel leg holder

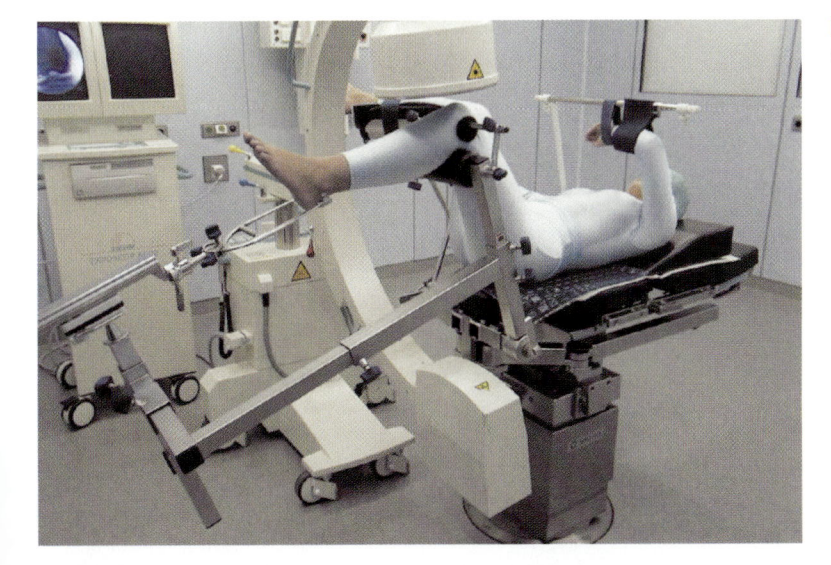

Fig. 19.10. Tibia device is lowered to optimise anteroposterior fluoroscopy

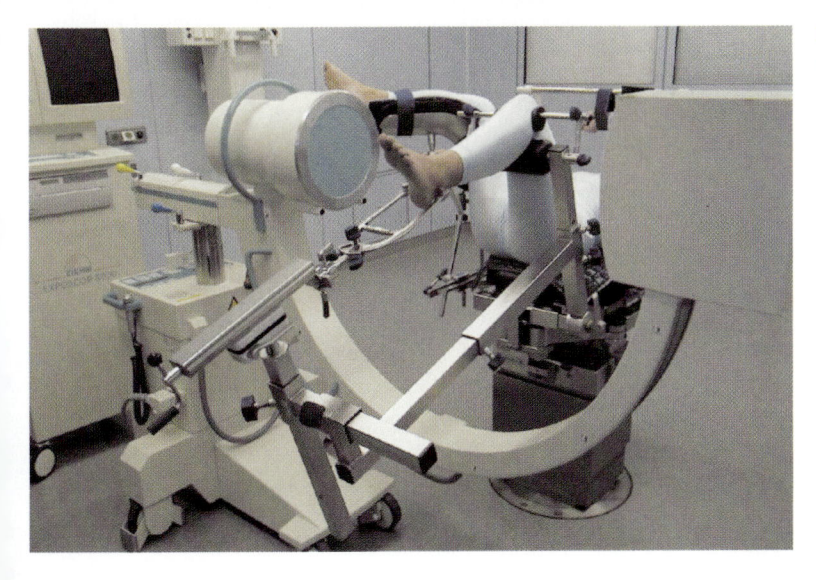

Fig. 19.11. Image intensifier in lateral position

20 Arthroscopic procedures

20.1 Shoulder – 268
20.1.1 Beach-chair position – 268
20.1.2 Lateral position – 270

20.2 Hips – 272
20.2.1 Supine position on the extension table – 272

20.3 Knee – 274
20.3.1 Supine position – 274

20.4 Foot/ankle – 276
20.4.1 Supine position – 276

20.1 Shoulder

20.1.1 Beach-chair position

Figs. 20.1–20.5.

Indications

Diagnostic and therapeutic arthroscopy procedures for impingement syndrome, rotator cuff rupture, tendinosis calcarea, shoulder instability, arthrosis/osteolysis of the acromioclavicular joint and synovitis.

Preparations
- Arm positioning devices
- Horseshoe-shaped headrest
- Remove the Gilchrist bandage
- Shaving in the area of the incision and preoperative skin cleansing

Positioning
- Beach-chair operating table position 2 or universal operating table with shoulder plate
- Anaesthetic preparation and induction in supine position with 2 adapted arm positioning devices
- Crosswise positioning of the operating table in the theatre
- When positioning the patient, take appropriate measures to prevent decubitus at areas which are subjected to pressure
- The patient's shoulders end at the upper edge of the operating table
- Bring the operating table gradually to the half-sitting (beach-chair) position
- Raise the back plate and alternately lower the head of the complete operating table until the final position is reached
- Change the Bowden cable over and lower the legs to the horizontal (system 1120)
- Position the head on a horseshoe-shaped headrest and fix with transparent plaster right across the forehead or use a head holder for shoulder operation (U-shaped helmet)
- Position the infusion arm on an arm positioning device
- Cover the arm on the side being operated while leaving it free to move and position it at the body with arm protection or place it on the arm positioning device
- Apply the neutral electrode and connect to the HF surgery device
- Fit the thorax support to the rail of the shoulder plate
- Arrange self-adhesive covers for preoperative skin disinfection
- Position the operating lights
- Patient warming system

Risks
- Nerve injuries (brachial plexus)

20.1 · Shoulder

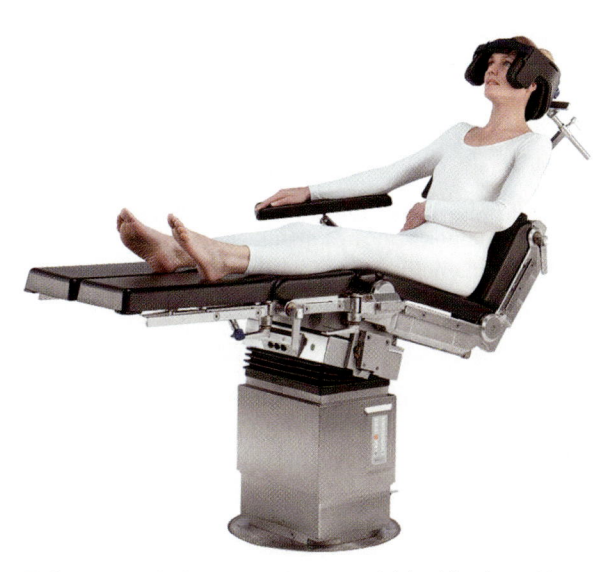

Fig. 20.1. Beach-chair positioning on special shoulder plate with helmet for safe positioning of the head

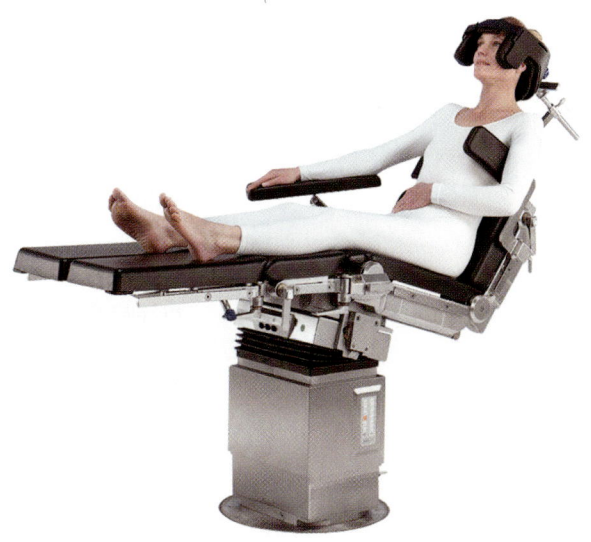

Fig. 20.2. The thorax support offers additional safety

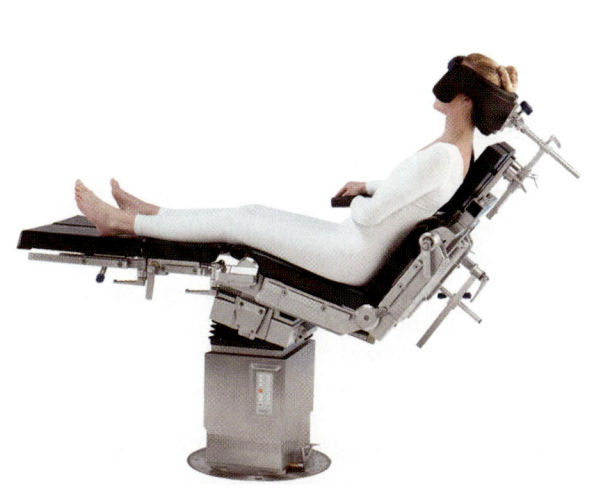

Fig. 20.3. The universal operating table with special shoulder plate is adapted to the body

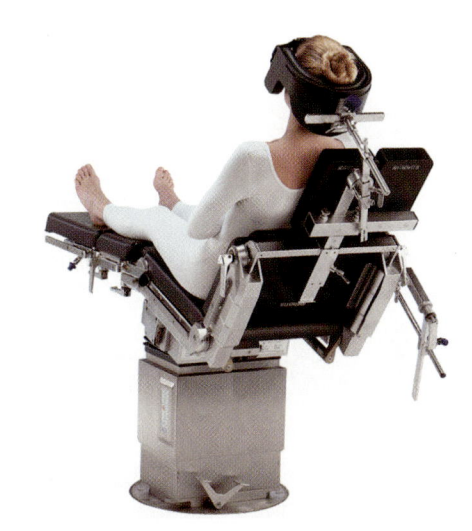

Fig. 20.4. A segment is removed to leave free access to the rear shoulder

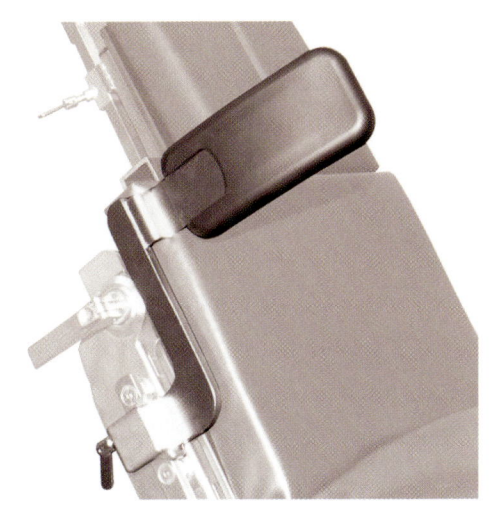

Fig. 20.5. Thorax support

20.1.2 Lateral position

◧ Figs. 20.6, 20.7.

Indications

Diagnostic and therapeutic arthroscopy procedures for impingement syndrome, rotator cuff rupture, tendinosis calcarea, shoulder instability, arthrosis/osteolysis of the acromioclavicular joint and synovitis.

Preparations

- Arm positioning devices
- Gel ring, gel cushion, Goepel leg holder, side supports, radial adjusting clamps, padded cushions (normal and flat) and wedge cushions, tunnel cushions, body belts
- Gallows for arm extension
- Shaving in the area of the incision and preoperative skin cleansing

Positioning

- Standard operating table position 1, position 2 or universal operating table
- Anaesthetic preparation and induction in supine position with 2 adapted arm positioning devices
- Crosswise positioning of the operating table in the theatre
- When positioning the patient, take appropriate measures to prevent decubitus at areas which are subjected to pressure
- **1st possibility:** fit the radial adjusting clamp to the side rail of the head plate and position the Goepel leg holder
- **2nd possibility:** fit gallows for suspending the arm being operated with counterweight (extension) to the foot end of the operating table
- Spread out the arm on the side not being operated
- Move the patient onto the healthy side
- Move the lower arm forwards so that the weight of the upper body does not lie directly on the shoulder
- Fit the body supports to the side rails and brace on the level of the sacrum and symphysis
- **1st possibility:** position the legs with the padded cushions (normal and flat) and possibly wedge cushions
- Fix the lower leg and the positioning aids with the body belts
- **2nd possibility:** position the legs with the tunnel cushion
- Apply the neutral electrode and connect to the HF surgery device
- Arrange absorbent drapes or self-adhesive covers for preoperative skin disinfection
- Position the operating lights without switching on
- Patient warming system

20.1 · Shoulder

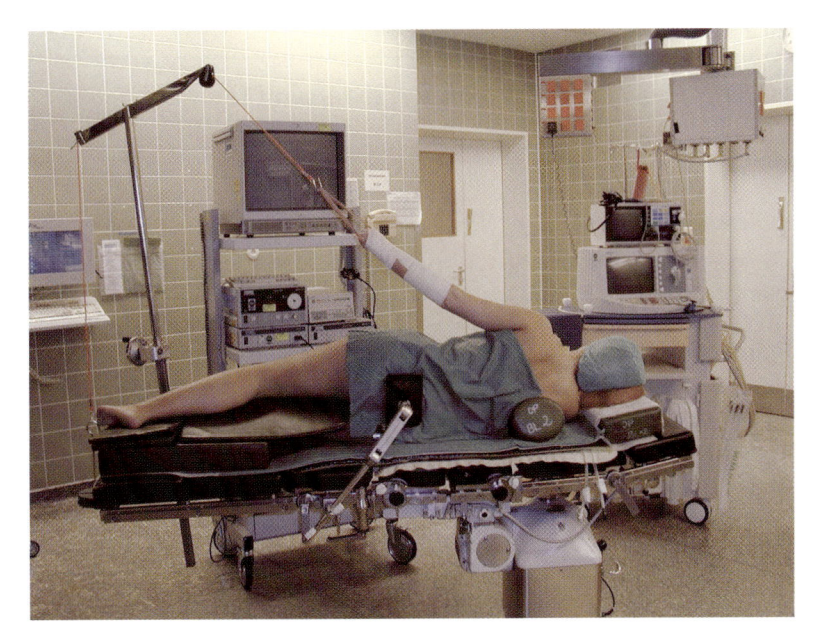

Fig. 20.6. Lateral position with arm extension

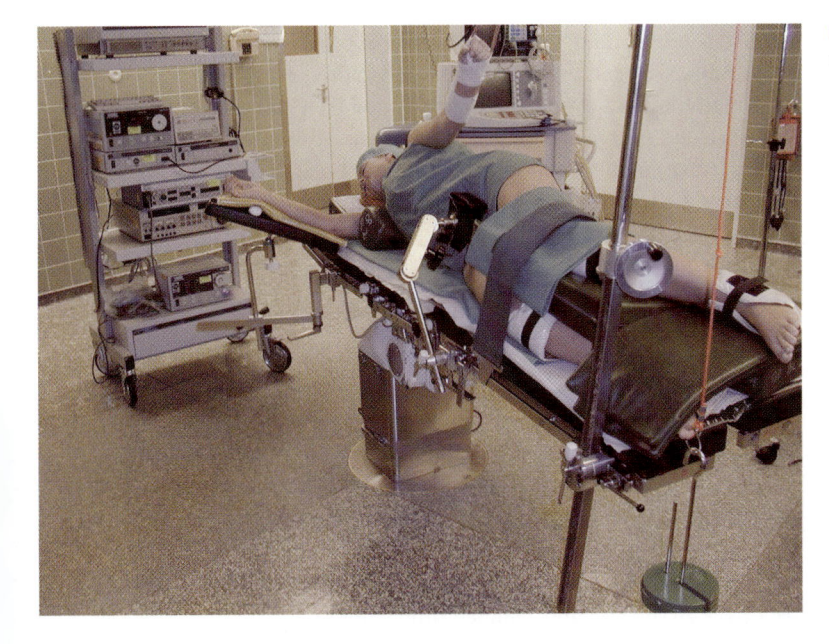

Fig. 20.7. Arm extension (gallows) can be swivelled and adjusted in height

20.2 Hips

20.2.1 Supine position on the extension table

◘ Figs. 20.8, 20.9.

Indications

Diagnostic and therapeutic arthroscopic procedures for floating cartilage, synovitis, fractures, labrum lesions and arthrosis.

Preparations
- Arm positioning devices
- Extension table accessories
- Shaving in the area of the incision and preoperative skin cleansing
- G-arm, alternatively 1 or 2 C-arms

Positioning
- Universal operating table for traumatology and orthopaedic procedures (extension table)
- Anaesthetic preparation and induction in supine position with 2 adapted arm positioning devices
- If necessary, diagonal positioning of the operating table in the theatre
- When positioning the patient, take appropriate measures to prevent decubitus at areas which are subjected to pressure
- Longitudinal adjustment of the operating table towards the feet (1150.20)
- Swivel the extension bars in a V-shape towards the feet
- Insert the countertraction bar on the side being treated
- Insert the long telescopic bar in the extension bar on the side not being operated
- Insert the short telescopic bar in the extension bar on the side being operated
- Fit the foot plate adapter
- Fit the screw tension device
- Fit the rotation tilt clamp to the screw tension device
- Position the foot plates
- Fit the positioned foot plates to the screw tension device and foot plate adapter, constantly pulling the legs at the rotation and tilting clamp
- Remove the (extension table) leg plates
- Position the arms
- Position the legs and set up the image intensifier
- Check all screwed and clamped connections
- Apply the neutral electrode and connect to the HF surgery device
- Arrange self-adhesive covers for preoperative skin disinfection
- Position the operating lights without switching on
- Patient warming system

Risks
- Nerve injuries (pudendal nerve)

20.2 · Hips

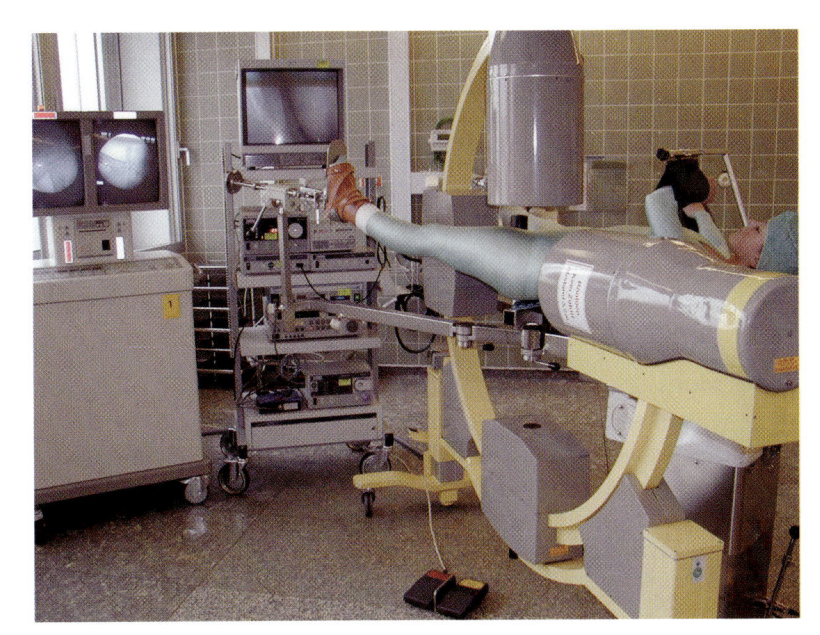

Fig. 20.8. Supine position on extension table with G-arm

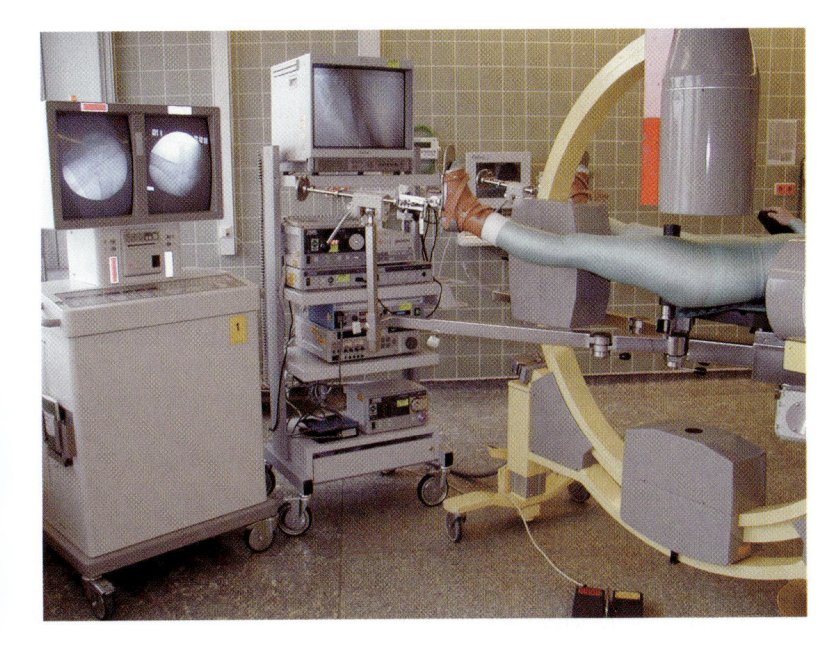

Fig. 20.9. Positioning the monitors at the foot end; foot holder closure is located on the inside for better padding of the feet on the outside

20.3 Knee

20.3.1 Supine position

◘ Figs. 20.10–20.15.

Indications

Diagnostic and therapeutic arthroscopic procedures for ligament injuries, meniscus lesions, cartilage damage, arthrosis, floating cartilage, synovitis, fractures and osteochondrosis dissecans.

Preparations
- Arm positioning devices
- Tourniquet, cotton wool padding, elastic bandages, perforated rubber sheet knee holder, special positioning cushion
- Shaving in the area of the incision and preoperative skin cleansing
- Apply a tourniquet in position

Positioning
- Standard operating table position 1, position 2 or universal operating table
- Anaesthetic induction in the supine position, padding under the shoulders
- Normal positioning of the operating table in the theatre
- When positioning the patient, take appropriate measures to prevent decubitus at areas which are subjected to pressure
- Position both arms on the arm positioning devices in 45° abduction position
- Fit the knee holder with radial adjusting clamp to the small rail of the leg plate on the operation side
- Fix the thigh in the knee holder
- Position the leg not being operated on the special positioning cushion (MHH), with abduction of the leg and swing down the leg plate
- Apply the neutral electrode and connect to the HF surgery device
- Connect the compressed air supply to the tourniquet
- Preoperative skin disinfection as far as the perforated rubber sheet
- Position the operating lights without switching on
- Patient warming system

Risks
- Dislocation in the leg holder
- Injury to the femoral nerve under hyperextension of the other hip, therefore positioning cushion (black) under the other thigh

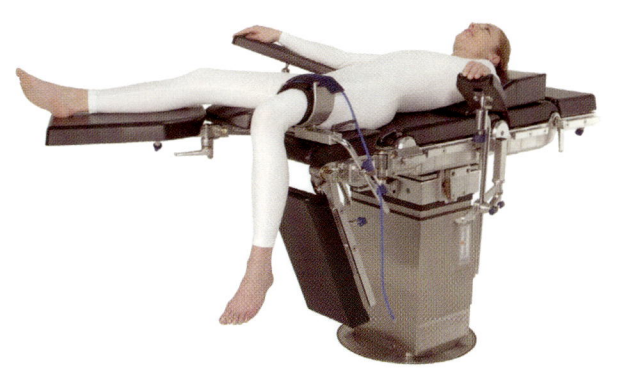

Fig. 20.10. Supine position on universal operating table with 4-section leg plates

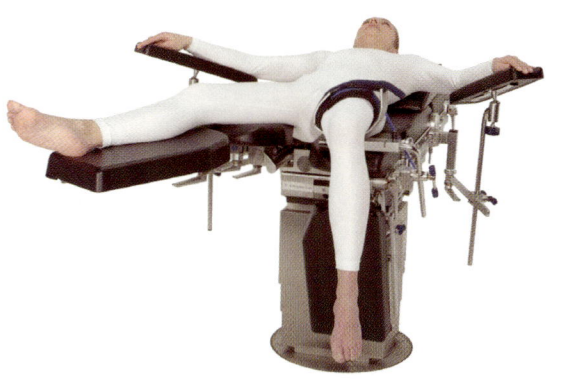

Fig. 20.11. Lower segment of the leg plate folded down and thigh fixed in a knee holder

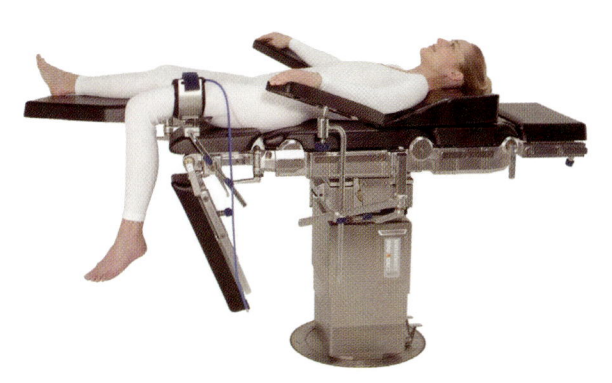

Fig. 20.12. Thigh padded to prevent pressure from the knee holder, at the same time this acts as tourniquet

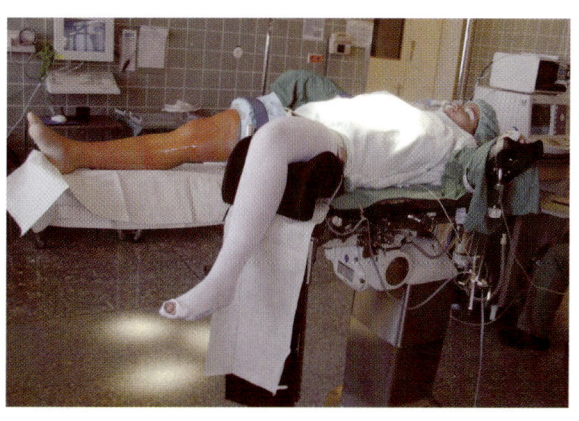

Fig. 20.13. Healthy leg lowered and abducted, thigh padded/raised with special positioning cushion (MHH) to prevent hyperextension in the hip joint

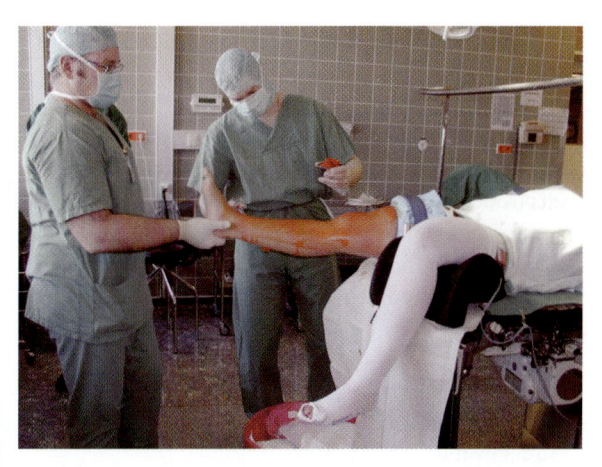

Fig. 20.14. Preoperative skin disinfection up to the perforated rubber sheet

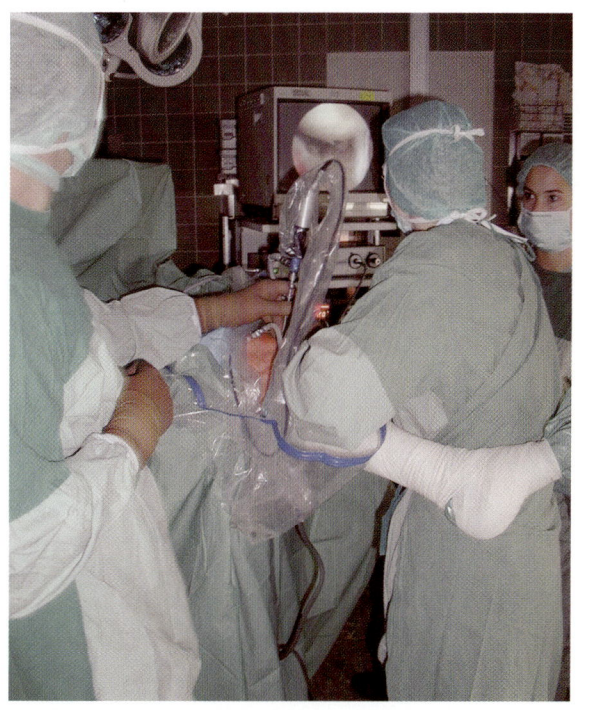

Fig. 20.15. Special covering for arthroscopy of the knee

20.4 Foot/ankle

20.4.1 Supine position

◻ Figs. 20.16–20.20.

Indications

Diagnostic and therapeutic arthroscopic procedures for ligament injuries, cartilage damage, arthrosis, floating cartilage, synovitis, fractures and osteochondrosis dissecans.

Preparations
- Arm positioning devices
- Shaving in the area of the incision and preoperative skin cleansing
- 1 to 2 tourniquets, cotton wool padding, elastic bandages, perforated rubber sheet, knee holder, special positioning cushion

Positioning
- Standard operating table position 1, position 2 or universal operating table
- Anaesthetic induction in the supine position, padding under the shoulders
- Normal positioning of the operating table in the theatre
- When positioning the patient, take appropriate measures to prevent decubitus at areas which are subjected to pressure
- Position both arms on the arm positioning devices in 45° abduction position
- Apply the tourniquets in position:
- **1st possibility:** lower leg only, here padding and tourniquet
- **2nd possibility:** thigh for tourniquet and lower leg for padding
- Lower the leg plate on the operation side by about 30° and fit the knee holder with the radial adjusting clamp to the rail of the leg plate in a raised position at the middle of the calf, so that the leg being operated is in a horizontal position as far as possible
- Fix the lower leg in the leg holder
- Position the leg not being operated on the special positioning cushions, with abduction of the leg and swing down the leg plate
- Apply the neutral electrode and connect to the HF surgery device
- Connect the compressed air supply to the tourniquet
- Preoperative skin disinfection as far as the perforated rubber sheet
- Position the operating lights without switching on
- Patient warming system

Risks
- Nerve lesions caused by the arthroscopy
- Pressure injuries caused by the tourniquet

20.4 · Foot/ankle

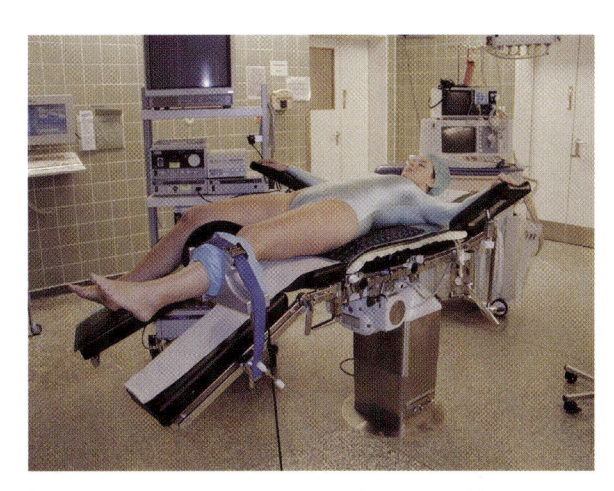

Fig. 20.16. Supine position on universal operating table with 4-section leg plates

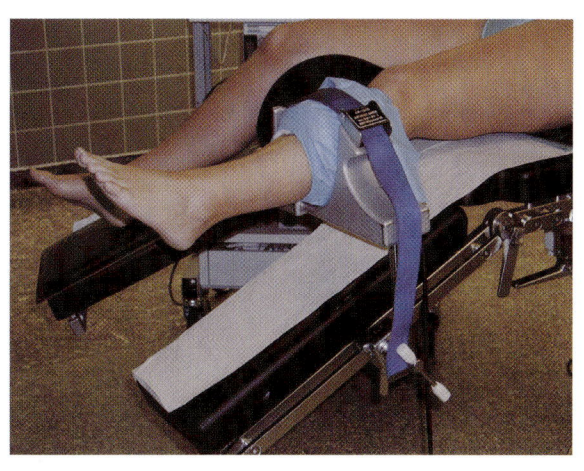

Fig. 20.17. Knee holder fitted to the side rail of the lower segment of the leg plate lowered through about 30°; a tourniquet is fitted to the lower leg

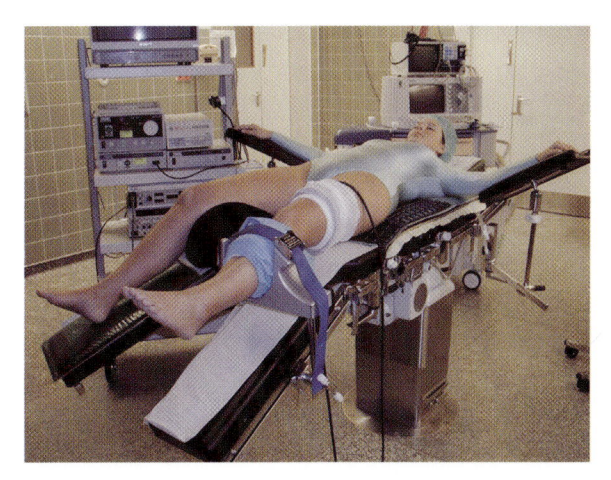

Fig. 20.18. Two tourniquets are positioned; the tourniquet at the lower leg is only for padding

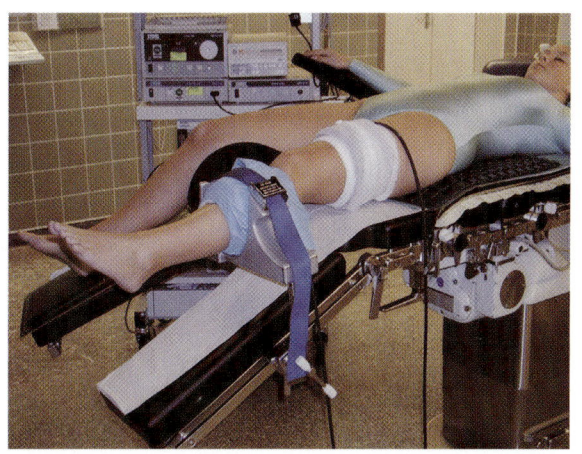

Fig. 20.19. Healthy leg lowered and abducted, thigh padded/raised with special positioning cushion (MHH) to prevent hyperextension in the hip joint

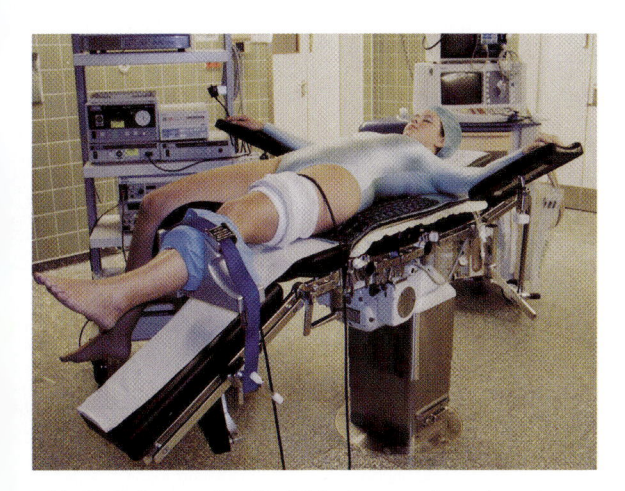

Fig. 20.20. Preoperative skin disinfection up to the perforated rubber sheet

21 Paediatric surgery

21.1 Various positions – 280
21.1.1 Supine position – 280
21.1.2 Prone position – 282
21.1.3 Lateral position – 284
21.1.4 Lithotomy position – 286

While there are no essential differences in the positioning of older children and adults for surgical procedures, there are certain special aspects to be taken into consideration for infants, newborn babies and premature babies. The temperature in the operating theatre should be more than 25°C and the small patient should be kept warm with a warming mat and a warming lamp before and after the operation. A temperature sensor on the surface of the patient's body is mandatory to protect from burning. There is no need to spread out the arms of small children, the arms are positioned close to the body and fixed with a compress. Small foam pads are placed under the knees and feet to pad the lower extremities. Infants legs are fixed with a plastic strip instead of the belt.

Basically there are differences in the following positionings: supine, prone, lateral, lithotomy and special positions, e.g. for minimally invasive procedures where the surgeon stands at the foot end or between the patient's legs.

21.1 Various positions

21.1.1 Supine position

◘ Figs. 21.1–21.6.

Indications
All open and minimally invasive procedures to the intra-abdominal and thoracic organs for congenital deformities (e.g. gastroschisis, omphalocele, diaphragmatic hernia), emergency operations (e.g. volvulus, necrotising enterocolitis, trauma), forms of cancer (e.g. Wilms' tumour, hepatoblastoma, neuroblastoma), urological procedures, hernia operations, funnel chest, placing a port catheter and procedures to the neck (neck cyst).

Preparations
- Padding for knees, feet and under the buttocks (for hernia/undescended testicle)
- Padding under the abdomen important during open laparotomies, not for laparoscopic procedures
- Warming mat, warming lamp
- Arm positioning device only for older children

Positioning
- Children's operating table in the neutral position
- X-ray apron depending on the procedure
- Connect the warming mat and lamp, affix the temperature sensor
- Prepare and induce the anaesthetic in the supine position
- Spread out and pad the arms for older children
- Abduct the arms laterally (90°) for funnel chest operations
- Padding at the feet, knees and pelvis/abdomen depending on the operation
- Apply the neutral electrode, connect to the HF surgery device
- Fix the legs with body belt for older children or plastic strips in younger children
- Use compresses to protect the electrode during disinfection
- Position the operating lamps
- Spread the legs, Trendelenburg position of the head depending on the operation

Risks
- Plexus injuries on overstretching the arms when spread out
- Positioning injuries from lacking or inadequate padding
- Burns from lacking moisture protection for the neutral electrode

21.1 · Various positions

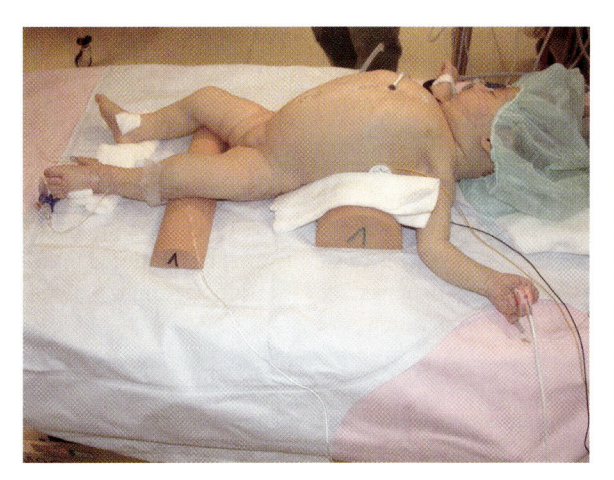

Fig. 21.1. Infant with imperforate bile duct

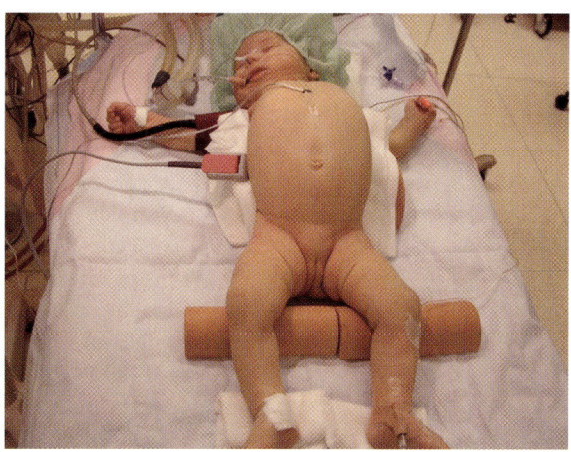

Fig. 21.2. Padding under the back for optimum exposure

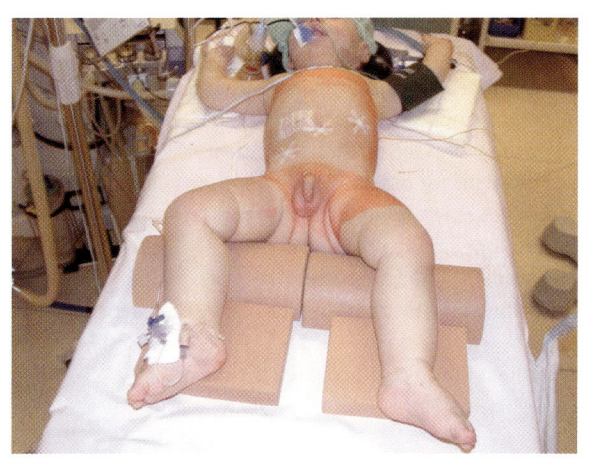

Fig. 21.3. Laparoscopic procedure on an infant without padding under the thorax

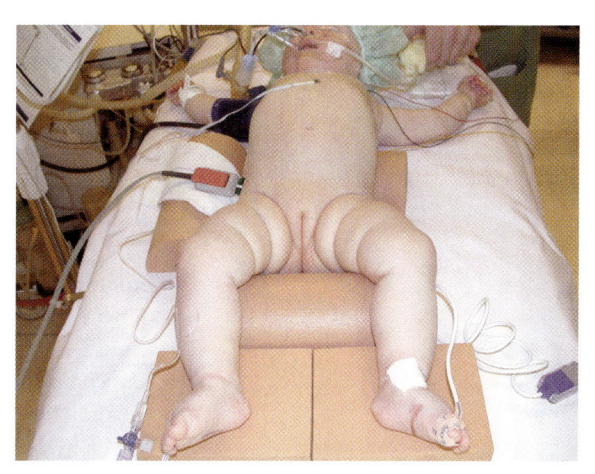

Fig. 21.4. Padding under the legs and feet

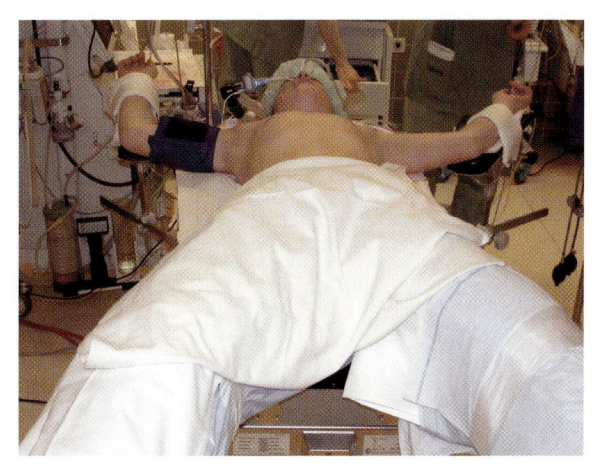

Fig. 21.5. Legs in abduction for laparoscopic fundoplication

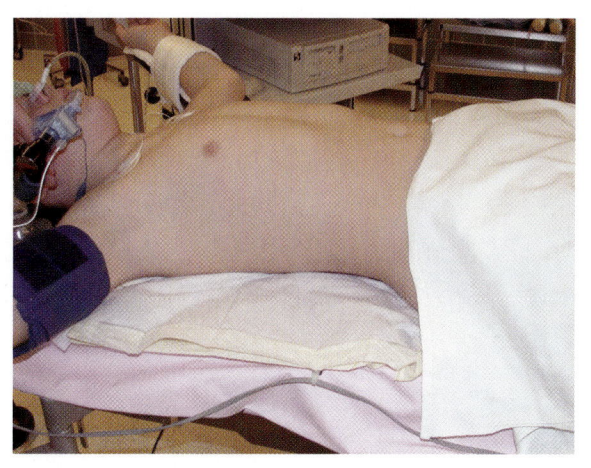

Fig. 12.6. Arms in abduction

21.1.2 Prone position

◨ Figs. 21.7–21.10.

Indications

All procedures to the skin and lower soft tissues on the back, buttocks and backside of the legs (haemangioma, tumours, sacrococcygeal teratoma). For anal atresia, the legs are sterile but mobile, a sterile towel roll is placed under the pelvis. In the high form, the patient has to be transferred from the supine to the prone position during the operation.

Preparations

- Padding for the face, genitals, knees and feet, and under the pelvis (for anal atresia)
- Warming mat, warming lamp
- Arm positioning device only for older children

Positioning

- Children's operating table in the neutral position
- Connect the warming mat and lamp, affix the temperature sensor
- Prepare and induce the anaesthetic in the supine position
- Transfer to the prone position in the operating theatre, for older children using a second operating table (see adults), it necessary
- Spread out and pad the arms for older children
- Padding for the face (gel ring), genitals, knees and feet, and under the pelvis/abdomen, depending on the procedure
- Apply the neutral electrode, connect to the HF surgery device
- Fix the legs with body belt for older children or plastic strips for younger children
- Use compresses to protect the electrode during disinfection
- Position the operating lamps

Risks

- Positioning injuries from lacking or inadequate padding (particularly for the face and genitals)
- Burns from lacking moisture protection for the neutral electrode

21.1 · Various positions

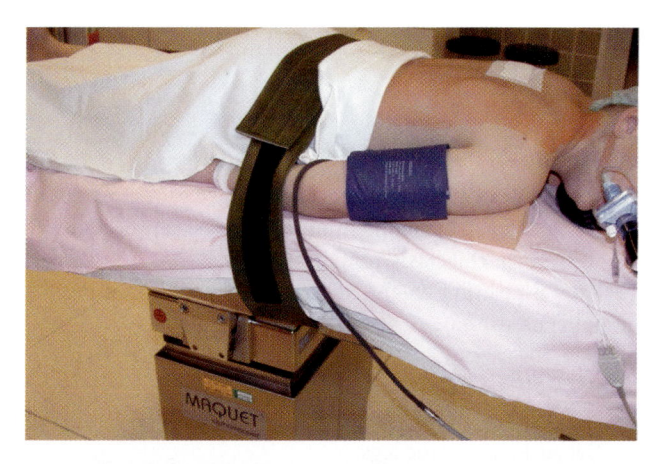

Fig. 21.7. Prone position with arms positioned under the body

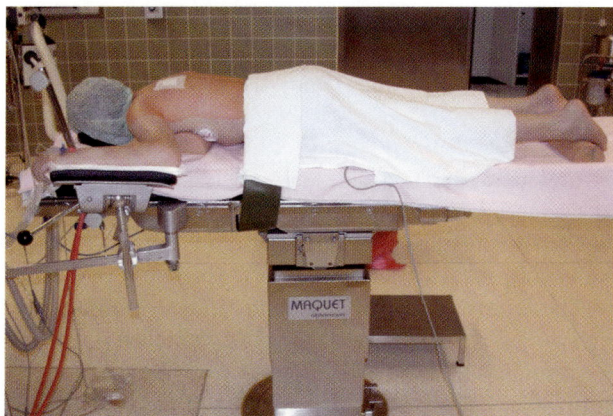

Fig. 21.8. Padding for the legs and thorax

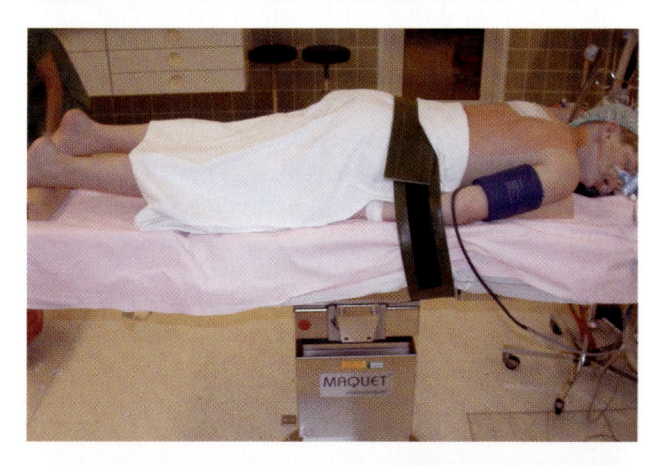

Fig. 21.9. Padding for the face to prevent positioning injuries

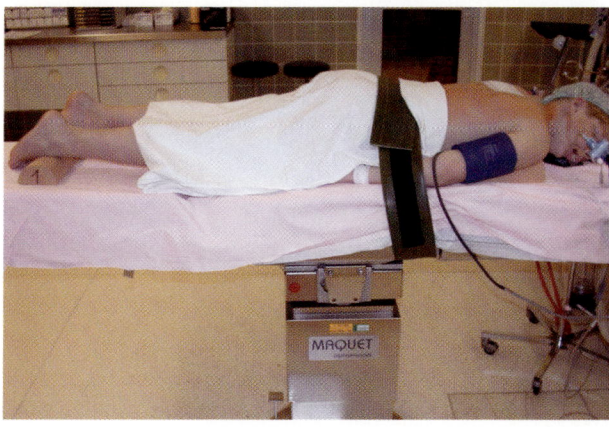

Fig. 21.10. Prone position, fixed with a belt

21.1.3 Lateral position

◘ Figs. 21.11–21.16.

Indications

Congenital deformities to the oesophagus (e.g. oesophagus atresia, oesophagus duplications), open and minimally invasive procedures to the lungs (e.g. sequestra, bronchiectasis, tumours).

Lateral position on the healthy side, position on the left-hand side for oesophagus atresia

Preparations
- Gel cushions/sandbags, possibly wedge cushion
- Gel cushions for the legs
- Leg holders (only for larger children)
- Padding for the legs and feet
- Warming mat, warming lamp

Positioning
- Children's operating table in the neutral position
- Connect the warming mat and lamp, affix the temperature sensor
- Prepare and induce the anaesthetic in the supine position
- Transfer to the lateral position in the operating theatre
- The upper arm is positioned in the cranial direction, padded and fixed in a cloth sling to the anaesthetic screen, for infants the arm is fixed in a lying position at the head with plaster strips
- In larger children, pull the lower arm so that the body weight does not lie directly on the shoulder and extend in this position
- Stabilise the body with sandbags or gel cushions, possibly wedge cushions
- Fix the lower leg with body belts for older children and plaster strips for younger children
- Pad the parts of the body at risk from pressure
- Apply the neutral electrode, connect to the HF surgery device
- Use compresses to protect the electrode during disinfection
- Position the operating lamps

Risks
- Positioning injuries from lacking or inadequate padding (particularly for the face and genitals)
- Burns from lacking moisture protection for the neutral electrode

21.1 · Various positions

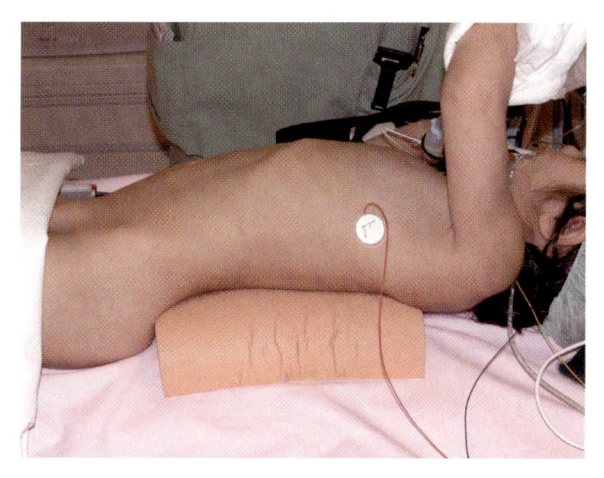

Fig. 21.11. Modified lateral position for thoracoscopy

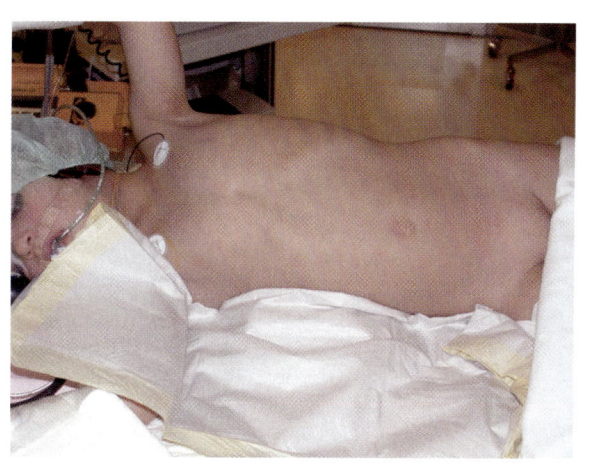

Fig. 21.12. Arm spread out, fixed to the anaesthesia screen

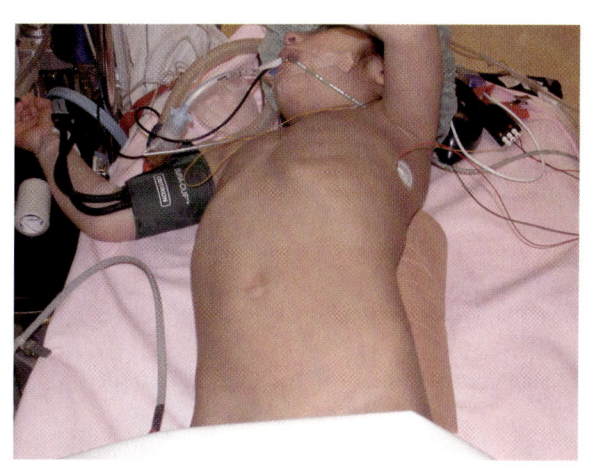

Fig. 21.13. Padding under the back

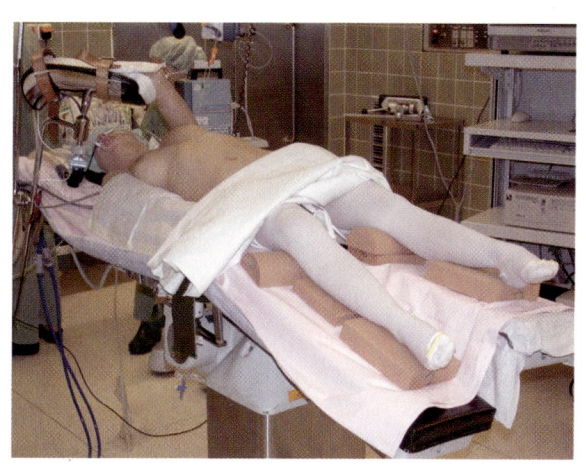

Fig. 21.14. Padding under the legs

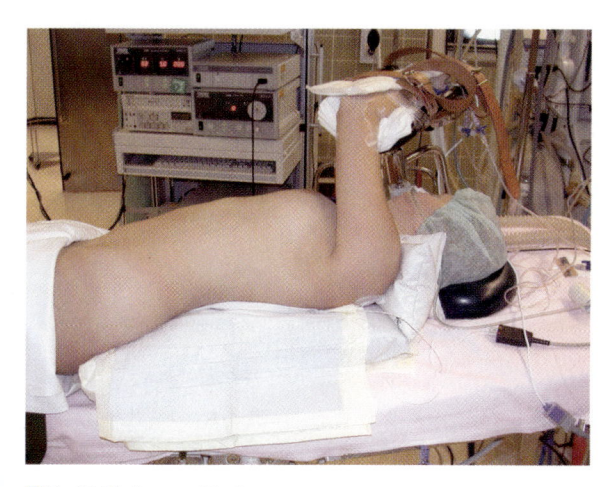

Fig. 21.15. Arm positioning

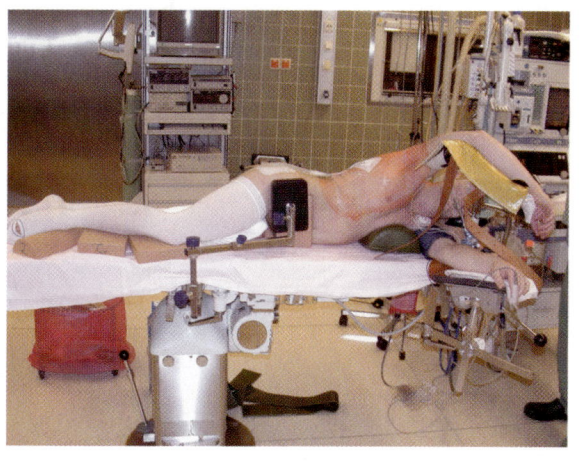

Fig. 21.16. Lateral position for lower lobe resection

21.1.4 Lithotomy position

◘ Figs. 21.17–21.21.

Indications
Rectoscopy, cystoscopy and procedures to the anus and rectum (e.g. abscesses, perianal vein thrombosis).

Preparations
- Two leg holders, pads for the legs
- Warming mat, warming lamp
- Arm position device only for older children

Positioning
- Children's operating table in the neutral position
- Connect the warming mat and lamp, affix the temperature sensor
- Prepare and induce the anaesthetic in the supine position
- Spread out and pad the arms of older children
- Fit the leg holders to the corresponding clamps
- Position the legs and remove the leg plates
- For infants, the legs can be hung in slings or from the anaesthesia screen
- Position the pelvic just above the edge of the buttocks plate
- Lower the still raised legs until the thighs are almost horizontal
- Pad the parts of the body at risk from pressure
- Position the operating lamps

Risks
- Positioning injuries from lacking or inadequate padding (particularly for the face and genitals)
- Burns from lacking moisture protection for the neutral electrode

21.1 · Various positions

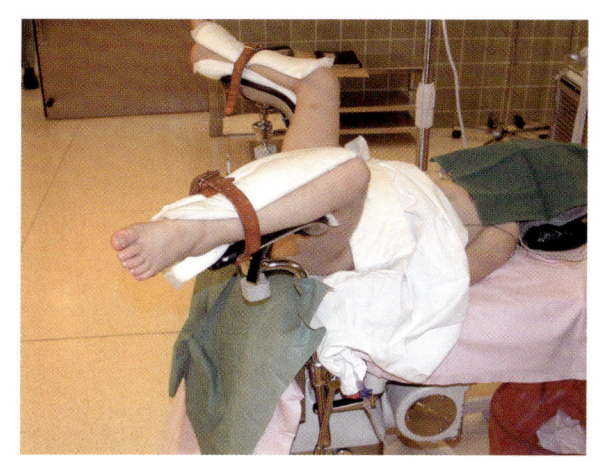

Fig. 21.17. Cystoscopy, padded leg holders

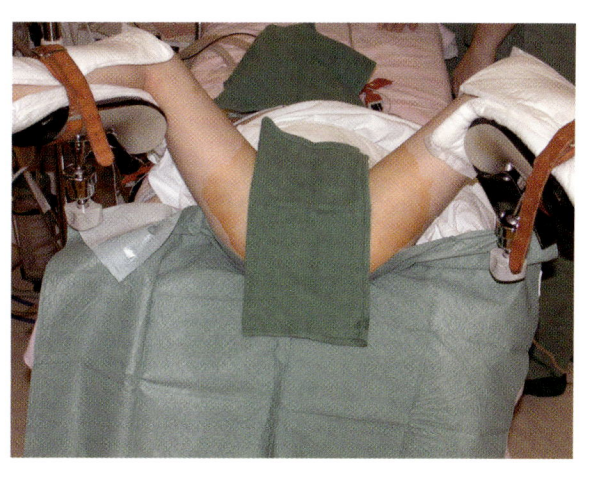

Fig. 21.18. Spreading the legs out at right angles

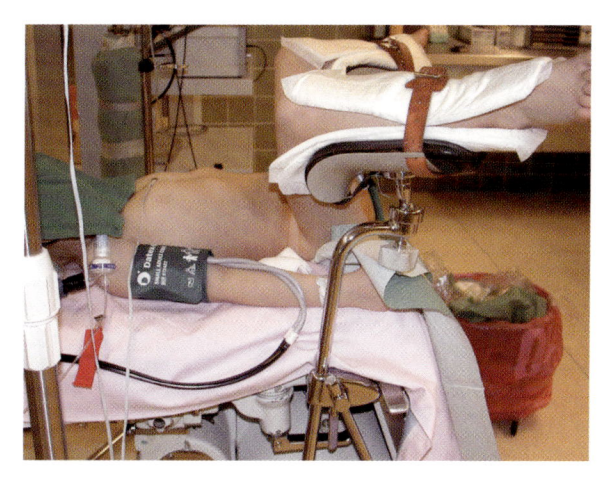

Fig. 21.19. Lateral view of the positioning

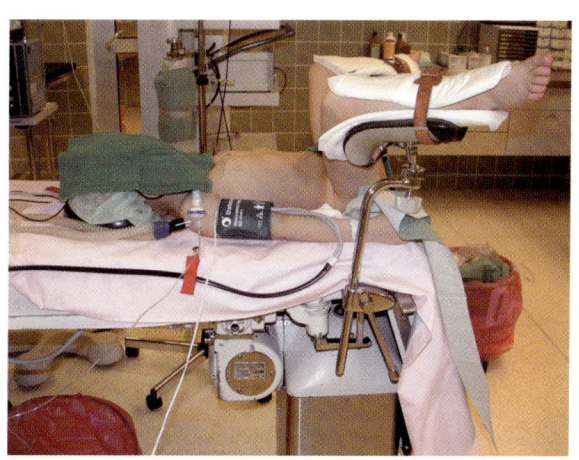

Fig. 21.20. Lateral view of the positioning

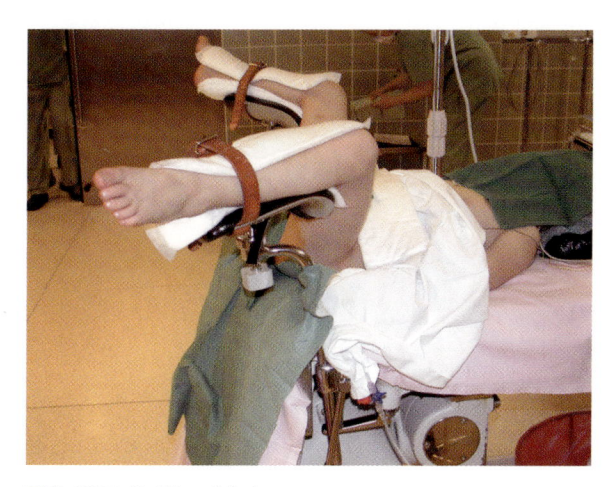

Fig. 21.21. Padding of the legs

22 Special aspects of Iso-C3D and navigation applications

22.1 Iso-C3D applications with and without navigation – 290
22.1.1 Vertebral column – 290
22.1.2 Pelvis/acetabulum – 294
22.1.3 Elbow/wrist – 296
22.1.4 Hips/DHS/neck of the femur: screwed solutions – 298
22.1.5 Head of the tibia and lower leg – 300
22.1.6 Ankle/pilon/talus – 302
22.1.7 Calcaneus fractures – 304

22.1 Iso-C3D applications with and without navigation

Basic ISC-C3D applications. During operations to the extremities, the extremity not being operated does not disturb much in the ray path, only the cube in the Iso centre (12×12×12 cm) is calculated and displayed.

A carbon operating table should always be used whenever possible. If an operating table contains metal bracing, the region being scanned must be positioned centrally on the table, or in the case of the hand or feet, the extremity can be allowed to hang over the edge of the table.

The Iso C-arm is covered with special sterile foil. In addition, the operation site should also be covered with sterile sheets. One useful method consists of wrapping the extremity in a stockinette. It is also advisable to wrap the table in a sterile sheet so that the device can rotate around the table.

In the case of the VIWAS table (single-section carbon operating table top), care must be taken to ensure that the duplex columns are as far as possible from the position of the C-arm.

Losses in quality can be caused above all when the region being examined is not positioned exactly in the central ray path. Such a central position should be correctly adjusted and verified in both levels before starting the scan. Bumping into the C-arm during the automatic orbital movement always means that the scan has to be aborted.

Navigation. The specific set-up must be known already before beginning the operation, and started before the operation or parallel to positioning the patient. Particular attention should be given to the position of the camera.

The units/camera positions described here are rated specifically for systems with autonomous camera as autonomous unit (e.g. Optotrack/Medivision).

22.1.1 Vertebral column

◘ Figs. 22.1–22.6.

Iso-C3D imaging
Prone position
- Position the patient in the middle of the table, pay attention to table top height and patient height, because the C-arm gap is limited.
- Choose a flat carbon table top (e.g. 1150.16) for obese patients.
- Do not use metallic bolsters (MHH), cushions should be the preferred positioning aids.
- In the single-section carbon VIWAS table, the gap in the C-arm is too small in some cases.
- When scanning the thoracic vertebral column, as far as possible use the respiratory standstill in expiration to avoid movement artefacts.
- In the case of dorsal instrumentation, proceed with the scan before applying the longitudinal and transfer connectors to reduce the artefacts.

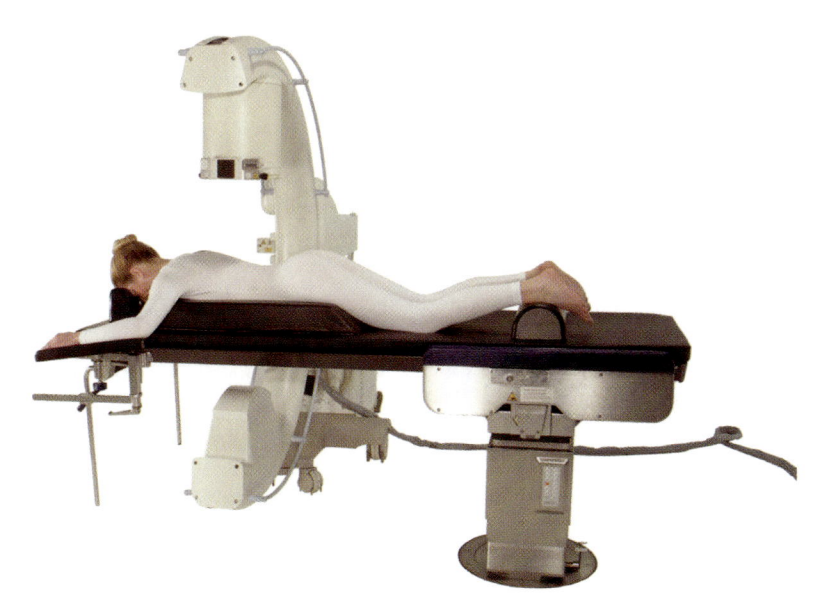

22.1 · Iso-C3D applications with and without navigation

Fig. 22.1. CRP operating table 1150.16, prone position and use of the image intensifier

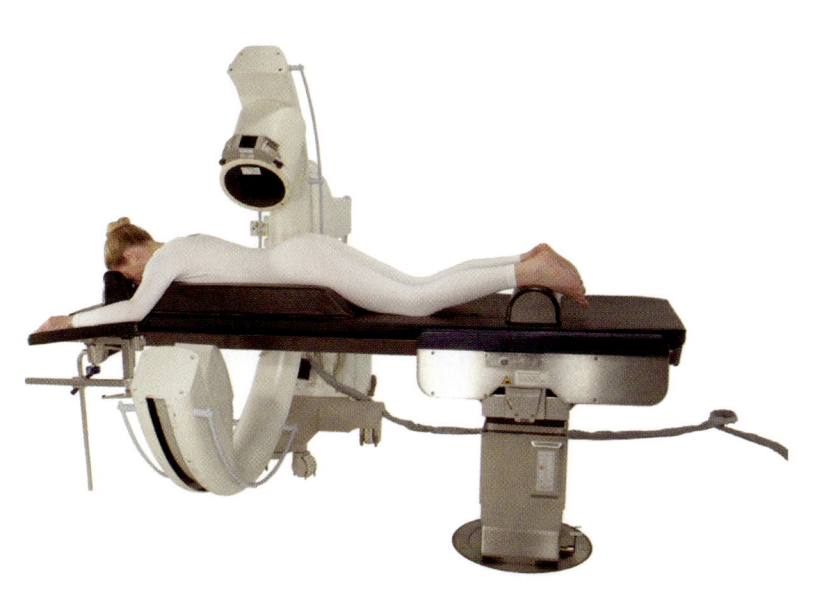

Fig. 22.2. CRP operating table 1150.16, prone position on padding cushions

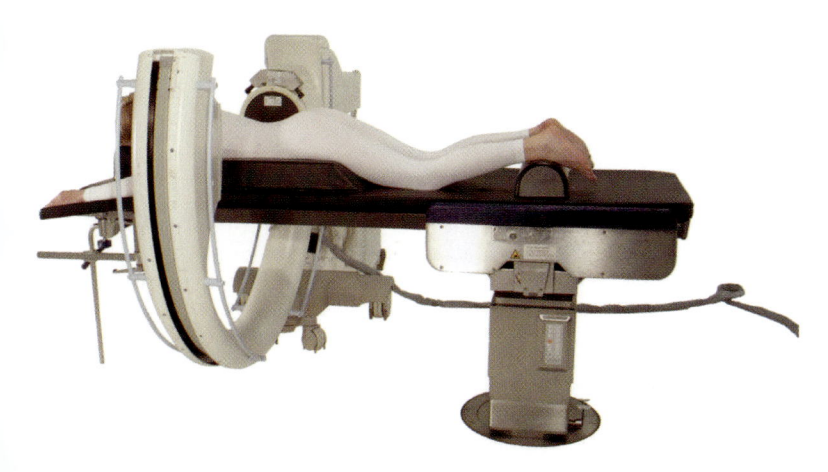

Fig. 22.3. Maximum longitudinal displacement of the CRP operating table 1150.16 towards the head

Positioning

The side positioning is not really relevant, but coordination and exact positioning is better from the side opposite the surgeon.

Iso-C3D navigation

- The Iso C assisted spinal operation is only possible on a carbon tabletop.
- The Iso C-arm comes from the side opposite the surgeon, just like the navigation device.
- Cover the operating site with sterile sheets, and also the Iso C.
- The reference base (RB) must protrude out of the sterile covering.
- In addition, a covering of sheets can be placed under the table as complete protection.
- The Iso C can be used as a normal image converter in the lateral position.
- The camera is placed at the end of the table or foot end.
- The reference base (RB) points to the foot end or to the camera.
- The monitor, C-arm and navigation device are positioned next to each other opposite the surgeon.

Fluoroscopic navigation
Prone position

- Use a carbon table top.
- Fluoroscopy scans at the start of the operation. To do so, cover the C-arm with sterile foil.
- Positioning cushions should be given preference over bolsters.
- The C-arm comes from the side opposite the surgeon.
- During the operation, the C-arm remains in the lateral position and is covered with sterile sheets.
- The camera is placed at the end of the table or foot end.
- The reference base (RM) points to the foot end or to the camera.
- The monitor, C-arm and navigation device are preferably positioned next to each other opposite the surgeon.

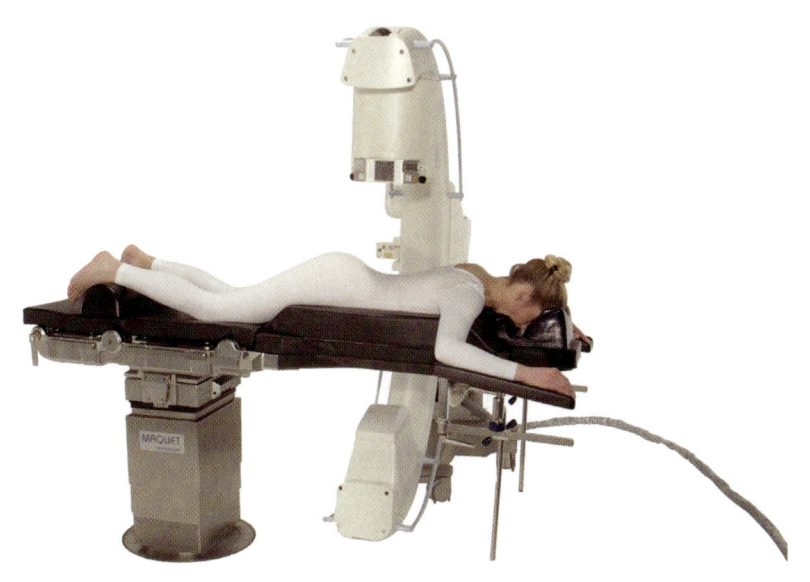

22.1 · Iso-C3D applications with and without navigation

Fig. 22.4. Universal operating table 1150.30, CRP back plate 1150.45, prone position

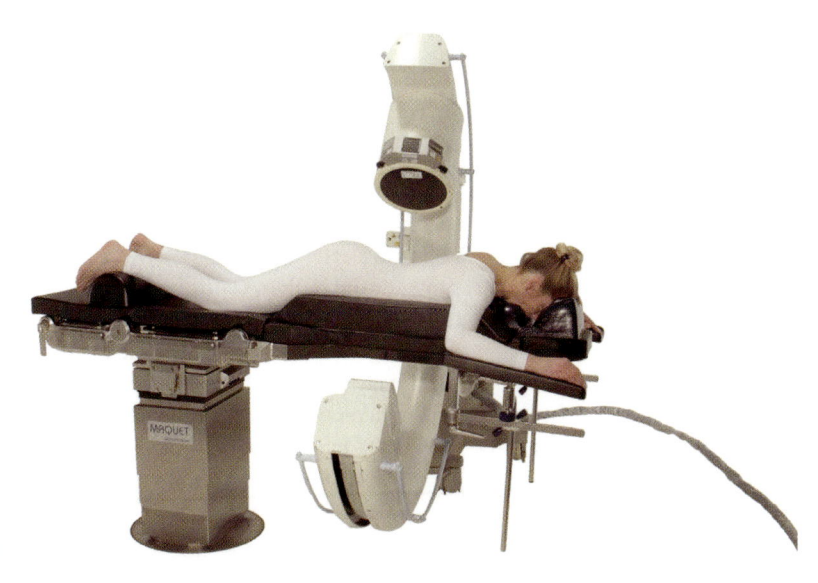

Fig. 22.5. Universal operating table 1150.30, prone position on padding cushions

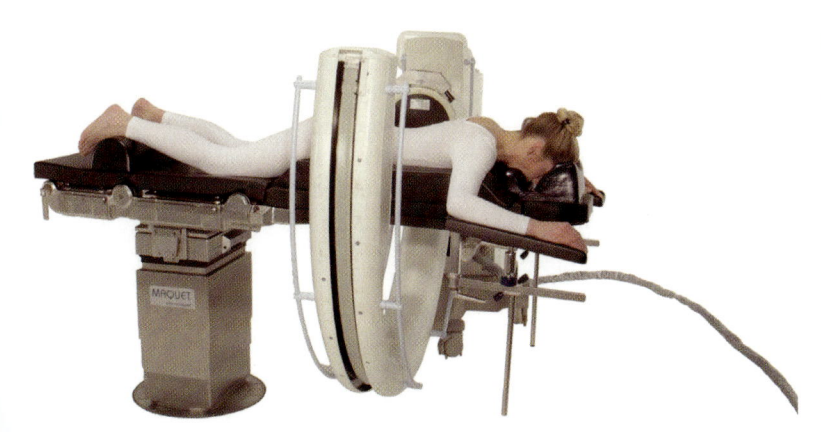

Fig. 22.6. Maximum longitudinal displacement of the universal operating table 1150.30 towards the feet

22.1.2 Pelvis/acetabulum

◘ Figs. 22.7–22.12.

Iso-C3D imaging
Supine position
- For scanning, position the »region of interest« in the middle of the table as far as possible.
- Pay attention to the C-arm gap in obese patients.

Lateral position
- Position the patient in the middle of the table, pay attention to table top height and patient height, because the C-arm gap is limited.
- Choose a flat carbon table top (e.g. 1150.16) for obese patients.
- In the VIWAS table with single-section carbon tabletop, the gap in the C-arm is too small, therefore always use another carbon tabletop.
- The body supports must be moved in the thoracic direction, side stability must be guaranteed without metal braces in the ray path.

Positioning
The side positioning is not really relevant, but coordination and exact positioning is better from the surgeon's side.

Iso-C3D navigation
- Use a carbon table top.
- Iso C-arm and navigation unit on the side opposite the surgeon.
- Cover the operating site and Iso C with sterile sheets.
- The reference base (RB) must protrude out of the sterile covering.
- In addition, a covering of sheets can be placed under the table as complete protection.
- The Iso C can be used as a normal image converter in the lateral position.
- Differentiate between the supine and lateral position. In the lateral position, the limited C-arm gap at the VIWAS table with single-section carbon table top means that the complete orbital movement is only possible for extremely slender patients.

Fluoroscopic navigation
Supine position
- Use a carbon table top.
- Fluoroscopy scans at the start of the operation. To do so, cover the C-arm with sterile foil.
- The C-arm is pushed in from the side opposite the surgeon.
- The camera is placed at the end of the table or foot end.
- The reference base (RM) points to the foot end or to the camera.
- The monitor, C-arm and navigation device are positioned next to each other opposite the surgeon.

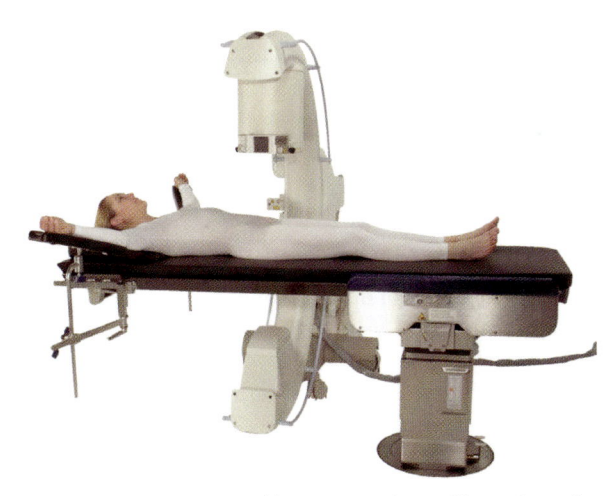

22.1 · Iso-C3D applications with and without navigation

Fig. 22.7. CRP operating table 1150.16, supine position and use of the image intensifier

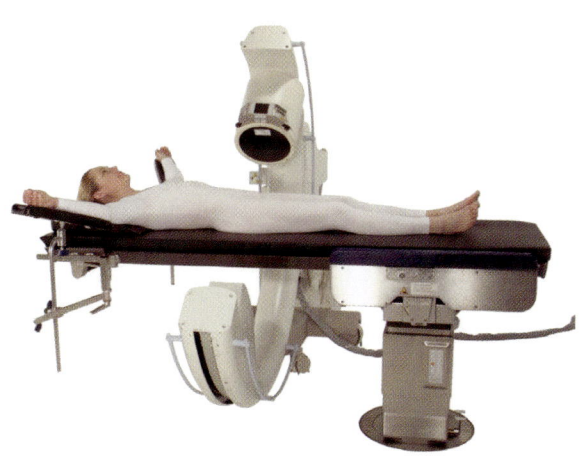

Fig. 22.8. CRP operating table 1150.16, arms positioned in maximum 90° abduction and supination position

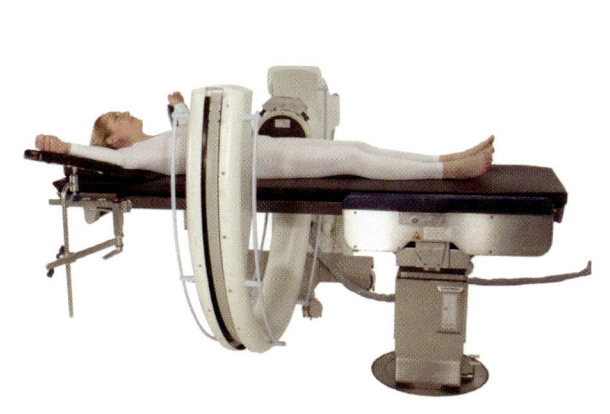

Fig. 22.9. Maximum longitudinal displacement of the CRP operating table 1150.16 towards the head

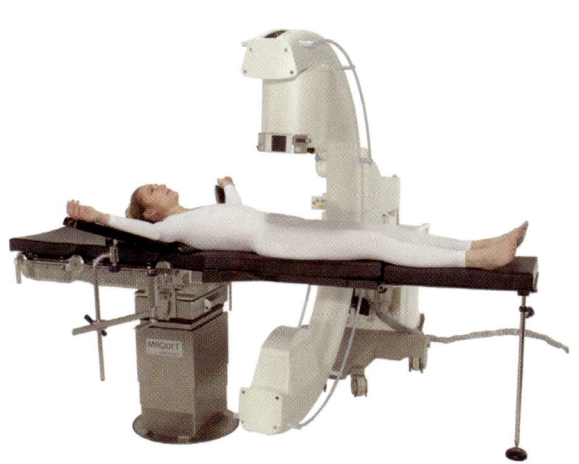

Fig. 22.10. Universal operating table 1150.30, CRP back plate 1150.45, extension plate with support, supine position

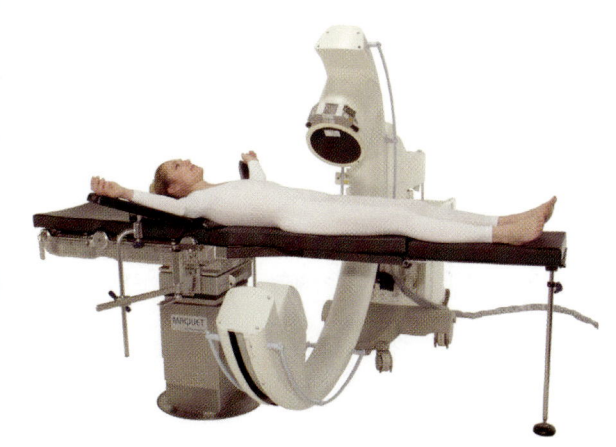

Fig. 22.11. Universal operating table 1150.30, arms positioned in maximum 90° abduction and supination position

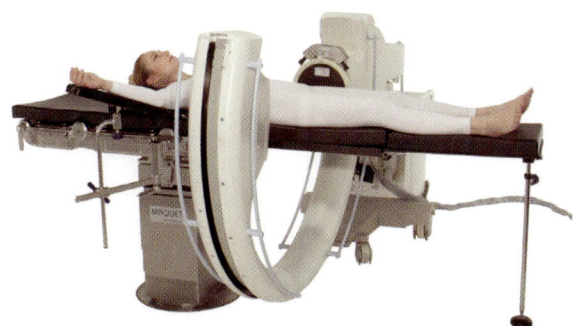

Fig. 22.12. Maximum longitudinal displacement of the universal operating table 1150.30 towards the feet

22.1.3 Elbow/wrist

◘ Figs. 22.13–22.16.

Iso-C3D imaging
Supine position with arm table
- Position the arm in the middle of the table for scanning.
- If a carbon arm table is not available or metal braces interfere with the ray path, let the arm hang over the edge of the table for scanning.

Positioning
Brought in from the assistant's side, so that the Iso C-arm can also be used as normal image converter during the operation.

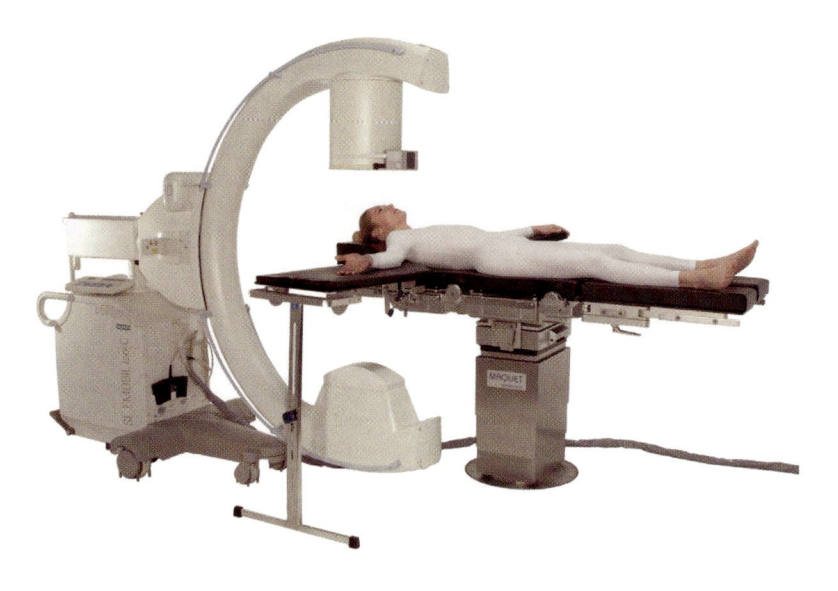

◘ **Fig. 22.13.** Universal operating table 1150.30, large arm table, supine position

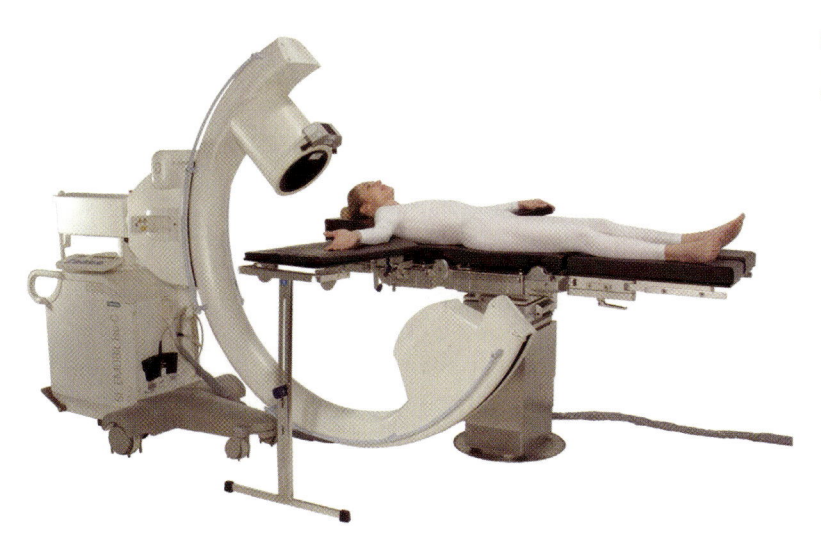

22.1 · Iso-C3D applications with and without navigation

Fig. 22.14. Universal operating table 1150.30, large arm table without lateral rail in the ray path

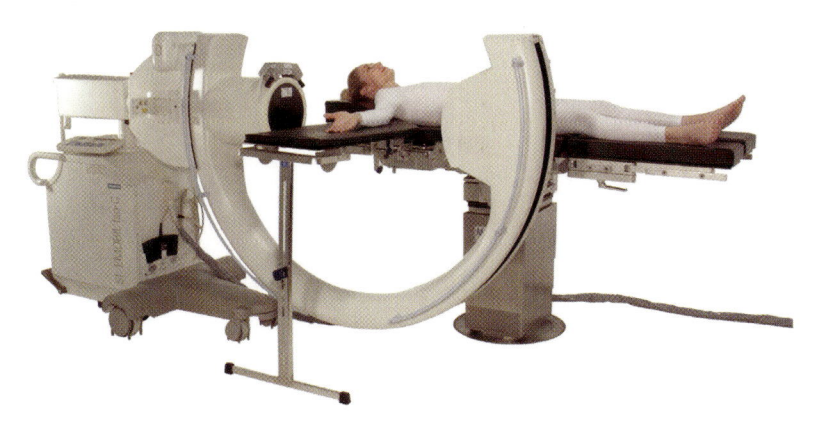

Fig. 22.15. Universal operating table 1150.30, use of the image intensifier from the head side

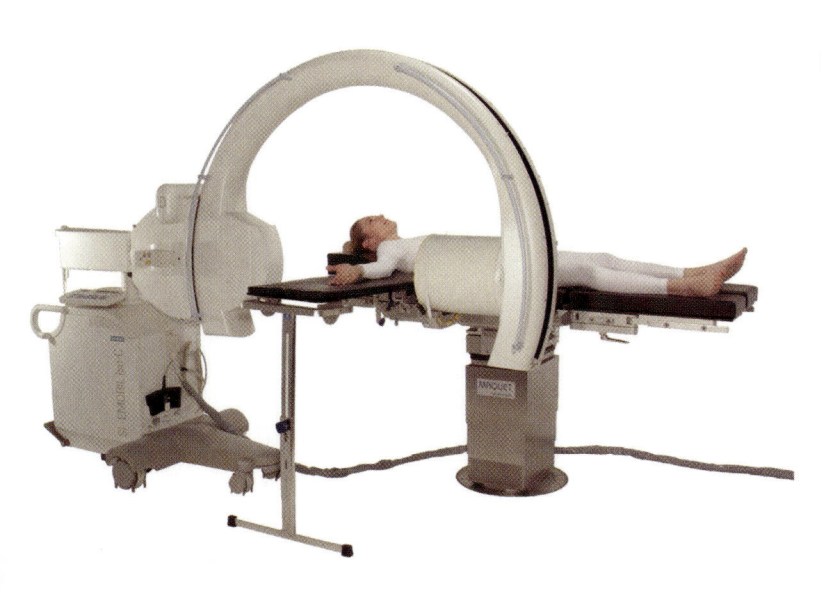

Fig. 22.16. Universal operating table 1150.30, optimum swivel range

22.1.4 Hips/DHS/neck of the femur: screwed solutions

◘ Figs. 22.17, 22.18.

Fluoroscopic navigation
- Classical extension table, legs spread.
- The C-arm is positioned between the legs, brought in from the direction of the feet. Only one C-arm is used.
- The surgeon is seated, looking towards the head.
- The RB is positioned on the side of the thigh.
- The camera, navigation system and fluoroscopy monitor are positioned at the head end on the operation side, at an angle of about 45° to the operating table.
- After making the registration adjustments, the C-arm remains in the anteroposterior position for further control scans during the operation.
- Cover the operation site with foil, preferably without holding clips.

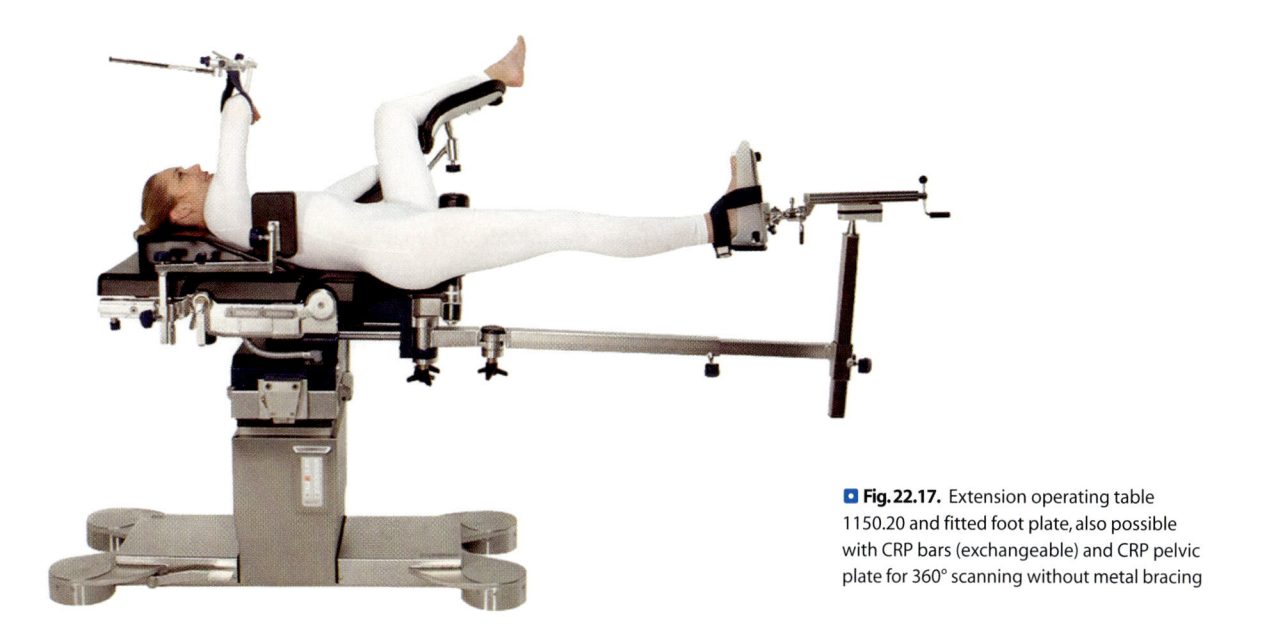

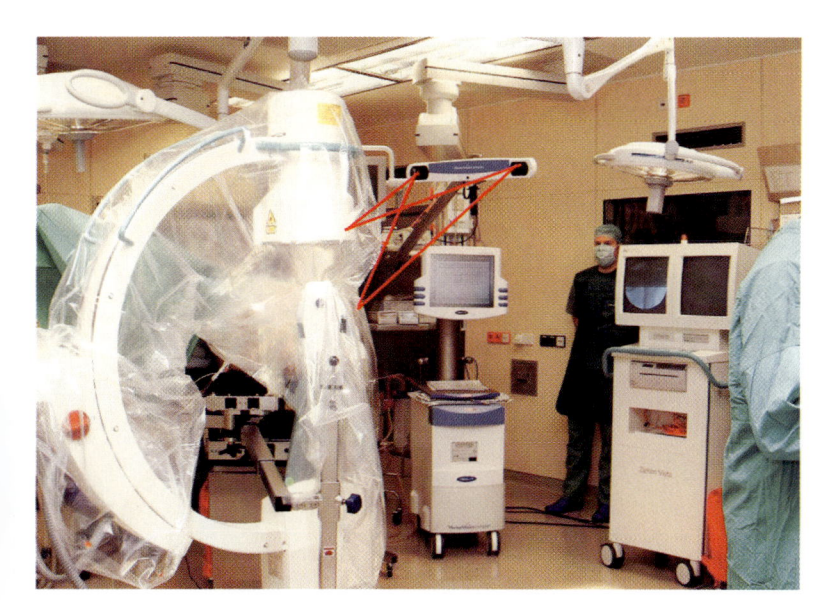

22.1 · Iso-C3D applications with and without navigation

Fig. 22.17. Extension operating table 1150.20 and fitted foot plate, also possible with CRP bars (exchangeable) and CRP pelvic plate for 360° scanning without metal bracing

Fig. 22.18. Patient in supine position on extension operating table 1150.20, fitted foot plates and use of the navigation system

22.1.5 Head of the tibia and lower leg

◘ Figs. 22.19–22.24.

Iso-C3D imaging
Supine position
- Position the leg in the middle of the table for scanning, with the other leg moved to the side or position in parallel.
- If necessary, the opposite side can also be positioned onto a Goepel leg holder for scanning.

Positioning

The side positioning is not really relevant, but coordination and exact positioning is better from the extremity being operated.

Fluoroscopic navigation
Supine position
- Camera always at the foot end.
- Cover with sterile sheets for Iso C, for fluoroscopy it is sufficient if the C-arm itself is covered with foil.
- The RB points to the foot end or camera.
- Position the monitors and navigation device on the opposite side to the surgeon.

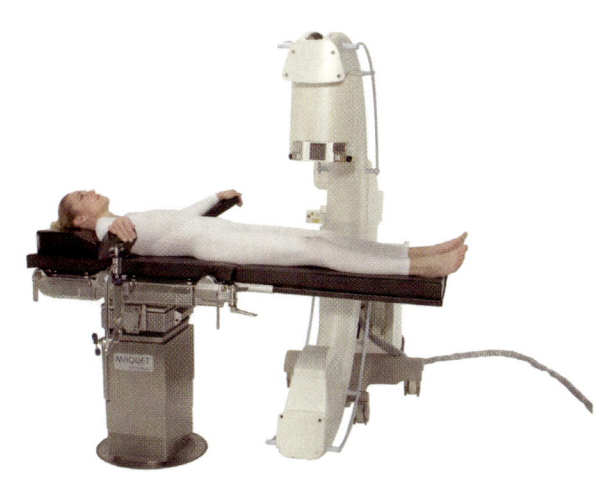

22.1 · Iso-C3D applications with and without navigation

Fig. 22.19. Universal operating table 1150.30, supine position, legs on divided CRP leg plates 1150.67

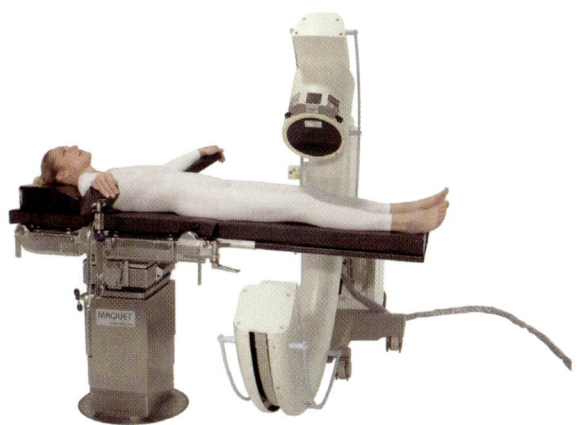

Fig. 22.20. Universal operating table 1150.30, divided CRP leg plates 1150.67

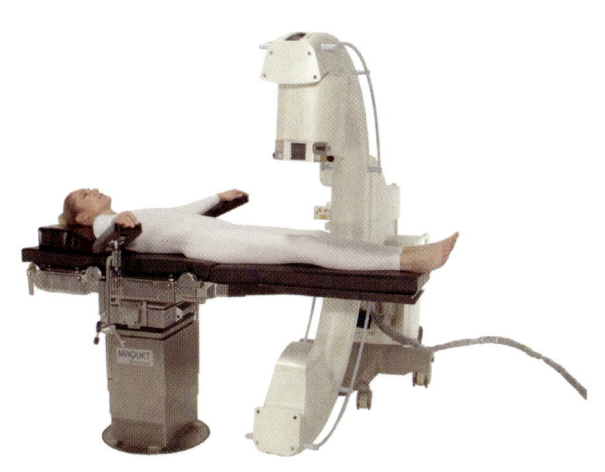

Fig. 22.21. Universal operating table 1150.30, supine position, legs on CRP module 1150.45

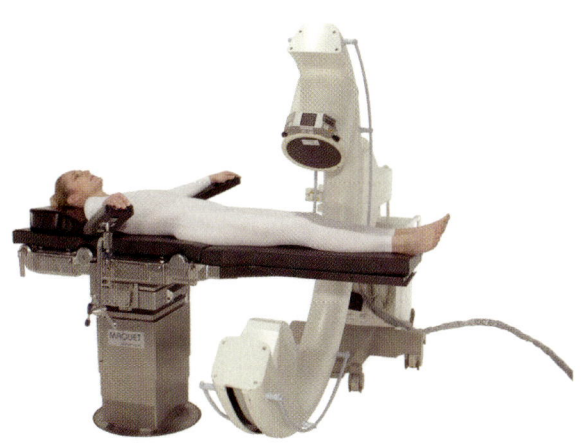

Fig. 22.22. Universal operating table 1150.30, CRP module 1150.45

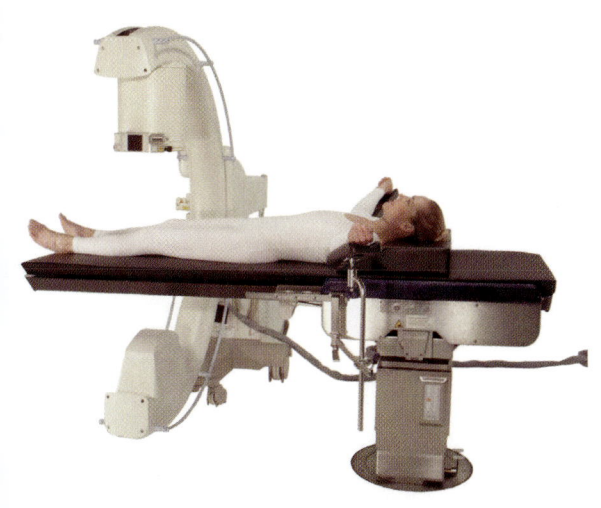

Fig. 22.23. CRP operating table 1150.16, supine position, maximum longitudinal displacement towards the feet

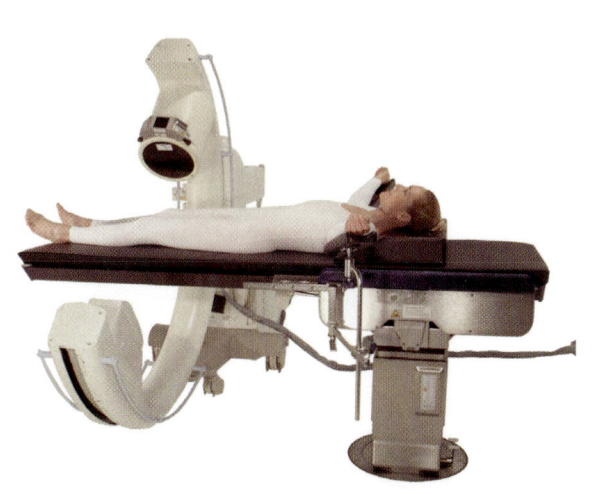

Fig. 22.24. CRP operating table 1150.16, supine position

22.1.6 Ankle/pilon/talus

◘ Figs. 22.25–22.27.

Iso-C3D imaging
Supine position
- Position the leg in the middle of the table for scanning, with the other leg moved to the side or position in parallel.
- If no carbon table top is available, pull the extremity down for scanning so that the foot hangs over the edge of the table.

Positioning
The side positioning is not really relevant, but coordination and exact positioning is better from the extremity being operated.

Iso-C3D navigation
Supine position
- Use a carbon table top.
- Iso C-arm and navigation device on the side opposite the surgeon.
- Cover the operation site and Iso C with sterile sheets.
- The RB should protrude from the sterile covering.
- In addition, a covering of sheets can be placed under the table as complete protection.
- The Iso C can be used as a normal image intensifier.

Fluoroscopic navigation
Supine position
- Use a carbon table top.
- If necessary, let the extremity hang over the end of the table.
- Fluoroscopy scans at the start of the operation. To do so, cover the C-arm with sterile foil.
- The C-arm comes from the side opposite the surgeon.
- The camera is placed at the end of the table or foot end.
- The RB points to the foot end or to the camera.
- The monitor, C-arm and navigation device are positioned next to each other opposite the surgeon.

22.1 · Iso-C3D applications with and without navigation

Fig. 22.25. Universal operating table 1150.30, supine position, legs on divided CRP leg plates 1150.67

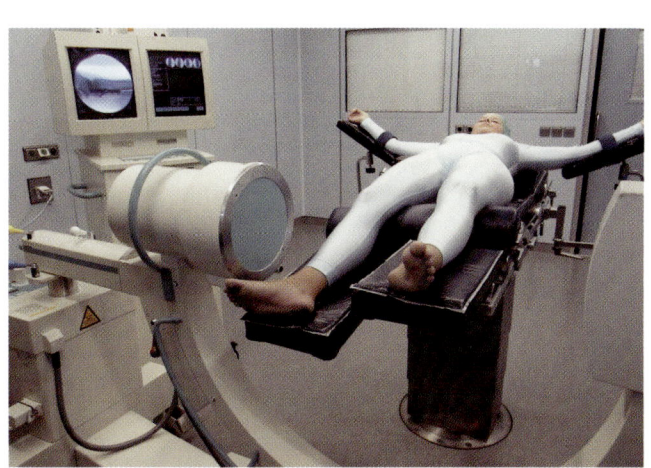

Fig. 22.27. Universal operating table 1150.30, right leg plate lowered

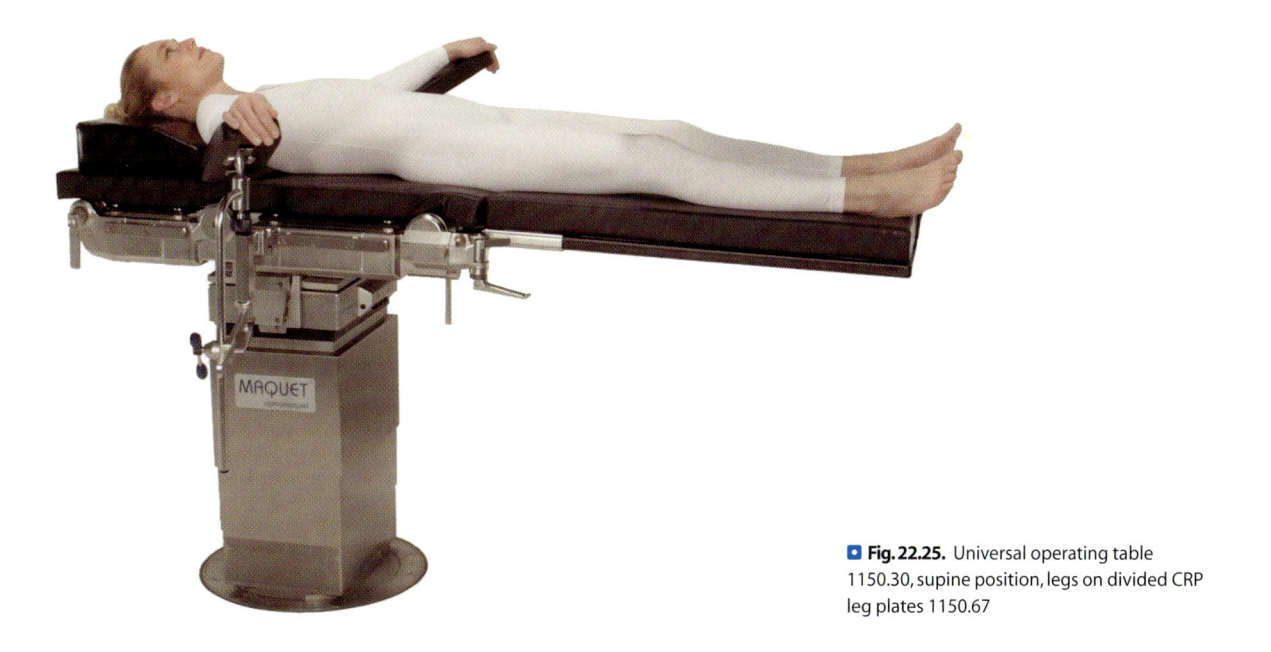

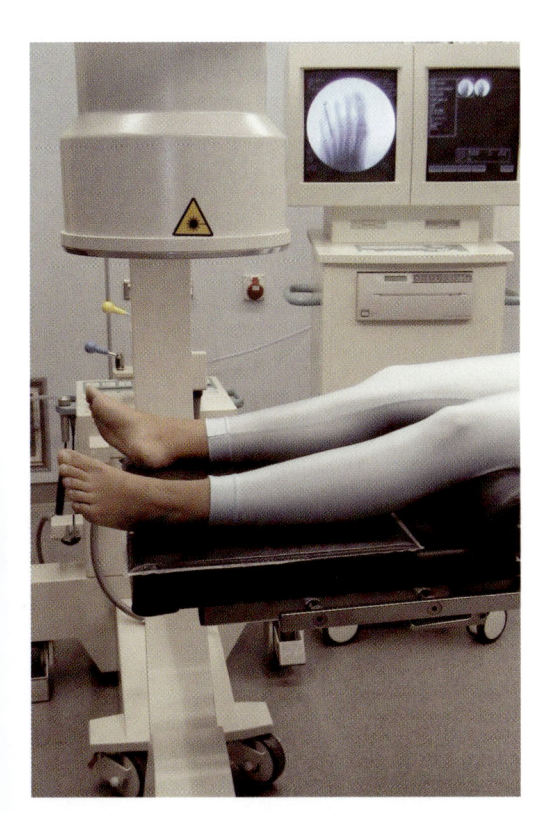

Fig. 22.26. Universal operating table 1150.30, divided standard leg plates, scanning range without side rails

22.1.7 Calcaneus fractures

◘ Figs. 22.28–22.33.

Iso-C3D imaging
Lateral position
Carbon table. During the operation, both legs are bent. For scanning, stretch the operated leg slightly, but the leg can remain on the table. Preferably the leg is placed centrally in the middle of the table.

Normal table. Position the leg before the operation so that for scanning, the leg is stretched so that it hangs over the end of the table.

Positioning
The side positioning is not relevant.

Supine position
- Position the leg in the middle of the table for scanning, with the other leg moved to the side or position it parallel.
- If no carbon table top is available, pull the extremity down for scanning so that the foot hangs over the edge of the table.

22.1 · Iso-C3D applications with and without navigation

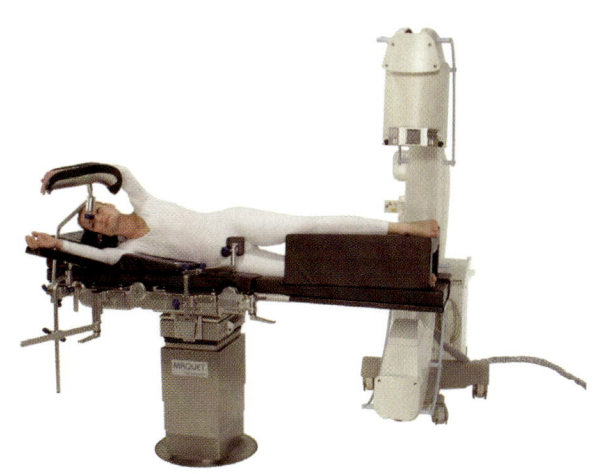

Fig. 22.28. Universal operating table 1150.30, divided leg plates 1150.67, lateral position with tunnel cushion

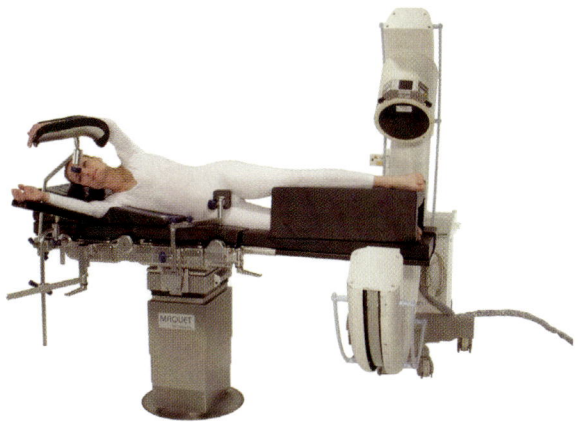

Fig. 22.29. Universal operating table 1150.30, swivelling movement of the Iso-C3D

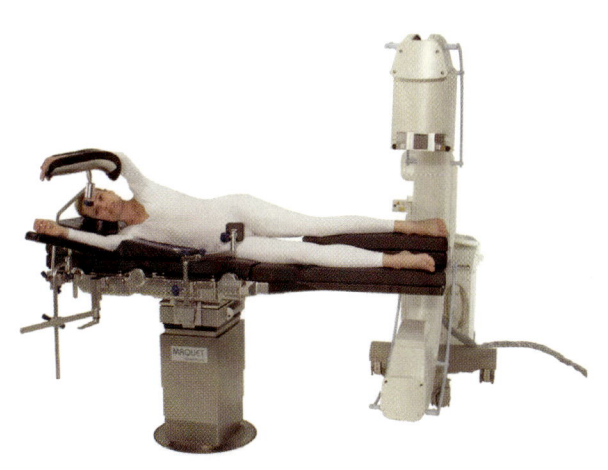

Fig. 22.30. Universal operating table 1150.30, CRP module 1150.45, lateral position with 2 flat padding cushions

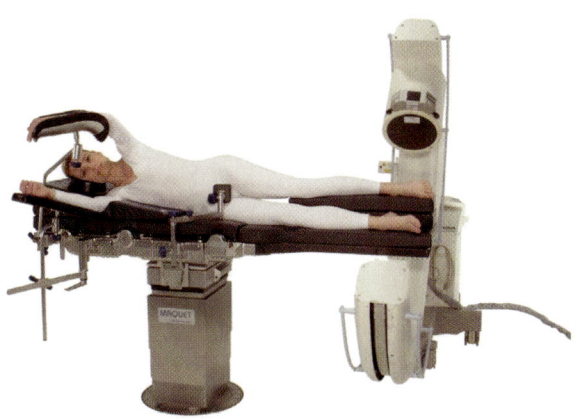

Fig. 22.31. Universal operating table 1150.30, CRP module 1150.45, swivelling movement of the Iso-C3D

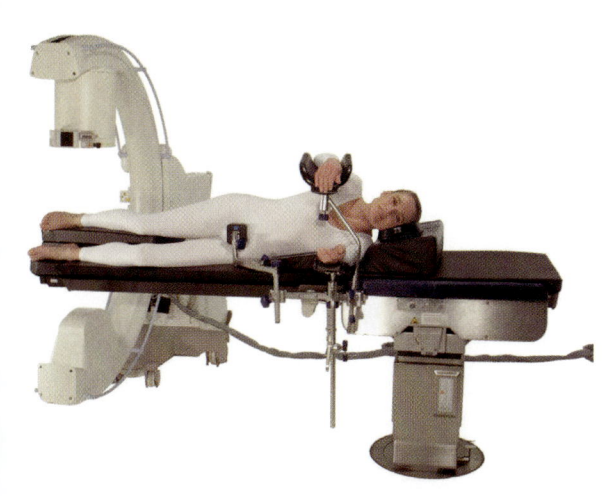

Fig. 22.32. CRP operating table 1150.16, lateral position with 2 flat padding cushions and maximum longitudinal displacement towards the feet

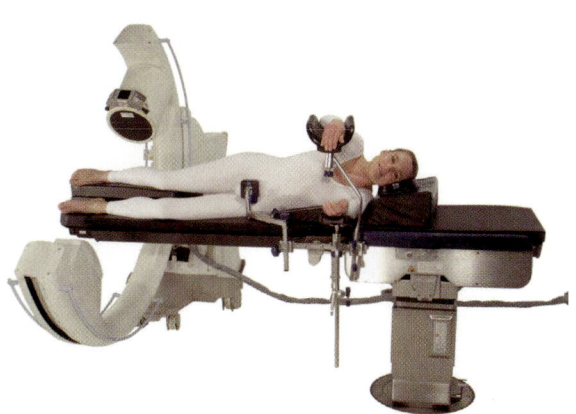

Fig. 22.33. CRP operating table 1150.16, swivelling movement of the Iso-C3D

Subject Index

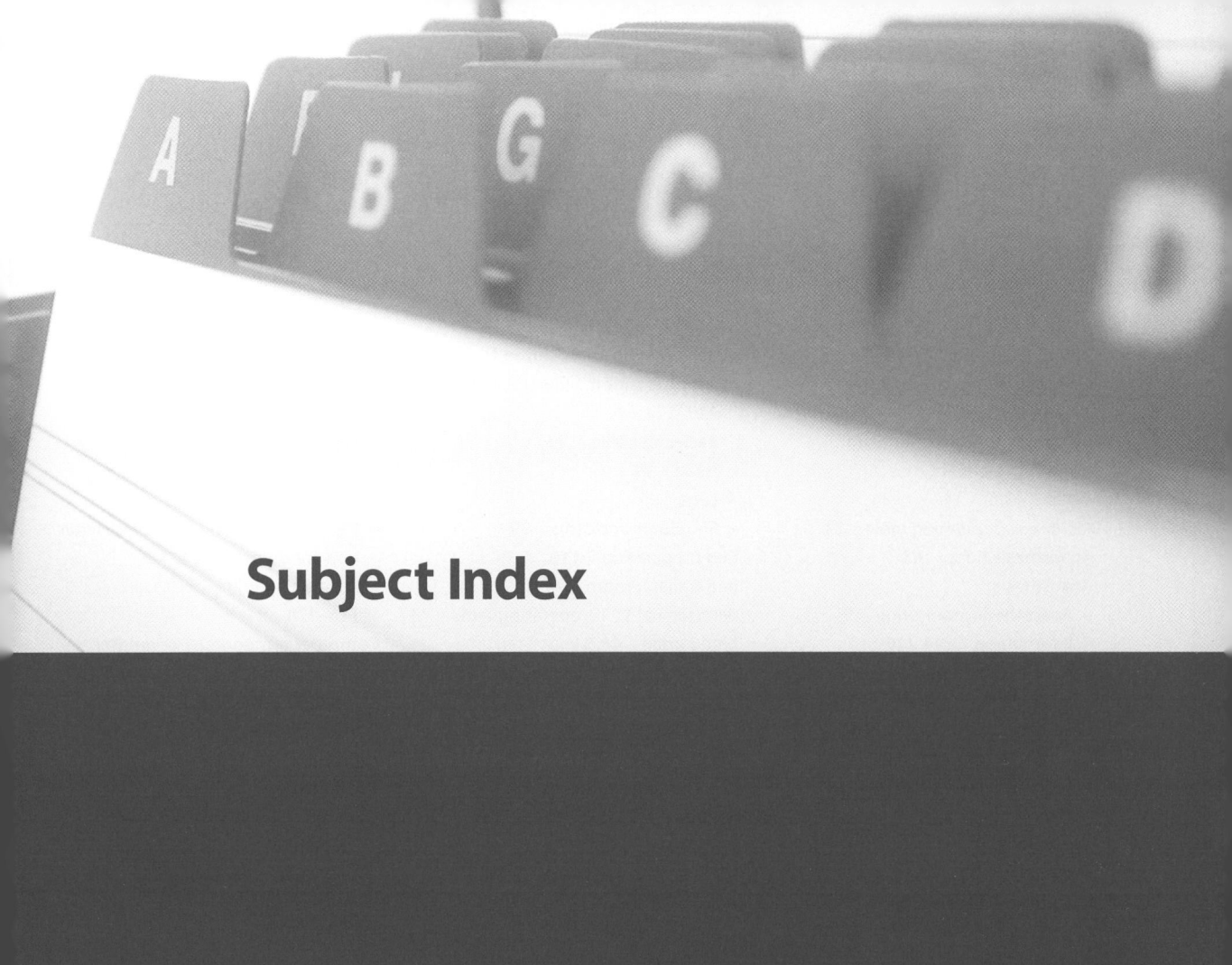

A

Accessory stand 88
Acetabulum 210–214
– -Navigation (Iso-C3D general and with navigation) 294–295
ADR (automatic service/dose control) 35–36
Agreement on cooperation in operative patient care (ArztRecht 1983, 43ff.) 14
Alphamaxx, operating table 73
Anaesthesia hoop 83
Anaesthesia
– Anaesthetic monitoring 15
– Information 144, 116
– Positioning injuries as seen by the anaesthetist (*see there*) 116–124
– Surgery/anaesthesia 116
– – Distribution of tasks 116
– – Shared responsibility 116
– Transport into the anaesthetising room 5
Anaesthetic (see anaesthesia)
Anaesthetising room, patient preparation 108–109
Anaesthetist, positioning responsibility 14–15
Angiography 65
Ankle (*see* Foot/Ankle) 252–256, 276
Ankle/pilon/talus 302–303
Application principles of § 25 X-ray Ordinance § 25 23
Arm positioning device 82
Arm protection 83
Arthroscopic procedures 268–276
– Foot/ankle 276
– Hips 272–274
– Knee 274–275
– Shoulder 268–271
Atomic Energy Law 21
AWIGS (image-assisted surgery) 60–67
– AWIGS transfer table turned 64
– Definition 60
– »Touchscreen« and IR remote control 64
– VIWAS (*see there*) 66–67
Axonotmesis 125

B

Back plate for shoulder operations 84
Back/buttocks support 85
Backache 120
Beach-chair position/sitting, half-sitting position 98–100, 121–122, 220–222
– Back and pelvis 99
– Head 99
– Legs 99
– Shoulders and arms 99
Bed preparation 110
Bed transfer room 74
Betastar 11131.12, operating table 73
blend (mix) 43, 51
– Gating with the slot or iris diaphragm 37
– Restrict the effective variable field 31
Blend cutting 44
Bodily harm, negligent 14
Body belt 85
Body dose 25
Body supports 84–85
Bolster (MHH) 81
Burden of proof 15
Burns from neutral electrode 47–48

C

Calcaneus fractures, navigation (Iso-C3D general and with navigation) 304
Calf 250–251
– Extension table 264
– Supine position 250–251, 264
Capacitive coupling, definition 52
Capacity 52
C-arm 56
Cauterisation 42
Cervical spine 186–196
Change in position 15, 116
Check-up, occupational health 25
Children
– Information 5
– Premedication 5
– Psychological management 4–6
– Specific fears 4
– Transfer 5–6
– Transport in the anaesthetising room 5
– Transport to the operating suite 5

Circulation concept in the operating suite 76
Circulation 74–75
Cleanmaquet 75, 77
Clothing in the operating suite 8
Coagulate/coagulation 43, 44
– Contact coagulation 44
– Definition 52
Compartment syndrome 126
– Position-related 121, 128
Compensation 14
Complications 116–128
– Patient positioning under resuscitation conditions 124–125
– Positioning injury (*see there*) 116–128
Computer tomography/computer tomograph (CT) 60
– Intraoperative CT scan 65
Constancy testing, X-ray/radiation protection 29–30
Contact coagulation 44
Control area, X-ray/radiation protection 21, 24–26
– Using radiation during the operation 21
Counter tension rod 86
Coupling, HF-surgery 48
– Capacitive 48, 52
– Cross coupling 52
– Direct 48, 51
Cross coupling 52
Crushed kidney (rhabdomyolysis) 126
Cushions for positioning 80–82
Cutting 43–44
– Blend cut 44
– Definition 53
– Smooth cut (»pure cut«) 43, 45

D

Depilation 111
Desiccation 43–45
– Definition 51
DGHM list 10
DHS, navigation (Iso-C3D general and with navigation) 298–299
Diagnostic reference values (DRW) 21
Digital image saving and processing 20
Disinfectant 11

Subject Index

Disinfection 10
- Cleaning hands and disinfection (*see there*) 9–10
- Procedure 10

Distribution of tasks surgery/anaesthesia 116

Division of labour, horizontal 14

Documentation
- Operation report 17
- Positioning documentation 16–17, 116
- Recording obligations 21

Dosage/dose/dose ranges 25–26
- Body dose 25
- Limit dose 25
- Limit values 26
- mSv (dose limit values) 22
- Official dosimeter (film badges) 28
- Personal dosmietry 25–26
- Rod dosimeter 25

Dose control, automatic (ADR) 35
Dose surface product (DFP) 29
Double wedge cushion 80

E

Effective radiation field 31–35
- Gating recommendation 33
- Restriction 31

Effective voltage 51

Elbows, navigation (Iso-C3D general and with navigation) 304–305

Electrode
- Active 50
- Definition 51

Electrosurgery (see high-frequency surgery) 42–54

Emergency transporter 63

Emergency, operation preparation (under time pressure) 110–111

End of the operation, measures 110

Euratom directives 21

Evaluation/viewing 30

Expert know-how
- According to the X-ray ordinance/medicine 20, 28
- In radiation protection 20, 23, 28

Expert test 36

Exposure for X-ray pictures
- Brief 20
- Continuous 20

Extension bars 86

Extension table 72, 121, 260–264
- Accessories 86–88
- Positioning injuries 121
- Proximal femur 260–261
- Thigh 262–264

Extremities
- Lower (*see there*) 154, 236–246
- Upper (*see there*) 152–154, 218–232

Extubation 110

Eyes, position-related injuries 119
- Loss of vision 119

F

Fasciotomy 128

Femur, proximal, extension table 260–261
- Supine position 260–261

Film badges (official dosimeter) 25, 28

Flank position
- Urology 178–180
- Visceral and transplantation surgery 170

Fluoroscopy 56

Focus/object distance 34

Foot plate adapter 87

Foot plate for extension table 88

Foot/ankle 252–256
- Arthroscopic procedures 276
- Lateral position 254
- Prone position 256
- Supine position 252–253

Fracture, open, preparation 111–113

Frequency 51

Fulguration 43, 45, 49, 51

Function workflow in the operating suite 108–113
- Preparations for open fractures 111–113
- Preparations in an emergency (under time pressure) 110–111
- Standard steps in the elective programme 108–110

G

Gel cushion 81

Gloves, discharges through 43, 48–49

Goepel leg holder 85

H

Hand cleaning and disinfection 9–10
- Hygienic 9–10
- Procedure 10
- Surgical 10

Hand operating table 84

Hand, supine position 232

Head cushions 80–82
- For supine position 82

Head extension, spine holding unit 89

Head plate adjustment, motor-driven 89

Head ring 80–81

Heart massage 124

Heidelberg position (position for *Kraske* access) 168–169

Height adjustment operating table 68

Helpers/helping persons, radiation protection 23

High-frequency surgery (HF surgery) 42–54
- General 42–45
- Monopolar 53
- Neutral electrode (*see there*) 46–48
- Pacemaker patients 49
- Rules for safe use 48–50

Hips 236
- Arthroscopic procedures 272–273
- Lateral position 238
- Navigation (Iso-C3D general and with navigation) 298–299
- Supine position 236–237

Horseshoe headrest, 2-part 83

Hygiene aspects 8–11
- Hand disinfection, hygienic 9
- Perioperative hygiene in accident surgery 8

Hygiene rules 8

Hypotension 126

Hypothermia 126

I

ICRP recommendations 21

Image intensifiers, surgical 35–41

Image quality 21, 29–30
- Diagnostic 30
- Focus-object distance 34
- Physical 29

Image receiving system of surgical image intensifiers   31–33
– Correct positioning   34
Image saving and processing, digital   20
Image-assisted surgery (see also AWIGS/VIWAS)   60–67
Implementation responsibility   15
Indication, justifying   21, 23, 28
Infection   8
– Nosocomial   8
– Prevention   9
– Wound infection (see there)   8, 10, 111
Information   108, 116
– for parents and children   5
Infusion arm   17
Instruction, annual, X-ray/radiation protection   28
Instruction, X-ray machine   24
Intensive care unit   110
International Commission on Radiological Protection (ICRP)   23
Interrupt circuit   33, 35
Iso C-arm   56
Iso-C3D general and with navigation   57–60, 289–304
– Ankle/pilon/talus   302–303
– Calcaneus fractures   304
– Elbows/wrist   296–297
– Head of the tibia and lower leg   300–301
– Hips/DHS/neck of the femur – screwed solutions   298–299
– Pelvis/acetabulum   294–295
– Spine   290–293
Isolation error, HF surgery   48

K

Kidney, rhabdomyolysis (crush kidney)   126
Kinesiology   103
Knee positioning unit
– Manual   86
– Motor-driven   89
Knee supports   86
Knee   246–248
– Arthroscopic procedures   274–275
– Prone position   248
– Supine position   2460–247
Kraske access, Heidelberg position   168–169

L

Laparoscopic procedures   174–176
Laparotomy, open   162–164
Lateral position padding   81–82
Lateral position   103–105
– Head   103
– Legs   104–105
– Paediatric surgery   284–285
– Positioning injuries   122
– Shoulder and arms   103–104
– Thoracic/lumbar spine   198–199
– Thorax and pelvis   104
– With vacuum mat   103
– Without vacuum mat   103
Law of the distance square   26, 31
Lead equivalent value   29
Leakage current   50
Leaking radiation   33, 36–37
Leg holder
– Goepel leg holder   85
– with one-hand control   85
Legal aspects   14–17
Limit dose   25
Lithotomy position   96–98
– Back and pelvis   96–97
– Head, shoulders, arms   96
– Legs   97–98
– Paediatric surgery   286
– Positioning injuries   121
– Urology   176–178
Loss of vision, position-related   119
Lower arm and hand, supine position   232
Lower extremity   236–246
– Calf   250–251
– Foot   252–256
– Hips   236
– Knee   246–248
– Thigh   240–244
– Vascular surgery   154

M

Mandatory information, X-ray/radiation protection   29
Maquet 1120 (1964), operating table system   71, 74
Medical product law (MPG)   22, 48, 79
Medical product owner ordinance (MPBetreibV)   48, 79
Meniscus rod   86
Minimally invasive surgery   44, 48–49
Mix (»blend«)   43, 51
Monitoring area, radiation protection   24
MPBetreibV (Medical product owner ordinance)   48, 79

N

Navigation   56–60, 289–304
– Ankle/pilon/talus   302–303
– Calcaneus fractures   304
– Elbows/wrist   296–297
– Equipment, erection and modalities   56
– Head of the tibia and lower leg   300–301
– Hips/DHS/neck of femur – screwed solutions   298–299
– Isomatic (non-image)-based   56
– – Iso-C3D general   57–60, 289–304
– – Iso-C3D navigation   60, 289–304
– Neuronavigation   65
– Pelvis/acetabulum   294–295
– Solid carbon table   57
– Spine   290–293
Neck of femur screwed solutions, navigation (Iso-C3D general and with navigation)   298–299
Neck, vascular surgery   150–152, 158–160
Nerve injuries, position   117–118, 125–128
– Brachial nerve   118
– Median nerve   118
– Pathophysiology   125
– Peroneal nerve   118, 127
– Plexus
– – Brachial   118, 126–127
– – Lumbosacral   127–128
– Prognosis   126
– Pudendal nerve   128
– Radial nerve   118
– Saphenus nerve   118
– Sciatic nerve   118
– Ulnar nerve   127
Neurology, positioning injuries as seen by the neurologist   125–128
– Frequency   125
– Pathophysiology   125
Neuronavigation   65
Neuropraxia   125
Neurosurgery   64

Subject Index

Neutral electrode 109
- High-frequency surgery 46–48, 53
- – Burns from 47–48
- – Coupling (*see there*) 48
- – Definition 53
- – Positioning 47
- – Safety systems 46–47
- – Task 46

Nursing staff, positioning responsibility 14–15

O

Occupational exposure to radiation, persons with 25–26
Occupational health check-up 25
One-stop shop 63
Operating suite/protective clothing 8–9
- sterile 9

Operating table column 75
- Mobile 75
- Rolling 75
- Stationary 75

Operating table preparations 92–93
Operating tables 68–79
- Accessories 82–86
- Models
- – *Alphamaxx* 73
- – *Betastar* 1131.12 73
- – Extension table 72, 121
- – Hand operating table 84
- – *Maquet 1120* (1964) 71, 74
- – Mobile tables 75
- – Special operating tables 68, 78
- – Universal operating tables 78
- Normal or in reverse direction 72
- Position 15
- Properties and requirements (*overview*) 68
- Table adjustments (*overview*) 69

Operation circulation concept 76
Operation preparations
- For open fractures 111–113
- In an emergency (under time pressure) 110–111

Operation report 17
Operative patient care, agreement on cooperation (ArztRecht 1983, 43ff.) 14
Output current/voltage/power 50
Output, bipolar 50

P

Pacemaker patients, HF surgery 48
Padding (SFC), operating table 68
Padding cushions 80
Paediatric surgery 280–286
- Lateral position 284–285
- Lithotomy position 286
- Prone position 282–283
- Supine position 280–282

Patient circulation concept 74–75
Patient positioning under resuscitation conditions (*see also* resuscitation) 124–125
Patient preparation, preoperative 10
Patient protection, X-ray 28
Patient reception 108
Patient sluice 108
Patient transfer system 108
Patient warming system 90, 109
Pelvic girdle 204–209
Pelvis 204–214
- Acetabulum 210–214
- Navigation (Iso-C3D general and with navigation) 294–295

Personal dosimetry 25–26
Plaster cast, postoperative 110
Plexus, position-related
- Brachial plexus 118, 126–127
- Lumbosacral plexus 127–128

Polyneuropathy 125
Positioning accessories and aids 79–89
- Bolster 79–82

Positioning bolster 79–82
Positioning injuries 14
- As seen by the anaesthetist 116–124
- – Frequency 116–117
- – Incidence 117
- – Type of injury 117–119
- As seen by the neurologist (*see also* nerve injuries) 125–128

Positioning responsibility 14–15, 116
- Anaesthetist 14–15
- Nursing staff 14–15
- Surgeon 14–15

Positioning
- Documentation of 16–17, 116
- Heidelberg position (position for *Kraske* access) 168–169
- Lateral position 178
- Of the arm 17
- On the extension table 260–264
- On the operating table 15
- Procedural instructions for 16
- Pronation on supination position (Texas position) 93
- Standard positioning (*see there*) 92–105
- Under resuscitation conditions 124–125
- Upper arm 224–226

Power 52
Premedication, children 5
Pressure points 92, 116
Procedural instructions for positioning 16
Pronation to supination position (Texas position) 93
Prone position 100–103, 222–224
- Arms 101–102
- Cervical spine (*see there*) 192–194
- Elbows 230–231
- Head 100–101
- Legs 102–103
- Paediatric surgery 282–283
- Positioning injuries 120–121
- Thoracic/lumbar spine 196–197
- Thorax and pelvis 102
- Upper arm 226–227
- Urology 182

Psychological management of children 4–6
Pure cut (smooth cut) 43, 45

Q

Quality assurance according to the X-ray Ordinance 29–30

R

Radial adjusting clamp 83
Radiation application 28
Radiation card 26
Radiation exposure 25, 28
- Category A 25

Radiation protection (*see also* X-ray) 20–41
- Constancy test 29–30
- Control area 24–26
- Diaphragms (*see there*) 31, 37
- Dosage/dose/dose range (*see there*) 21–22, 25–26
- Effective radiation area 33, 35

Radiation protection
- Expert know-how in radiation protection   20, 23, 28
- Expert test   36
- Helpers/helping persons   23, 28
- In the operating suite   20–35
- Instruction, annual   28
- Knowledge   20
- Knowledge   23
- Leaking radiation   33, 36–37
- Mandatory information   29
- Monitoring area   24
- Occupational exposure – persons with   25–26
- Patient protection   28

Radiation protection accessories   29
Radiation protection clothing   35
Radiation protection gloves   33
Radiation protection manager   24–25, 28
Radiation protection officer   24–25, 28
Radiation Protection Ordinance (StrlSchV)   21, 23
Radiation protection principles   21
Radiation protection test   29
Radiation times   35
Radiation user   29

Radiology
- Radiation protection (see there)   20–35
- X-ray (see there)   20–41

Radiolucent padding (SFC), operating table   68
Reaction time   11
Recording obligations   21
Recovery room   110
Reference base (RB)   56
REM contact quality monitoring system   53
Resistance   54
Responsible, shared   116

Resuscitation
- Intraoperative   125
- Measures   124
- Patient positioning under resuscitation conditions   124–125

Rhabdomyolysis (crush kidney)   126
Rod dosimeter   25
Rolls and half rolls for positioning   80
Röntgen, W.C.   20, 30, 35

S

Scanning times   35
Screw tension device   87
Scrub room   10
Shaving   10, 111
Shoulder luxation   120

Shoulder operations
- Arthroscopic procedures   268–271
- Back plate for   84
- Positioning   218

Shunt arms, position-related   119
Skin and soft tissue injuries, positioning   117
Skin disinfection   113
Skull clamp   123
Sliding gantry (see also VIWAS)   66–67
Sliding rail extension   86
Sluice for patients   108
Soft tissue damage, positioning   117
Solid carbon table   57
Special head cushion   80
Special leg plates   88
Special operating tables   68
Special units   89

Spinal column   186–200, 290–293
- Cervical spine (see there)   186–196
- – Lateral position   198–199
- – Prone position   196–197
- – Supine position   200
- Thoracic/lumbar spine (see there)   196–200
- – Prone position/CRP horseshoe headrest   192
- – Prone position/spine holding device/skull holding device   194–196
- – Supine position/CRP horseshoe headrest   186–187
- – Supine position/skull clamp   188–189
- – Supine position/spine holding device MAQUET T554.0000   190–191

Spine holding unit/ head extension   89
Spray coagulation   43, 45, 49
- Definition   53

Staff sluice   8
Standard positioning (see also Positioning)   92–105
- Beach-chair position/sitting, half-sitting position (see there)   98–100, 123–124, 220–222
- Lateral position (see there)   103–105, 122, 198–199, 284–285
- Lithotomy position (see there)   96–98, 121, 286
- Operating table preparation   92–93
- Prone position (see there)   100–103, 122–123, 182, 192–194, 196–197, 222–224, 226–227, 230–231, 282–283
- Supine position (see there)   93–95, 119–120, 186–191, 200, 218, 224–225, 228–230, 232, 280–281

Stereotactic operation   65
Sterility   8
Sternotomy (median thoracotomy)   134–136
Struma position   121
Supine position   93–95, 119–120, 218, 224–226
- Back and pelvis   95
- Cervical spine (see there)   190–194
- Elbows   228–229
- Head   93
- Legs   95
- Lower arm and hand   232
- Paediatric surgery   280–281
- Positioning injuries   119–120
- Shoulders and arms   93–95
- Thoracic/lumbar spine   200
- Upper arm   224–226
- Urology   174–176, 180–182

Surgeon, positioning responsibility   14–15

Surgery/anaesthesia
- Distribution of tasks   116
- Joint responsibility   116

Surgical gloves   9

T

Texas position (pronation to supination position)   93
Thigh counter tension bar   88
Thigh   240–244
- Extension table   262–263
- Lateral position   244
- Supine position   240–241, 262–263
- – Modified   242–243

Subject Index

Thoracic/lumbar spine 196–200
- Lateral position 197–199
- Prone position 196–197
- Supine position 198–199

Thoracic-outlet syndrome, position-related 119

Thoracotomy 134–144
- Bilateral 136–138
- Lateral 138–142
- Median (sternotomy) 134–136

Thorax support 84

Tibia, head of and lower leg 300–301

Tilt, operating table 68

Tilting (right/left), operating table 68

Tortious liability 16

Tourniquet 109, 117

Transfer board 62

Transplantation surgerye 166–178

Transport to the operating suite – children 5

Transporter 75

Trauma concept 62

Tunnel cushion 81

U

Ultrasound dissection 42

Units 86–89
- Knee positioning unit (see there) 86, 89
- Special units 89
- Spindle unit 87

Upper arm, position 224–226
- Prone position 226
- Supine position 224–226

Upper extremity 217–232
- Beach-chair position 120–222
- Prone position 222–223
- Shoulder 218
- Supine position (see there) 218
- Upper arm 224–226
- Vascular surgery 152–154

Urology 174–182
- Lateral position 178–180
- Lithotomy position 176–178
- Prone position 182
- Supine position 174–176
- – Modified 180–181

Used equipment, X-ray 30

V

Vacuum mats 89, 96
- Lateral position 103

Vascular surgery 150–154
- Lower extremity 162
- Neck 150–152
- Upper extremity 152–154

Vessels, position-related injuries 118–119
- Shunt arms 119
- Thoracic-outlet syndrome 119

Visceral and transplantation surgery 158–170
- Heidelberger position (position for *Kraske* access) 168–169
- Laparoscopic procedures 166–168
- Laparotomy, open 162–164
- Neck 158–160

VIWAS (image-assisted surgery) 66–67
- AWIGS (see there) 60–67
- In combination with a »sliding gantry 66–67
- In combination with an angiography machine 66

W

Warming system for patients 90, 109

Wedge cushion 80

Whole-body scan 60

Wound cleaning 112

Wound infection 8, 10
- Measures 8
- Shaving 10, 111

Wrist, navigation (Iso-C3D general and with navigation) 196–197

X

X-ray card 29

X-ray Ordinance 21, 29
- Principles of application of § 25 X-ray Ordinance 23

X-ray pictures/machine (see also radiation protection) 20–41
- Annual instruction 28
- Constancy test 29–30
- Control area 24–26
- Diaphragms 31, 37
- Dosage/dose/dose ranges (see there) 21–22, 25–26
- Effective radiation field (see there) 31–35
- Evaluation/viewing 30
- Expert know-how according to the X-ray Ordinance/Medicine 20, 28
- Exposure (see there) 20
- Helpers/helping persons 23, 28
- Image intensifiers, surgical 35–41
- Image quality (see there) 21, 29–30
- Indication, justifying 21, 23, 28
- Instructions, X-ray machine 24
- Leakage radiation 33, 36–37
- Mandatory information 29
- Monitoring area 24
- Obligations when operating an X-ray machine 24
- Postoperative X-rays 110
- Quality assurance as per X-ray Ordinance 29–30
- Scanning times 35
- Used machines 30

X-ray radiation in the operating suite 20–41

X-ray tube 31